Learning Disabilities Sourcebook, 3rd Edition

Leukemia Sourcebook

Liver Disorders Sourcebook

Lung Disorders Sourcebook

Medical Tests Sourcebook, 3rd Edition

Men's Health Concerns Sourcebook, 2nd
    Edition

Mental Health Disorders Sourcebook, 4th
    Edition

Mental Retardation Sourcebook

Movement Disorders Sourcebook, 2nd Edition

Multiple Sclerosis Sourcebook

Muscular Dystrophy Sourcebook

Obesity Sourcebook

Osteoporosis Sourcebook

Pain Sourcebook, 3rd Edition

Pediatric Cancer Sourcebook

Physical & Mental Issues in Aging Sourcebook

Podiatry Sourcebook, 2nd Edition

Pregnancy & Birth Sourcebook, 2nd Edition

Prostate Cancer Sourcebook

Prostate & Urological Disorders Sourcebook

Reconstructive & Cosmetic Surgery
    Sourcebook

Rehabilitation Sourcebook

Respiratory Disorders Sourcebook, 2nd
    Edition

Sexually Transmitted Diseases Sourcebook,
    3rd Edition

Sleep Disorders Sourcebook, 2nd Edition

Smoking Concerns Sourcebook

Sports Injuries Sourcebook, 3rd Edition

Stress-Related Disorders Sourcebook, 2nd
    Edition

Stroke Sourcebook, 2nd Edition

Surgery Sourcebook, 2nd Edition

Thyroid Disorders Sourcebook

Transplantation Sourcebook

Traveler's Health Sourcebook

Urinary Tract & Kidney Diseases & Disorders
    Sourcebook, 2nd Edition

Vegetarian S[...]

Women's Hea[...]
    Edition

Workplace He[...]

Worldwide Health Sourcebook

Teen Health Series

Abuse & Violence Information for
    Teens

Accident & Safety Information for Teens

Alcohol Information for Teens, 2nd
    Edition

Allergy Information for Teens

Asthma Information for Teens

Body Information for Teens

Cancer Information for Teens

Complementary & Alternative
    Medicine Information for Teens

Diabetes Information for Teens

Diet Information for Teens, 2nd Edition

Drug Information for Teens, 2nd Edition

Eating Disorders Information for Teens,
    2nd Edition

Fitness Information for Teens, 2nd
    Edition

Learning Disabilities Information for
    Teens

Mental Health Information for Teens,
    2nd Edition

Pregnancy Information for Teens

Sexual Health Information for Teens,
    2nd Edition

Skin Health Information for Teens, 2nd
    Edition

Sleep Information for Teens

Sports Injuries Information for Teens,
    2nd Edition

Stress Information for Teens

Suicide Information for Teens

Tobacco Information for Teens

Contagiou
Diseases
SOURCEBOOI

Second Edition

Health Reference Series

Second Edition

Contagious
Diseases
SOURCEBOOK

RC 113 .C664 2010

Contagious diseases
  sourcebook

*Basic Consumer Health Information about Diseases
Spread from Person to Person through Direct Physical
Contact, Airborne Transmissions, Sexual Contact, or
Contact with Blood or Other Body Fluids, Including
Pneumococcal, Staphylococcal, and Streptococcal
Diseases, Colds, Influenza, Lice, Measles,
Mumps, Tuberculosis, and Others*

*Along with Facts about Self-Care and Over-the-
Counter Medications, Antibiotics and Drug
Resistance, Disease Prevention, Vaccines, and
Bioterrorism, a Glossary, and a Directory
of Resources for More Information*

Edited by
Joyce Brennfleck Shannon

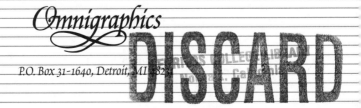

Omnigraphics

P.O. Box 31-1640, Detroit, MI 48231

Bibliographic Note

Because this page cannot legibly accommodate all the copyright notices, the Bibliographic Note portion of the Preface constitutes an extension of the copyright notice.

Edited by Joyce Brennfleck Shannon

Health Reference Series

Karen Bellenir, *Managing Editor*
David A. Cooke, MD, FACP, *Medical Consultant*
Elizabeth Collins, *Research and Permissions Coordinator*
Cherry Edwards, *Permissions Assistant*
EdIndex, Services for Publishers, *Indexers*

* * *

Omnigraphics, Inc.
Matthew P. Barbour, *Senior Vice President*
Kevin M. Hayes, *Operations Manager*

* * *

Peter E. Ruffner, *Publisher*

Copyright © 2010 Omnigraphics, Inc.

ISBN 978-0-7808-1075-4

Library of Congress Cataloging-in-Publication Data

Contagious diseases sourcebook : basic consumer health information about diseases spread from person to person ... / edited by Joyce Brennfleck Shannon. -- 2nd ed.
  p. cm.
  Summary: "Provides basic consumer health information about the transmission and treatment of diseases spread from person to person, along with facts about prevention, self-care, and drug resistance. Includes index, glossary of related terms, and other resources"--Provided by publisher.
  Includes bibliographical references and index.
  ISBN 978-0-7808-1075-4 (hardcover : alk. paper) 1. Communicable diseases--Popular works. I. Shannon, Joyce Brennfleck.
  RC113.C664 2010
  362.196'9--dc22
                                                        2009041846

Table of Contents

Visit www.healthreferenceseries.com to view *A Contents Guide to the Health Reference Series*, a listing of more than 15,000 topics and the volumes in which they are covered.

Part II: Types of Contagious Diseases

Part III: Self-Treatment for Contagious Diseases

Part IV: Medical Diagnosis and Treatment of Contagious Diseases

Part V: Preventing Contagious Diseases

Part VI: Additional Help and Information

Preface

About This Book

Contagious diseases occur when microbes—bacteria, viruses, and fungi—are passed from person to person. While vaccination programs and other prevention measures have been successful in reducing the number of new cases of many contagious diseases, the National Center for Health Statistics reports that the incidence rates for others, including pertussis, chlamydia, and human immunodeficiency virus (HIV) infections, have been rising in recent years. Also, newly recognized infectious agents, including the H1N1 flu (swine flu), and some particularly virulent or drug-resistant strains of well-known microbial infections, such as methicillin-resistant *Staphylococcus aureus* (MRSA), have emerged and caused substantial concern.

Contagious Diseases Sourcebook, Second Edition provides updated information about microbes that are spread from person to person and the diseases they cause, including influenza, lice infestation, pneumonias, staphylococcal and streptococcal infections, tuberculosis, and others. The types of diagnostic tests and treatments available from medical professionals are explained, and self-care practices for familiar symptoms—such as the sniffles and sore throat that often accompany the common cold—are described. Other topics addressed include antibiotic resistance, the role of handwashing in preventing the spread of disease, and recommendations and controversies surrounding vaccination programs. The book concludes with a glossary of related terms and a directory of additional resources.

How to Use This Book

This book is divided into parts and chapters. Parts focus on broad areas of interest. Chapters are devoted to single topics within a part.

Part I: What You Need to Know about Germs describes various types of microbes and different kinds of infections. It explains how the immune system responds to germs and how diseases can be transmitted from one person to another. Public health issues are also discussed, including the practice of screening internationally adopted children for contagious diseases and the threat of bioterrorism.

Part II: Types of Contagious Diseases provides facts about forty-eight specific diseases of concern—from adenovirus to whooping cough—in individual, alphabetically arranged chapters.

Part III: Self-Treatment for Contagious Diseases discusses frequently used remedies for common illnesses and disease symptoms. Facts about the proper use of over-the-counter (OTC) medications are included along with a chapter focusing on the dangers associated with drug interactions. The part concludes with information about the use of probiotics, herbal and dietary supplements, and other forms of complementary and alternative medicine.

Part IV: Medical Diagnosis and Treatment of Contagious Diseases explains the tests and procedures used to identify the presence of microbial infection, including *Streptococcus* and *Staphylococcus* bacteria and viruses associated with colds, influenza, and other diseases. Antibiotic and antiviral medications are discussed, and the growing problem of antimicrobial resistance—the way microbes change to counteract the effectiveness of drug treatments—is explained.

Part V: Preventing Contagious Diseases begins with information about a simple practice that is a key element in the fight against the spread of germs—handwashing. It continues with facts about vaccines, another effective tool for halting the proliferation of disease. Information about vaccine recommendations for children, adolescents, and adults is included, and this part also addresses problems associated with vaccines, the vaccine adverse event reporting system, and the difficulties that can arise as a result of vaccine misinformation.

Part VI: Additional Help and Information provides a glossary of terms related to contagious diseases and a directory of resources for additional information.

Bibliographic Note

This volume contains documents and excerpts from publications issued by the following U.S. government agencies: Agency for Healthcare Research and Quality (AHRQ); Centers for Disease Control and Prevention (CDC); National Center for Complementary and Alternative Medicine (NCCAM); National Heart, Lung, and Blood Institute (NHLBI); National Institute of Allergy and Infectious Diseases (NIAID); National Institute of Diabetes and Digestive and Kidney Diseases (NIDDK); National Institute of Neurological Disorders and Stroke (NINDS); U.S. Department of Health and Human Services (HHS); U.S. Department of State; U.S. Food and Drug Administration (FDA); and the Women's Health Information Center.

In addition, this volume contains copyrighted documents from the following individuals and organizations: A.D.A.M., Inc.; American Academy of Family Physicians; American Association for Clinical Chemistry; American Association of Blood Banks; American College Health Association; American Lung Association; American Social Health Association; Association for Professionals in Infection Control and Epidemiology; Immunization Action Coalition; National Foundation for Infectious Diseases; National Network for Immunization Information; Nemours Foundation; Organization of Teratology Information Specialists; Soap and Detergent Association; Vinay N. Reddy, MD; and Trust for America's Health.

Full citation information is provided on the first page of each chapter or section. Every effort has been made to secure all necessary rights to reprint the copyrighted material. If any omissions have been made, please contact Omnigraphics to make corrections for future editions.

Acknowledgements

In addition to the listed organizations, agencies, and individuals who have contributed to this *Sourcebook*, special thanks go to managing editor Karen Bellenir, research and permissions coordinator Liz Collins, and document engineer Bruce Bellenir for their help and support.

About the Health Reference Series

The *Health Reference Series* is designed to provide basic medical information for patients, families, caregivers, and the general public.

Each volume takes a particular topic and provides comprehensive coverage. This is especially important for people who may be dealing with a newly diagnosed disease or a chronic disorder in themselves or in a family member. People looking for preventive guidance, information about disease warning signs, medical statistics, and risk factors for health problems will also find answers to their questions in the *Health Reference Series*. The *Series*, however, is not intended to serve as a tool for diagnosing illness, in prescribing treatments, or as a substitute for the physician/patient relationship. All people concerned about medical symptoms or the possibility of disease are encouraged to seek professional care from an appropriate health care provider.

A Note about Spelling and Style

Health Reference Series editors use *Stedman's Medical Dictionary* as an authority for questions related to the spelling of medical terms and the *Chicago Manual of Style* for questions related to grammatical structures, punctuation, and other editorial concerns. Consistent adherence is not always possible, however, because the individual volumes within the *Series* include many documents from a wide variety of different producers and copyright holders, and the editor's primary goal is to present material from each source as accurately as is possible following the terms specified by each document's producer. This sometimes means that information in different chapters or sections may follow other guidelines and alternate spelling authorities. For example, occasionally a copyright holder may require that eponymous terms be shown in possessive forms (Crohn's disease *vs.* Crohn disease) or that British spelling norms be retained (leukaemia *vs.* leukemia).

Locating Information within the Health Reference Series

The *Health Reference Series* contains a wealth of information about a wide variety of medical topics. Ensuring easy access to all the fact sheets, research reports, in-depth discussions, and other material contained within the individual books of the *Series* remains one of our highest priorities. As the *Series* continues to grow in size and scope, however, locating the precise information needed by a reader may become more challenging.

A *Contents Guide to the Health Reference Series* was developed to direct readers to the specific volumes that address their concerns. It presents an extensive list of diseases, treatments, and other topics of general interest compiled from the Tables of Contents and major index headings. To access *A Contents Guide to the Health Reference Series*, visit www.healthreferenceseries.com.

Medical Consultant

Medical consultation services are provided to the *Health Reference Series* editors by David A. Cooke, MD, FACP. Dr. Cooke is a graduate of Brandeis University, and he received his MD degree from the University of Michigan. He completed residency training at the University of Wisconsin Hospital and Clinics. He is board-certified in Internal Medicine. Dr. Cooke currently works as part of the University of Michigan Health System and practices in Ann Arbor, MI. In his free time, he enjoys writing, science fiction, and spending time with his family.

Our Advisory Board

We would like to thank the following board members for providing guidance to the development of this *Series*:

- Dr. Lynda Baker, Associate Professor of Library and Information Science, Wayne State University, Detroit, MI
- Nancy Bulgarelli, William Beaumont Hospital Library, Royal Oak, MI
- Karen Imarisio, Bloomfield Township Public Library, Bloomfield Township, MI
- Karen Morgan, Mardigian Library, University of Michigan-Dearborn, Dearborn, MI
- Rosemary Orlando, St. Clair Shores Public Library, St. Clair Shores, MI

Health Reference Series *Update Policy*

The inaugural book in the *Health Reference Series* was the first edition of *Cancer Sourcebook* published in 1989. Since then, the *Series* has been enthusiastically received by librarians and in the medical community. In order to maintain the standard of providing high-quality health information for the layperson the editorial staff at Omnigraphics felt it was necessary to implement a policy of updating volumes when warranted.

Medical researchers have been making tremendous strides, and it is the purpose of the *Health Reference Series* to stay current with the most recent advances. Each decision to update a volume is made on an individual basis. Some of the considerations include how much new information is available and the feedback we receive from people who use the books. If there is a topic you would like to see added to the update list, or an area of medical concern you feel has not been adequately addressed, please write to:

Editor
Health Reference Series
Omnigraphics, Inc.
P.O. Box 31-1640
Detroit, MI 48231-1640
E-mail: editorial@omnigraphics.com

Part One

What You Need to Know about Germs

Chapter 1

Understanding Microbes (Germs)

Chapter Contents

Section 1.1

What Are Microbes?

Text in this section is excerpted from "Understanding Microbes in Sickness and in Health," National Institute of Allergy and Infectious Diseases (NIAID), NIH Publication No. 06–4914, January 2006.

Microbes are tiny organisms—too tiny to see without a microscope, yet they are abundant on Earth. They live everywhere—in air, soil, rock, and water. Some live happily in searing heat, while others thrive in freezing cold. Some microbes need oxygen to live, but others do not. These microscopic organisms are found in plants and animals as well as in the human body. Some microbes cause disease in humans, plants, and animals. Others are essential for a healthy life, and we could not exist without them. Indeed, the relationship between microbes and humans is delicate and complex.

Most microbes belong to one of four major groups: bacteria, viruses, fungi, or protozoa. A common word for microbes that cause disease is germs. Some people refer to disease-causing microbes as bugs. "I've got the flu bug," for example, is a phrase you may hear used to describe an influenza virus infection.

Since the 19th century, we have known microbes cause infectious diseases. Near the end of the 20th century, researchers began to learn that microbes also contribute to many chronic diseases and conditions. Mounting scientific evidence strongly links microbes to some forms of cancer, coronary artery disease, diabetes, multiple sclerosis, and chronic lung diseases.

Bacteria

Microbes belonging to the bacteria group are made up of only one cell. Under a microscope, bacteria look like balls, rods, or spirals. Bacteria are so small that a line of 1,000 could fit across the eraser of a pencil. Life in any form on Earth could not exist without these tiny cells.

Bacteria can inhabit a variety of environments, including extremely hot and cold areas. Many bacteria prefer the milder temperature of the healthy human body. Like humans, some bacteria (aerobic bacteria) need oxygen to survive. Others (anaerobic bacteria), however, do not. Amazingly, some can adapt to new environments by learning to survive with or without oxygen.

Like all living cells, each bacterium requires food for energy and building materials. There are countless numbers of bacteria on Earth—most are harmless and many are even beneficial to humans. In fact, less than one percent of bacteria cause diseases in humans. For example, harmless anaerobic bacteria, such as *Lactobacilli acidophilus*, live in our intestines, where they help to digest food, destroy disease-causing microbes, fight cancer cells, and give the body needed vitamins. Healthy food products, such as yogurt, sauerkraut, and cheese, are made using bacteria. Some bacteria produce poisons called toxins, which also can make us sick.

Are toxins always harmful?

Certain bacteria give off toxins that can seriously affect your health. Botulism, a severe form of food poisoning, affects the nerves and is caused by toxins from *Clostridium botulinum* bacteria. Under certain circumstances, however, bacterial toxins can be helpful. Several vaccines that protect us from getting sick are made from bacterial toxins. One type of pertussis vaccine, which protects infants and children from whooping cough, contains toxins from *Bordetella pertussis* bacteria. This vaccine is safe and effective and causes fewer reactions than other types of pertussis vaccine.

Viruses

Viruses are among the smallest microbes, much smaller even than bacteria. Viruses are not cells. They consist of one or more molecules of deoxyribonucleic acid (DNA) or ribonucleic acid (RNA), which contain the genes from the virus surrounded by a protein coat. Viruses can be rod-shaped, sphere-shaped, or multisided. Some viruses look like tadpoles.

Unlike most bacteria, most viruses do cause disease because they invade living, normal cells, such as those in your body. They then multiply and produce other viruses like themselves. Each virus is very particular about which cell it attacks. Various human viruses specifically attack particular cells in your body's organs, systems, or tissues, such as the liver, respiratory system, or blood.

Although types of viruses behave differently, most survive by taking over the machinery that makes a cell work. Briefly, when a piece of a virus, called a virion, comes in contact with a cell it likes, it may attach to special landing sites on the surface of that cell. From there, the virus may inject molecules into the cell, or the cell may swallow the virion. Once inside the cell, viral molecules such as DNA or RNA direct the cell to make new virus offspring. That's how a virus infects a cell. Viruses can even infect bacteria. These viruses, called bacteriophages, may help researchers develop alternatives to antibiotic medicines for preventing and treating bacterial infections.

Many viral infections do not result in disease. For example, by the time most people in the United States become adults, they have been infected by cytomegalovirus (CMV). Most of these people, however, do not develop CMV-disease symptoms. Other viral infections can result in deadly diseases such as acquired immunodeficiency syndrome (AIDS) or Ebola hemorrhagic fever.

Fungi

A fungus is actually a primitive plant. Fungi can be found in air, in soil, on plants, and in water. Thousands, perhaps millions, of different types of fungi exist on Earth. The most familiar ones to us are mushrooms, yeast, mold, and mildew. Some live in the human body, usually without causing illness. Fungal diseases are called mycoses. Mycoses can affect your skin, nails, body hair, internal organs such as your lungs, and body systems such as your nervous system. *Aspergillus fumigatus*, for example, can cause aspergillosis, a fungal infection in your respiratory system.

Some fungi have made our lives easier. Penicillin and other antibiotics, which kill harmful bacteria in our bodies, are made from fungi. Other fungi, such as certain yeasts, also can be helpful. For example, when a warm liquid, such as water, and a food source are added to certain yeasts, the fungus ferments. The process of fermentation is essential for making healthy foods like some breads and cheeses.

Protozoa

Protozoa are a group of microscopic one-celled animals. Protozoa can be parasites or predators. In humans, protozoa usually cause disease.

Some protozoa, like plankton, live in water environments and serve as food for marine animals, such as some kinds of whales. Protozoa also can be found on land in decaying matter and in soil, but they must have a moist environment to survive. Termites would not be able to do such a good job of digesting wood without these microorganisms in their guts.

Malaria is caused by a protozoan parasite. Another protozoan parasite, *Toxoplasma gondii*, causes toxoplasmosis in humans. This is an especially troublesome infection in pregnant women because of its effects on the fetus, and in people with human immunodeficiency virus (HIV) infection or other immune deficiency disorders.

Table 1.1. Microbes in the Healthy Human Body*

Microbes found in

Ear (outer)	*Aspergillus* (fungus)
Skin	*Candida* (fungus)
Small intestine	*Clostridium*
Intestines	*Escherichia coli*
Vagina	*Gardnerella vaginalis*
Stomach	*Lactobacillus*
Urethra	*Mycobacterium*
Nose	*Staphylococcus aureus*
Mouth	*Streptococcus salivarius*
Large intestine	*Trichomonas hominis* (protozoa)

*A selection of usually harmless microbes, some of which help keep our bodies functioning normally. If their numbers become unbalanced, however, these microbes may make us sick. All are bacteria, unless otherwise noted.

Section 1.2

Microbes Can Cause Different Kinds of Infections

Text in this section is from "Microbes: Kinds of Infections, and Emerging and Re-Emerging Microbes," National Institute of Allergy and Infectious Diseases (NIAID), July 22, 2008; and "Microbes: Diseases and Infections Caused by Microbes," NIAID, July 14, 2008.

Some disease-causing microbes can make you very sick quickly and then not bother you again. Some can last for a long time and continue to damage tissues. Others can last forever, but you won't feel sick anymore, or you will feel sick only once in a while. Most infections caused by microbes fall into three major groups.

Acute Infections

Acute infections are usually severe and last a short time. They can make you feel very uncomfortable, with signs and symptoms such as tiredness, achiness, coughing, and sneezing. The common cold is such an infection. The signs and symptoms of a cold can last for 2–24 days (but usually a week), though it may seem like a lot longer. Once your body's immune system has successfully fought off one of the many different types of rhinoviruses or other viruses that may have caused your cold, the cold does not come back. If you get another cold, it is probably because you have been infected with other cold-causing viruses.

Chronic Infections

Chronic infections usually develop from acute infections and can last for days to months to a lifetime. Sometimes people are unaware they are infected but still may be able to transmit the germ to others. For example, hepatitis C, which affects the liver, is a chronic viral infection. In fact, most people who have been infected with the hepatitis C virus do not know it until they have a blood test that shows antibodies to the virus. Recovery from this infection is rare—about

85 percent of infected persons become chronic carriers of the virus. In addition, serious signs of liver damage, like cirrhosis or cancer, may not appear until as long as 20 years after the infection began.

Latent Infections

Latent infections are hidden or silent and may or may not cause symptoms again after the first acute episode. Some infectious microbes, usually viruses, can wake up—become active again but not always causing symptoms—off and on for months or years. When these microbes are active in your body, you can transmit them to other people. Herpes simplex viruses, which cause genital herpes and cold sores, can remain latent in nerve cells for short or long periods of time, or forever.

Chickenpox is another example of a latent infection. Before the chickenpox vaccine became available in the 1990s, most children in the United States got chickenpox. After the first acute episode, usually when children are very young, the *Varicella zoster* virus goes into hiding in the body. In many people, it emerges many years later when they are older adults and causes a painful disease of the nerves called herpes zoster, or shingles.

Emerging and Re-Emerging Microbes

By the mid-20th century, some scientists thought that medicine had conquered infectious diseases. With the arrival of antibiotics and modern vaccines, as well as improved sanitation and hygiene, many diseases that formerly posed an urgent threat to public health were brought under control or largely eliminated.

The emergence of new microbes and the re-emergence of old microbes has continued, however, as it has throughout history. Several pressures are contributing to the emergence of new diseases such as:

- rapidly changing human demographics;
- rapid global travel;
- changes in land use patterns; and
- ecological, environmental, and technological changes.

Even public health practices such as widespread antibiotic use are contributing to this emergence. These pressures are both shaping the evolution of microbes and bringing people into closer and more frequent contact with microbes.

Unsanitary conditions in animal agriculture and increasing commerce in exotic animals (for food and as pets) have also contributed to the rise in opportunity for animal microbes to jump from animals to humans. From time to time, with the right combination of selective pressures, a formerly harmless human or animal microbe can evolve into a pathogen that can cause a major outbreak of human disease. At times, changes in societal and environmental factors can also lead to re-emergence of diseases that were previously under control.

Table 1.2. Common Diseases and Infections and Their Microbial Causes

	Bacteria	Fungus	Protozoa	Virus
Athlete's foot		X		
Chickenpox				X
Common cold				X
Diarrheal disease	X		X	X
Flu (influenza)				X
Genital herpes				X
Malaria			X	
Meningitis	X			X
Pneumococcal pneumonia	X	X		X
Sinusitis	X	X		X
Skin diseases	X	X	X	X
Tuberculosis	X			
Urinary tract infection	X			
Vaginal infections	X	X		
Viral hepatitis				X

Section 1.3

Preventing Microbial Diseases

"Microbes: Prevention," National Institute of
Allergy and Infectious Diseases (NIAID), July 14, 2008.

Handwashing

Handwashing is one of the simplest, easiest, and most effective ways
to prevent getting or passing on many germs. Amazingly, it is also one
of the most overlooked. Health care experts recommend scrubbing your
hands vigorously for at least 15 seconds with soap and water, about as
long as it takes to recite the English alphabet. This will wash away cold
viruses and staph and strep bacteria as well as many other disease-
causing microbes. It is especially important to wash your hands:

- before preparing or eating food,
- after coughing or sneezing,
- after using the bathroom, and
- after changing a diaper.

Health care providers should be especially conscientious about
washing their hands before and after examining any patient. Workers in childcare and elder care settings, too, should be vigilant about
handwashing.

Medicines

There are medicines on the market that help prevent people from
getting infected by germs. For example, you can prevent getting the
flu (influenza) by taking an antiviral medicine. Vaccines, however, are
the best defense against influenza viruses.

Under specific circumstances, health care providers may prescribe
antibiotics to protect people from getting certain bacteria such as *Mycobacterium tuberculosis*, which causes tuberculosis (TB). Health care
experts usually advise people traveling to areas where malaria is
present to take antiparasitic medicines to prevent possible infection.

Vaccines

In 1796, Edward Jenner laid the foundation for modern vaccines by discovering one of the basic principles of immunization. He had used a relatively harmless microbe, cowpox virus, to bring about an immune response that would help protect people from getting infected by the related but deadly smallpox virus. Dr. Jenner's discovery helped researchers find ways to ease human disease suffering worldwide. By the beginning of the 20th century, doctors were immunizing patients with vaccines for diphtheria, typhoid fever, and smallpox. Today, safe and effective vaccines prevent childhood diseases, including measles, whooping cough, chickenpox, and the form of meningitis caused by *Haemophilus influenzae* type B, or HIB, virus.

Vaccines, however, are not only useful for young children. Adolescents and adults should get vaccinated regularly for tetanus and diphtheria. A vaccine to prevent meningococcal meningitis is now available and recommended for all adolescents. In addition, adults who never had diseases such as measles or chickenpox during childhood or who never received vaccines to prevent them should consider being immunized. Childhood diseases can be far more serious in adults.

More people travel all over the world today. So, finding out which immunizations are recommended for travel to your destination(s) is important. Vaccines also can prevent yellow fever, polio, typhoid fever, hepatitis A, cholera, rabies, and other bacterial and viral diseases that are more prevalent abroad than in the United States.

In the fall of the year, many adults and children may benefit from getting the flu vaccine. Your health care provider also may recommend immunizations for pneumococcal pneumonia and hepatitis B if you are at risk of getting these diseases.

How You Can Be Protected from Microbes

You can become immune, or develop immunity, to a microbe in several ways. The first time T cells and B cells in your immune system meet up with an antigen, such as a virus or bacterium, they prepare the immune system to destroy the antigen.

Naturally Acquired Immunity

Because the immune system often can remember its enemies, those cells become active if they meet that particular antigen again. This is called naturally acquired immunity. Another example of naturally acquired immunity occurs when a pregnant woman passes antibodies to her unborn baby. Babies are born with weak immune responses, but they are protected from some diseases for their first few months of life by antibodies received from their mothers before birth. Babies who are nursed also receive antibodies from breast milk that help protect their digestive tracts.

Artificial Immunity

Artificial immunity can come from vaccines. Immunization with vaccines is a safe way to get protection from germs. Some vaccines contain microorganisms or parts of microorganisms that have been weakened or killed. If you get this type of vaccine, those microorganisms (or their parts) will start your body's immune response, which will demolish the foreign invader but not make you sick. This is a type of artificially acquired immunity.

Immunity can be strong or weak and short- or long-lived, depending on the type of antigen, the amount of antigen, and the route by which it enters your body. When faced with the same antigen, some people's immune system will respond forcefully, others feebly, and some not at all.

The genes you inherit also can influence your likelihood of getting a disease. In simple terms, the genes you get from your parents can influence how your body reacts to certain microbes.

Section 1.4

General Symptoms, Diagnosis, and Treatment of Microbial Diseases

"Microbes: Symptoms, Diagnosis, and Treatment," National Institute of Allergy and Infectious Diseases (NIAID), July 14, 2008. The sections titled, "How Medicines Can Help," and "How Your Immune System Can Help," were updated July 7, 2009.

Symptoms

Generally, you should consult your health care provider if you have or think you may have an infectious disease. However, some infectious diseases, such as the common cold, usually do not require a visit to your doctor. They often last a short time and are not life-threatening, or there is no specific treatment. We have all heard the advice to rest and drink plenty of liquids to treat colds. Unless there are complications, most victims of colds find that their immune systems successfully fight off the viral culprits. In fact, the coughing and sneezing that make you feel miserable are part of your immune system's way of fighting off the culprits.

If you have other conditions in which your immune system does not function properly, you should be in contact with your health care provider whenever you suspect you have any infectious disease, even the common cold. Such conditions can include asthma and immune deficiency diseases like human immunodeficiency virus (HIV) infection and acquired immunodeficiency syndrome (AIDS). In addition, some common, usually mild infectious diseases, such as chickenpox or flu, can cause serious harm in very young children and the elderly.

You should call a health care provider immediately in the following situations:

- You have been bitten by an animal.
- You are having difficulty breathing.
- You have a cough that has lasted for more than a week.
- You have a fever higher than 100 degrees Fahrenheit.

- You have episodes of rapid heartbeat.
- You have a rash (especially if you have a fever at the same time).
- You have swelling.
- You suddenly start having difficulty with seeing (blurry vision, for example).
- You have been vomiting.

Diagnosis

Sometimes your health care provider can diagnose an infectious disease by listening to your medical history and doing a physical exam. For example, listening to you describe what happened and any symptoms you have noticed plays an important part in helping your doctor find out what is wrong.

Blood and urine tests are other ways to diagnose an infection. A laboratory expert can sometimes see the offending microbe in a sample of blood or urine viewed under a microscope. One or both of these tests may be the only way to determine what caused the infection, or they may be used to confirm a diagnosis that was made based on taking a medical history and doing a physical exam.

In another type of test, your health care provider will take a sample of blood or other body fluid, such as vaginal secretion, and then put it into a special container called a Petri dish to see if any microbe grows. This test is called a culture. Certain bacteria, such as chlamydia and strep, and viruses, such as herpes simplex, usually can be identified using this method. X-rays, scans, and biopsies (taking a tiny sample of tissue from the infected area and inspecting it under a microscope) are among other tools the doctor can use to make an accurate diagnosis.

All of the listed procedures are relatively safe, and some can be done in your doctor's office or a clinic. Others pose a higher risk to you because they involve procedures that go inside your body. One such invasive procedure is taking a biopsy from an internal organ. For example, one way a doctor can diagnose *Pneumocystis carinii* pneumonia, a lung disease caused by a fungus, is by doing a biopsy on lung tissue and then examining the sample under a microscope.

Treatment

How an infectious disease is treated depends on the microbe that caused it and sometimes on the age and medical condition of the person affected. Certain diseases are not treated at all, but are allowed to run their course, with the immune system doing its job alone. Some diseases, such as the common cold, are treated only to relieve the symptoms. Others, such as strep throat, are treated to destroy the offending microbe as well as to relieve symptoms.

How Medicines Can Help

For Bacteria

The last century saw an explosion in our knowledge about how microbes work and in our methods of treating infectious diseases. For example, the discovery of antibiotics to treat and cure many bacterial diseases was a major breakthrough in medical history. Doctors, however, sometimes prescribe antibiotics unnecessarily for a variety of reasons, including pressure from patients with viral infections. Patients may insist on being prescribed an antibiotic without knowing that it will not work on viruses. Colds and flu are two notable viral infections for which some doctors send their patients to the drugstore with a prescription for an antibiotic.

Because antibiotics have been overprescribed or inappropriately prescribed for many years, bacteria have become resistant to the killing effects of these drugs. This resistance, called antibiotic or drug resistance, has become a very serious problem, especially in hospital settings. Bacteria that are not killed by the antibiotic become strong enough to resist the same medicine the next time it is given. Because bacteria multiply so rapidly, changed or mutated bacteria that resist antibiotics will quickly outnumber those that can be destroyed by those same drugs.

For Viruses

Viral diseases can be very difficult to treat because viruses live inside your body's cells where they are protected from medicines in the bloodstream. Researchers developed the first antiviral drug in the late 20th century. The drug, acyclovir, was first approved by the Food and Drug Administration (FDA) to treat herpes simplex virus infections. Only a few other antiviral medicines are available to prevent and treat viral infections and diseases.

Health care providers treat human immunodeficiency virus (HIV) infection with a group of powerful medicines that can keep the virus in check. Known as highly active antiretroviral therapy, or HAART, this treatment has improved the lives of many suffering from this deadly infection.

Viral diseases should never be treated with antibiotics. Sometimes a person with a viral disease will develop a bacterial disease as a complication of the initial viral disease. Although safe and effective treatments and cures for most viral diseases have eluded researchers, there are safe vaccines to protect you from viral infections and diseases.

For Fungi

Medicines applied directly to the infected area are available by prescription and over the counter for treating skin and nail fungal infections. Unfortunately, many people have had limited success with them. During the 1990s, oral prescription medicines became available for treating fungal infections of the skin and nails. For many years, very powerful oral antifungal medicines were used only to treat systemic (within the body) fungal infections, such as histoplasmosis. Doctors usually prescribe oral antifungal medications cautiously because all of them, even the milder medicines for skin and nail fungi, can have very serious side effects.

For Protozoa

Diseases caused by protozoan parasites are among the leading causes of death and disease in tropical and subtropical regions of the world. Developing countries within these areas contain three-quarters of the world's population, and their people suffer the most from these diseases. Controlling parasitic diseases is a problem because there are no vaccines for any of them.

In many cases, controlling the insects that transmit these diseases is difficult because of pesticide resistance, concerns regarding environmental damage, and lack of adequate public health systems to apply existing insect-control methods. Thus, disease control relies heavily on the availability of medicines. Health care providers usually use antiparasitic medicines to treat protozoal infections. Unfortunately, there are very few medicines that fight protozoa, and some of those are either harmful to humans or are becoming ineffective.

How Your Immune System Can Help

Your immune system has an arsenal of ways to fight off invading microbes. Most begin with B and T cells and antibodies whose sole purpose is to keep your body healthy. Some of these cells sacrifice their lives to rid you of disease and restore your body to a healthy state. Some microbes normally present in your body also help destroy microbial invaders. For example, normal bacteria, such as lactobacillus in your digestive system, help destroy disease-causing microbes. Other important ways your body reacts to an infection include fever, coughing, and sneezing.

Fever

Fever is one of your body's special ways of fighting an infectious disease. Many microbes are very sensitive to temperature changes and cannot survive in temperatures higher than normal body heat, which is usually around 98.6 degrees Fahrenheit. Your body uses fever to destroy flu viruses.

Coughing and Sneezing

Another tool in your immune system's reaction to invading infection-causing microbes is mucus production. Coughing and sneezing helps mucus move those germs out of your body efficiently and quickly.

Other methods your body may use to fight off an infectious disease include the following:

- Inflammation
- Vomiting
- Diarrhea
- Fatigue
- Cramping

Chapter 2

The Immune System and Its Response to Infection

The immune system is a network of cells, tissues, and organs that work together to defend the body against attacks by "foreign" invaders. These are primarily microbes—tiny organisms such as bacteria, parasites, and fungi that can cause infections. Viruses also cause infections, but are too primitive to be classified as living organisms. The human body provides an ideal environment for many microbes. It is the immune system's job to keep them out or, failing that, to seek out and destroy them.

Self and Non-Self

The key to a healthy immune system is its remarkable ability to distinguish between the body's own cells, recognized as "self," and foreign cells, or "nonself." The body's immune defenses normally coexist peacefully with cells that carry distinctive "self" marker molecules. But when immune defenders encounter foreign cells or organisms carrying markers that say "nonself," they quickly launch an attack.

Anything that can trigger this immune response is called an antigen. An antigen can be a microbe such as a virus, or a part of a microbe such as a molecule. Tissues or cells from another person (except an identical twin) also carry nonself markers and act as foreign antigens. This explains why tissue transplants may be rejected.

Excerpted from "Understanding the Immune System," National Institute of Allergy and Infectious Diseases (NIAID), available online at http://www3.niaid .nih.gov/topics/immuneSystem, updated October 2008.

The Structure of the Immune System

The organs of the immune system are positioned throughout the body. They are called lymphoid organs because they are home to lymphocytes, small white blood cells that are the key players in the immune system. Bone marrow, the soft tissue in the hollow center of bones, is the ultimate source of all blood cells, including lymphocytes. The thymus is a lymphoid organ that lies behind the breastbone.

Lymphocytes known as T lymphocytes or T cells (T stands for thymus) mature in the thymus and then migrate to other tissues. B lymphocytes, also known as B cells, become activated and mature into plasma cells, which make and release antibodies.

Lymphocytes can travel throughout the body using the blood vessels. The cells can also travel through a system of lymphatic vessels that closely parallels the body's veins and arteries. Cells and fluids are exchanged between blood and lymphatic vessels, enabling the lymphatic system to monitor the body for invading microbes. The lymphatic vessels carry lymph, a clear fluid that bathes the body's tissues.

Small, bean-shaped lymph nodes are laced along the lymphatic vessels, with clusters in the neck, armpits, abdomen, and groin. Each lymph node contains specialized compartments where immune cells congregate, and where they can encounter antigens. Immune cells, microbes, and foreign antigens enter the lymph nodes via incoming lymphatic vessels or the lymph nodes' tiny blood vessels. All lymphocytes exit lymph nodes through outgoing lymphatic vessels. Once in the bloodstream, lymphocytes are transported to tissues throughout the body. They patrol everywhere for foreign antigens, then gradually drift back into the lymphatic system to begin the cycle all over again.

The spleen is a flattened organ at the upper left of the abdomen. Like the lymph nodes, the spleen contains specialized compartments where immune cells gather and work. The spleen serves as a meeting ground where immune defenses confront antigens.

Other clumps of lymphoid tissue are found in many parts of the body, especially in the linings of the digestive tract, airways, and lungs—territories that serve as gateways to the body. These tissues include the tonsils, adenoids, and appendix.

Immune Cells and Their Products

The immune system stockpiles a huge arsenal of cells, not only lymphocytes but also cell-devouring phagocytes and their relatives. Some immune cells take on all intruders, whereas others are trained on highly specific targets. To work effectively, most immune cells need the cooperation of their comrades. Sometimes immune cells communicate by direct physical contact, and sometimes they communicate releasing chemical messengers.

The immune system stores just a few of each kind of the different cells needed to recognize millions of possible enemies. When an antigen first appears, the few immune cells that can respond to it multiply into a full-scale army of cells. After their job is done, the immune cells fade away, leaving sentries behind to watch for future attacks.

All immune cells begin as immature stem cells in the bone marrow. They respond to different cytokines and other chemical signals to grow into specific immune cell types, such as T cells, B cells, or phagocytes. Because stem cells have not yet committed to a particular future, their use presents an interesting possibility for treating some immune system disorders.

Mounting an Immune Response

Infections are the most common cause of human disease. Disease-causing microbes (pathogens) attempting to get into the body must first move past the body's external armor, usually the skin or cells lining the body's internal passageways.

The skin provides an imposing barrier to invading microbes. It is generally penetrable only through cuts or tiny abrasions. The digestive and respiratory tracts—both portals of entry for a number of microbes—also have their own levels of protection. Microbes entering the nose often cause the nasal surfaces to secrete more protective mucus, and attempts to enter the nose or lungs can trigger a sneeze or cough reflex to force microbial invaders out of the respiratory passageways. The stomach contains a strong acid that destroys many pathogens that are swallowed with food.

If microbes survive the body's front-line defenses, they still have to find a way through the walls of the digestive, respiratory, or urogenital passageways to the underlying cells. These passageways are lined with tightly packed epithelial cells covered in a layer of mucus, effectively blocking the transport of many pathogens into deeper cell layers.

Mucosal surfaces also secrete a special class of antibody called immunoglobulin A (IgA), which in many cases is the first type of antibody to encounter an invading microbe. Underneath the epithelial layer a variety of immune cells, including macrophages, B cells, and T cells, lie in wait for any microbe that might bypass the barriers at the surface.

Next, invaders must escape a series of general defenses of the innate immune system, which are ready to attack without regard for specific antigen markers. These include patrolling phagocytes, natural killer T cells, and complement.

Microbes cross the general barriers then confront specific weapons of the adaptive immune system tailored just for them. These specific weapons, which include both antibodies and T cells, are equipped with singular receptor structures that allow them to recognize and interact with their designated targets.

Bacteria, Viruses, and Parasites

The most common disease-causing microbes are bacteria, viruses, and parasites. Each uses a different tactic to infect a person, and, therefore, each is thwarted by different components of the immune system.

Most bacteria live in the spaces between cells and are readily attacked by antibodies. When antibodies attach to a bacterium, they send signals to complement proteins and phagocytic cells to destroy the bound microbes. Some bacteria are eaten directly by phagocytes, which signal to certain T cells to join the attack.

All viruses, plus a few types of bacteria and parasites, must enter cells of the body to survive, requiring a different kind of immune defense. Infected cells use their major histocompatibility complex molecules to put pieces of the invading microbes on their surfaces, flagging down cytotoxic T lymphocytes to destroy the infected cells. Antibodies also can assist in the immune response by attaching to and clearing viruses before they have a chance to enter cells.

Parasites live either inside or outside cells. Intracellular parasites such as the organism that causes malaria can trigger T cell responses. Extracellular parasites are often much larger than bacteria or viruses and require a much broader immune attack. Parasitic infections often trigger an inflammatory response in which eosinophils, basophils, and other specialized granule-containing cells rush to the scene and release their stores of toxic chemicals in an attempt to destroy the invaders. Antibodies also play a role in this attack, attracting the granule-filled cells to the site of infection.

Immunity: Natural and Acquired

Long ago, physicians realized that people who had recovered from the plague would never get it again—they had acquired immunity.

This is because some of the activated T and B cells had become memory cells. Memory cells ensure that the next time a person meets up with the same antigen, the immune system is already set to demolish it.

Immunity can be strong or weak, short-lived or long-lasting, depending on the type of antigen it encounters, the amount of antigen, and the route by which the antigen enters the body. Immunity can also be influenced by inherited genes. When faced with the same antigen, some individuals will respond forcefully, others feebly, and some not at all.

An immune response can be sparked not only by infection but also by immunization with vaccines. Some vaccines contain microorganisms—or parts of microorganisms—that have been treated so they can provoke an immune response but not full-blown disease.

Immunity can also be transferred from one individual to another by injections of serum rich in antibodies against a particular microbe (antiserum). For example, antiserum is sometimes given to protect travelers to countries where hepatitis A is widespread. The antiserum induces passive immunity against the hepatitis A virus. Passive immunity typically lasts only a few weeks or months.

Infants are born with weak immune responses but are protected for the first few months of life by antibodies they receive from their mothers before birth. Babies who are nursed can also receive some antibodies from breast milk that help to protect their digestive tracts.

Immune Tolerance

Immune tolerance is the tendency of T or B lymphocytes to ignore the body's own tissues. Maintaining tolerance is important because it prevents the immune system from attacking its fellow cells. Tolerance occurs in at least two ways—central tolerance and peripheral tolerance.

Central tolerance occurs during lymphocyte development. Very early in each immune cell's life, it is exposed to many of the self molecules in the body. If it encounters these molecules before it has fully matured, the encounter activates an internal self-destruct pathway, and the immune cell dies. This process, called clonal deletion, helps ensure that self-reactive T cells and B cells, those that could develop the ability to destroy the body's own cells, do not mature and attack healthy tissues.

Because maturing lymphocytes do not encounter every molecule in the body, they must also learn to ignore mature cells and tissues.

In peripheral tolerance, circulating lymphocytes might recognize a self molecule but cannot respond because some of the chemical signals required to activate the T or B cell are absent. So-called clonal anergy, therefore, keeps potentially harmful lymphocytes switched off. Peripheral tolerance may also be imposed by a special class of regulatory T cells that inhibits helper or cytotoxic T-cell activation by self antigens.

Vaccines

Vaccination helps the body's immune system prepare for future attacks. Vaccines consist of killed or modified microbes, parts of microbes, or microbial deoxyribonucleic acid (DNA) that trick the body into thinking an infection has occurred.

A vaccinated person's immune system attacks the harmless vaccine and prepares for invasions against the kind of microbe the vaccine contained. In this way, the person becomes immunized against the microbe. Vaccination remains one of the best ways to prevent infectious diseases, and vaccines have an excellent safety record. Previously devastating diseases such as smallpox, polio, and whooping cough (pertussis) have been greatly controlled or eliminated through worldwide vaccination programs.

Chapter 3

Immunodeficiency and Contagious Diseases

Most of us are no strangers to infections. Just about everybody has had a cold, cough, infected cut, the flu, or chicken pox. Some people have had first-hand experience with infections that are even more serious—pneumonia and meningitis.

Usually, we expect to recover quickly from an infection. We count on our body's immune defenses (sometimes with the help of antibiotics) to get rid of any germs that cause infection, and to protect us against new germs in the future. Some people, however, are born with an immune defense system that is faulty. They are missing some or, in the worst cases, almost all of the body's immune defense weapons. Such people are said to have a primary immunodeficiency (PI).

There are over 70 different types of PIs. Each type has somewhat different symptoms, depending on which parts of the immune defense system are deficient. Some deficiencies are deadly, while some are mild. But they all have one thing in common: they may open the door to multiple infections.

Individuals with PI—many of them infants and children—get one infection after another. Ear, sinus, and other infections may not improve with treatment as expected, but keep coming back or occurring with less common but severe infections, such as recurrent pneumonia. Besides being painful, frightening, and frustrating, these constant

Text in this chapter is from "Primary Immunodeficiency: When the Body's Defenses Are Missing," National Institute of Child Health and Human Development (NICHD), updated April 7, 2008. The complete document is available online at http://www.nichd.nih.gov/publications/pubs/PrimaryImmunocover.cfm.

infections can cause permanent damage to the ears or to the lungs. In the more severe forms of PI, germs which cause only mild infections in people with healthy immune systems may cause severe or life-threatening infections.

Although infections are the hallmark of PIs, they are not always the only health problem, or even the main one. Some PIs are associated with other immune system disorders, such as anemia, arthritis, or autoimmune diseases. Other PIs involve more than the immune system; some, for instance, are associated with symptoms involving the heart, digestive tract, or the nervous system. Some PIs retard growth and increase the risk of cancer.

Today, thanks to rapid advances in medicine, many PI diseases can be successfully treated or even cured. With proper treatment, most people with PIs are not only surviving once-deadly diseases, they are usually able to lead normal lives. Children usually can go to school, mix with playmates, and take part in sports. Most adults with PI are leading productive lives in their communities.

Successfully combating PI, however, depends on prompt detection. Physicians, parents, and adult patients alike need to recognize when infections are more than ordinary, so that treatment can be started in time to prevent permanent damage or life-threatening complications.

What Is Primary Immunodeficiency?

A PI disease results whenever one or more essential parts of the immune system is missing or not working properly at birth because of a genetic defect. Since the immune system is tremendously complex, hundreds of things can go wrong during development and sometimes the backup systems cannot compensate for the defects.

A variety of developmental errors in the immune system create different types of PIs. They make people susceptible to different kinds of germs and create different sets of symptoms. PI diseases were once thought to be rare, mostly because only the more severe forms were recognized. Today physicians realize that PIs are not uncommon. They are sometimes relatively mild, and they can occur in teenagers and adults as often as in infants and children. Very serious inherited immunodeficiencies become apparent almost as soon as a baby is born. Many more are discovered during the baby's first year of life. Others—usually the milder forms—may not show up until people reach their twenties and thirties. There are even some inherited immune deficiencies that never produce symptoms.

The exact number of persons with PI is not known. It is estimated that each year about 400 children are born in the United States with a serious PI. The number of Americans now living with a primary immunodeficiency is estimated to be between 25,000 and 50,000. As new laboratory tests become more widely available, more cases of PIs are being recognized. At the same time, new types of PI are being discovered and described. Currently, the World Health Organization (WHO) lists over 70 PIs and the numbers are increasing.

Among the rarest forms of immune deficiency is severe combined immune deficiency (SCID). SCID has been reported in small numbers, while some deficiencies, like DiGeorge syndrome, are diagnosed more commonly. At the other extreme, an immune disorder called selective immunoglobulin A (IgA) deficiency may occur in as many as one in every 300 persons. This figure is an estimate, based on studies of blood from blood donors, since most people with IgA deficiency are healthy and never realize they have this disorder.

Signs and Symptoms

The most common problem in PI disease is an increased susceptibility to infection. For people with PI, infections may be common, severe, lasting, or hard to cure. Even healthy youngsters may get frequent colds, coughs, or earaches. For example, many infants and young children with normal immunity have one to three ear infections per year. Children with PI, however, can get one infection after another. Or, they get two or three infections at a time. Weakened by infection, the child may fail to gain weight or fall behind in growth and development.

Despite the usual antibiotics, the infections of PI often drag on and on, or they keep coming back—that is, they become chronic. One common problem is chronic sinusitis (infection and inflammation of the sinuses, air passages in bones of the cheeks, forehead, and jaw). Another common problem is chronic bronchitis (infection and inflammation of the airways leading to the lungs).

Serious infections, especially bacterial infections, may cause a youngster to be hospitalized repeatedly. Pneumonia is an infection of the smallest airways and air sacs in the lungs, which prevents oxygen from reaching the blood and makes breathing hard. Meningitis, an infection of the membranes that surround the brain and spinal cord, causes fever and severe headache, and can lead to seizures, coma, and even death. Osteomyelitis is an infection that invades and destroys bones. Cellulitis is a serious infection of connective tissues just beneath the skin. Some people with PI develop blood poisoning, an infection that flourishes in the bloodstream and spreads rapidly through the body. Some people may develop deep abscesses, pockets of pus that form around infections in the skin or in body organs.

Some children with PI are infected with germs that a healthy immune system would hold in check. These are known as opportunistic infections because the germs take advantage of the opportunity afforded by a weakened immune system. Such an unusual infection may be the tip-off to an immunodeficiency. For example, *Pneumocystis carinii* is a microscopic parasite that infects many healthy people without making them sick. But when the immune system is compromised, *Pneumocystis* can produce a severe form of pneumonia. *Toxoplasma* is another widespread parasite that usually produces no disease. In persons with a weakened immune system, it causes toxoplasmosis, which can be a life-threatening infection of the brain that can cause confusion, headaches, fever, paralysis, seizures, and coma.

Beyond all the infections, some immunodeficiency diseases produce other immune system problems, including autoimmune disorders. Autoimmune disorders develop when the immune system gets out of control and mistakenly attacks the body's own organs and tissues. In some autoimmune disorders, the faulty immune system targets a single type of cell or tissue. For example, an immune attack on blood cells can lead to anemia, and an attack on islet cells of the pancreas can lead to diabetes.

In other situations, the immune system strikes multiple cells and tissues, producing diseases such as rheumatoid arthritis or systemic lupus erythematosus (SLE). Rheumatoid arthritis targets primarily the joints, but it can also damage nerves, lungs, and skin. Lupus strikes skin, muscles, joints, kidneys, and other organs, causing rashes, joint pain, fatigue, and fever, among other things.

Finally, an immunodeficiency can be just one part of a complex syndrome, with a telltale combination of signs and symptoms. For example, children with DiGeorge syndrome not only have an underdeveloped thymus gland (and a corresponding lack of T cells); they typically have congenital heart disease; malfunctioning, or underdeveloped parathyroid glands; and characteristic facial features. Young boys with Wiskott-Aldrich syndrome, in addition to being prone to infections, develop bleeding problems and a skin rash.

The Ten Warning Signs of Primary Immunodeficiency*

1. Eight or more new ear infections within a year.

2. Two or more serious sinus infections within a year.

3. Two or more months on antibiotics with little effect.

4. Two or more pneumonias within a year.

5. Failure of an infant to gain weight or grow normally.

6. Recurrent deep abscesses in the skin or organs.

7. Persistent thrush in mouth or on skin, after the child is one year old.

8. Need for intravenous antibiotics to clear infections.

9. Two or more deep-seated infections such as meningitis, osteomyelitis, cellulitis, or sepsis.

10. A family history of primary immunodeficiency.

*Courtesy of The Jeffrey Modell Foundation and the American Red Cross.

Diagnosing PI

Sometimes the signs and symptoms of a PI are so severe, or so characteristic, that the diagnosis is obvious. In most cases, it is not clear if a long string of illnesses are just ordinary infections, or if they are the result of an immunodeficiency. Many conditions can produce an immunodeficiency, at least temporarily, and most children who seem to have too many infections are not, in fact, suffering from an immunodeficiency. Experts estimate that half of the children who see a doctor for frequent infections are normal. Another 30 percent may have allergies, and ten percent have some other type of serious disorder. Just ten percent turn out to have a primary or secondary immunodeficiency.

The Basics

When a pattern of frequent infections suggests an immunodeficiency, the doctor begins by exploring the patient's history and the family's history, and then conducts a physical examination.

Evaluating Immune Responses

To find out if illness can be traced to an immunodeficiency, laboratory tests are necessary. These tests, most of which can be performed on a sample of blood, probe the soundness of the various parts of the immune system. Are all the right immune cells present, in adequate numbers, and are they working properly? Are there normal amounts and types of antibodies?

Screening starts out with a few relatively simple and inexpensive routine tests. In fact, just two routine tests—complete blood count and quantitative immunoglobulins—will detect most, but not all, immunodeficiencies. If antibodies are normal—or if the patient's infections seem to be caused by viruses or fungi—the T cells should be checked. If the T cells are present in normal numbers and function normally, phagocyte function should be evaluated.

When screening tests indicate an immunodeficiency—or when they fail to explain a stubborn infection—additional tests will likely be needed. There are dozens of sophisticated tests that allow doctors to identify and count subsets of B cells and T cells, and to assess subtle abnormalities in antibodies, immune cells, and immune tissues. Tests can also probe the characteristics of infectious germs.

Evaluating Infections

If an infection proves resistant to standard treatments, the doctor will want to find out exactly what germs are involved. Samples of mucus, sputum, or stool, or sometimes a small sample of the infected tissue itself, removed surgically, can be cultured in the laboratory. This allows germs to grow until they are plentiful enough to study in detail. Once the germ is identified, it becomes possible to select the most effective treatment.

An experienced physician will also find clues in particular combinations of details, such as age and sex, along with the physical findings. For example, a young infant suffering from diarrhea, pneumonia, and thrush, and exhibiting failure to thrive, may well have SCID. A 4-year-old with swollen lymph glands, skin problems, pneumonia, and bone infections may have chronic granulomatous disease (CGD). A 10-year old with sinus and respiratory infections, an enlarged spleen, and signs of autoimmune problems is apt to have common variable immunodeficiency.

Treatments for PI

Treating PI involves not only curing infections but also correcting the underlying immunodeficiency. In addition, any associated conditions, such as autoimmune disorders or cancer, need special attention.

Treating Infections

The first goal of treatment is to clear up any current infection. Doctors can prescribe a wide range of infection-fighting antimicrobials. Some are broad-spectrum antibiotics that combat a range of germs. Others zero in on specific germs. When an infection fails to respond to standard medications, the patient may need to be hospitalized to be treated with antibiotics and other drugs intravenously.

For chronic infections, a variety of medicines can help relieve symptoms and prevent complications. These may include drugs like aspirin or ibuprofen to ease fever and general body aches; decongestants to shrink swollen membranes in the nose, sinuses, or throat; and expectorants to thin mucus secretions in the airways.

People who have chronic respiratory infections may be made more comfortable with a technique known as postural drainage (or bronchial drainage). Developed for persons with cystic fibrosis, postural drainage uses gravity, along with light blows to the chest wall, to help clear secretions from the lungs.

In bone marrow transplantation (BMT), bone marrow is taken from a healthy person and transferred to the patient. Because bone marrow is the source of all blood cells, including infection-fighting white blood cells, a successful bone marrow transplant amounts to getting a new, working immune system.

Preventing Infections

When the immune defenses are weak, it is essential to avoid germs. Precautions range from common sense practices like good hygiene (using mild soaps to keep the skin clean and brushing teeth twice a day) and good nutrition to elaborate measures to prevent all contact with infectious agents.

Anyone with an immunodeficiency needs to avoid unnecessary exposure to infectious agents. This means staying away from people with colds or other infections, and avoiding large crowds. (On the other hand, children are encouraged to attend school, to play in small groups, and to participate in sports.)

Antibiotics are important for preventing or controlling infections. If infections threaten to become chronic, the doctor may prescribe continuous long-term, low-dose antibiotics. Such preventive, or prophylactic, therapy may help prevent hearing loss or permanent breathing problems. When *Pneumocystis carinii* pneumonia is a danger—for instance, in children with a profound T cell deficiency—an appropriate prophylactic treatment may consist of a combination of two drugs, trimethoprim and sulfamethoxazole.

Important Precautions

Children with PI diseases, especially those with defective T cells, x-linked agammaglobulinemia, and ataxia telangiectasia should not receive live virus vaccines, such as the oral polio, measles, and chicken pox (varicella) vaccines. It is not even safe to give live virus vaccines to children suspected of immunodeficiency until a definitive diagnosis is rendered. There is a risk that such vaccines could cause serious illness or even death. Moreover, blood transfusions should not only be free of infectious viruses (for example, hepatitis or cytomegalovirus), but also—for T cell deficient children—irradiated to incapacitate mature donor T cells that might attack the tissues of the recipient and result in graft versus host disease (GVHD).

Chapter 4

Transmission of Contagious Disease

Chapter Contents

Section 4.1

Transmission of Microbes
That Cause Contagious Disease

This section includes text from "Understanding Microbes:
Transmission," National Institute of Allergy and Infectious Diseases
(NIAID), July 16, 2008.

Some Microbes Can Travel through the Air

You can transmit microbes to another person through the air by
coughing or sneezing. These are common ways to get viruses that
cause colds or flu, or the bacteria that cause tuberculosis (TB). Inter-
estingly, international airplane travel can expose you to germs not
common in your own country.

Close Contact Can Pass Germs to Another Person

Scientists have identified more than 500 types of bacteria that live
in our mouths. Some keep the oral environment healthy, while others
cause problems like gum disease. One way you can transmit oral bacteria is by kissing. Microbes such as human immunodeficiency virus
(HIV), herpes simplex virus, and gonorrhea bacteria are examples of
germs that can be transmitted directly during sexual intercourse.

You Can Pick Up and Spread Germs by Touching
Infectious Material

A common way for some microbes to enter the body, especially when
caring for young children, is through unintentionally passing feces from
hand to mouth or the mouths of young children. Infant diarrhea is often spread in this way. Daycare workers, for example, can pass diarrhea-causing rotavirus or *Giardia lamblia* (protozoa) from one baby to
the next between diaper changes and other childcare practices. It also
is possible to pick up cold viruses from shaking someone's hand or from
touching contaminated surfaces, such as a handrail or telephone.

A Healthy Person Can Carry Germs and Pass Them to Others

The story of "Typhoid Mary" is a famous example from medical history about how a person can pass germs on to others, yet not be affected by those germs. The germs in this case were *Salmonella typhi* bacteria, which cause typhoid fever and are usually spread through food or water.

In the early 20th century, Mary Mallon, an Irish immigrant, worked as a cook for several New York City families. More than half of the first family she worked for came down with typhoid fever. Through a clever deduction, a researcher determined that the disease was caused by the family cook. He concluded that although Mary had no symptoms of the disease, she probably had had a mild typhoid infection sometime in the past. Though not sick, she still carried the Salmonella bacteria and was able to spread them to others through the food she prepared.

Germs from Your Household Pet Can Make You Sick

You can catch a variety of germs from animals, especially household pets. The rabies virus, which can infect cats and dogs, is one of the most serious and deadly of these microbes. Fortunately, rabies vaccine prevents animals from getting rabies. Vaccines protect people from accidentally getting the virus from an animal. They also prevent people who already have been exposed to the virus, such as through an animal bite, from getting sick.

Dog and cat saliva can contain any of more than 100 different germs that can make you sick. *Pasteurella* bacteria, the most common, can be transmitted through bites that break the skin causing serious, and sometimes fatal, diseases such as blood infections and meningitis. Meningitis is the inflammation of the lining of the brain and spinal cord.

Warm-blooded animals are not the only ones that can cause you harm. Pet reptiles such as turtles, snakes, and iguanas can give *Salmonella* bacteria to their unsuspecting owners.

Some Microbes in Food or Water Could Make You Sick

Cryptosporidia are bacteria found in human and animal feces. These bacteria can get into lake, river, and ocean water from sewage spills, animal waste, and water runoff. Millions can be released from infectious fecal matter. People who drink, swim in, or play in infected water can get sick. People, including babies, with diarrhea caused by

Cryptosporidia or other diarrhea-causing microbes such as *Giardia* and *Salmonella*, can infect others while using swimming pools, water parks, hot tubs, and spas.

Section 4.2

Preventing the Transmission of Sexually Transmitted Disease

Excerpted from "Clinical Prevention Guidance-STD Treatment Guidelines 2006," Centers for Disease Control and Prevention (CDC), 2006.

The prevention and control of sexually transmitted diseases (STD) are based on the following five major strategies: 1) education and counseling of persons at risk on ways to avoid STD through changes in sexual behaviors; 2) identification of asymptomatically infected persons and of symptomatic persons unlikely to seek diagnostic and treatment services; 3) effective diagnosis and treatment of infected persons; 4) evaluation, treatment, and counseling of sex partners of persons who are infected with STD; and 5) pre-exposure vaccination of persons at risk for vaccine-preventable STD.

Client-Initiated Interventions to Reduce Sexual Transmission of STD/Human Immunodeficiency Virus (HIV), and Unintended Pregnancy

Abstinence and Reduction of Number of Sex Partners

The most reliable way to avoid transmission of STD is to abstain from sex (oral, vaginal, or anal sex) or to be in a long-term, mutually monogamous relationship with an uninfected partner.

Pre-Exposure Vaccination

Pre-exposure vaccination is one of the most effective methods for preventing transmission of some STD. For example, because hepatitis B virus (HBV) infection is frequently sexually transmitted, HBV vaccination is recommended for all unvaccinated, uninfected persons being evaluated for an STD. In addition, hepatitis A vaccine is licensed and is recommended for men who have sex with men (MSM) and illicit drug users (both injecting and non-injecting). A quadrivalent vaccine against human papillomavirus (HPV types 6, 11, 16, 18) is now available and licensed for females aged 9–26 years. Vaccine trials for other STD are being conducted.

Male Condoms

When used consistently and correctly, male latex condoms are highly effective in preventing the sexual transmission of HIV infection and can reduce the risk for other STD, including chlamydia, gonorrhea, and trichomoniasis, and might reduce the risk of women developing pelvic inflammatory disease (PID). Condom use might reduce the risk for transmission of herpes simplex virus-2 (HSV-2), although data for this effect are more limited. Condom use might reduce the risk for HPV-associated diseases (for example, genital warts and cervical cancer) and mitigate the adverse consequences of infection with HPV, as their use has been associated with higher rates of regression of cervical intraepithelial neoplasia (CIN) and clearance of HPV infection in women, and with regression of HPV-associated penile lesions in men. A limited number of prospective studies have demonstrated a protective effect of condoms on the acquisition of genital HPV; one recent prospective study among newly sexually active college women demonstrated that consistent condom use was associated with a 70% reduction in risk for HPV transmission.

Patients should be advised that condoms must be used consistently and correctly to be effective in preventing STD, and they should be instructed in the correct use of condoms.

Female Condoms

Laboratory studies indicate that the female condom (Reality™), which consists of a lubricated polyurethane sheath with a ring on each end that is inserted into the vagina, is an effective mechanical barrier to viruses, including HIV, and to semen. A limited number of clinical studies have evaluated the efficacy of female condoms in providing protection from STD, including HIV. If used consistently and correctly, the female condom might substantially reduce the risk for STD.

Vaginal Spermicides and Diaphragms

Vaginal spermicides containing nonoxynol-9 (N-9) are not effective in preventing cervical gonorrhea, chlamydia, or HIV infection. Furthermore, frequent use of spermicides containing N-9 has been associated with disruption of the genital epithelium, which might be associated with an increased risk for HIV transmission. Therefore, N-9 is not recommended for STD/HIV prevention. In case-control and cross-sectional studies, diaphragm use has been demonstrated to protect against cervical gonorrhea, chlamydia, and trichomoniasis. On the basis of all available evidence, diaphragms should not be relied on as the sole source of protection against HIV infection. Diaphragm and spermicide use have been associated with an increased risk for bacterial urinary tract infections in women.

Condoms and N-9 Vaginal Spermicides

Condoms lubricated with spermicides are no more effective than other lubricated condoms in protecting against the transmission of HIV and other STD, and those that are lubricated with N-9 pose the concerns that have been discussed previously.

Rectal Use of N-9 Spermicides

Recent studies indicate that N-9 might increase the risk for HIV transmission during vaginal intercourse. Although similar studies have not been conducted among men who use N-9 spermicide during anal intercourse with other men, N-9 can damage the cells lining the rectum, which might provide a portal of entry for HIV and other sexually transmissible agents. Therefore, N-9 should not be used as a microbicide or lubricant during anal intercourse.

Non-Barrier Contraception, Surgical Sterilization, and Hysterectomy

Sexually active women who are not at risk for pregnancy might incorrectly perceive themselves to be at no risk for STD, including HIV infection. Contraceptive methods that are not mechanical barriers offer no protection against HIV or other STD.

Partner Management

Partner notification, previously referred to as "contact tracing" but recently included in the broader category of partner services, is the process by which providers or public health authorities learn from persons with STD about their sex partners and help to arrange for the evaluation and treatment of sex partners. Providers can seek this information and help to arrange for evaluation and treatment of sex partners, either directly or with assistance from state and local health departments. The intensity of partner services and the specific STD for which they are offered vary among providers, agencies, and geographic areas. Ideally, such services should be accompanied by health counseling and might include referral of patients and their partners for other services, whenever appropriate.

Many persons individually benefit from partner notification. When partners are treated, index patients have reduced risk for reinfection. At a population level, partner notification can disrupt networks of STD transmission and reduce disease incidence. Therefore, providers should encourage their patients with STD to notify their sex partners and urge them to seek medical evaluation and treatment, regardless of whether assistance is available from health agencies.

Reporting and Confidentiality

The accurate and timely reporting of STD is integrally important for assessing morbidity trends, targeting limited resources, and assisting local health authorities in partner notification and treatment. STD/HIV and acquired immunodeficiency syndrome (AIDS) cases should be reported in accordance with state and local statutory requirements. Syphilis, gonorrhea, chlamydia, chancroid, HIV infection, and AIDS are reportable diseases in every state.

Section 4.3

Risk of Infectious Disease from Blood Transfusion

Text in this section is from "What Is a Blood Transfusion?" and "What Are the Risks of a Blood Transfusion?" National Heart, Lung, and Blood Institute (NHLBI), September 2007. The citation for Table 4.1, © 2008 American Association of Blood Banks, is located at the bottom of the table.

What Is a Blood Transfusion?

A blood transfusion is a safe, common procedure in which blood is given to you through an intravenous (IV) line in one of your blood vessels. Blood transfusions are done to replace blood lost during surgery or a serious injury. A transfusion also may be done if your body cannot make blood properly because of an illness.

During a blood transfusion, a small needle is used to insert an IV line into one of your blood vessels. Through this line, you receive healthy blood. The procedure usually takes 1–4 hours, depending on how much blood you need.

Blood transfusions are very common. Each year, almost five million Americans need a blood transfusion. Most blood transfusions go well. Mild complications can occur. Very rarely, serious problems develop.

Important Information about Blood

The heart pumps blood through a network of arteries and veins throughout the body. Blood has many vital jobs. It carries oxygen and other nutrients to your body's organs and tissues. Having a healthy supply of blood is important to your overall health.

Blood is made up of various parts, including red blood cells, white blood cells, platelets, and plasma. Blood is transfused either as whole blood (with all its parts) or, more often, as individual parts.

Blood Types

Every person has one of the following blood types: A, B, AB, or O. Also, every person's blood is either Rh-positive or Rh-negative. So, if you have type A blood, it's either A positive or A negative.

The blood used in a transfusion must work with your blood type. If it doesn't, antibodies (proteins) in your blood attack the new blood and make you sick. Type O blood is safe for almost everyone. About 40 percent the population has type O blood. People with this blood type are called universal donors. Type O blood is used for emergencies when there's no time to test a person's blood type. People with type AB blood are called universal recipients. This means they can get any type of blood. If you have Rh-positive blood, you can get Rh-positive or Rh-negative blood. But if you have Rh-negative blood, you should get only Rh-negative blood. Rh-negative blood is used for emergencies when there's no time to test a person's Rh type.

Blood Banks

Blood banks collect, test, and store blood. They carefully screen all donated blood for possible infectious agents, such as viruses that could make you sick. Blood bank staff also screen each blood donation to find out whether it's A, B, AB, or O and whether it's Rh-positive or Rh-negative.

To prepare blood for a transfusion, some blood banks remove white blood cells. Although rare, some people are allergic to white blood cells in donated blood. Removing these cells makes allergic reactions less likely. A blood bank will store your blood for your use if you have surgery scheduled and have time to store blood prior to the surgery.

What Are the Risks of a Blood Transfusion?

Most blood transfusions go very smoothly. However, mild problems and, very rarely, serious problems can occur.

Allergic Reaction

Some people have allergic reactions to the blood given during transfusions. This can happen even when the blood given is the right blood type. A transfusion is stopped at the first signs of an allergic reaction. The health care team determines how mild or severe the reaction is, what treatments are needed, and if the transfusion can safely be restarted.

Viruses and Infectious Diseases

Some infectious agents, such as human immunodeficiency virus (HIV), can survive in blood and infect the person receiving the blood transfusion. To keep blood safe, blood banks carefully screen donated blood.

Fever

You may get a sudden fever during or within a day of your blood transfusion. This is usually your body's normal response to white blood cells in the donated blood. Over-the-counter fever medicine will usually treat the fever.

Iron Overload

Getting many blood transfusions can cause too much iron to build up in your blood (iron overload). People with a blood disorder like thalassemia, which requires multiple transfusions, are at risk of iron overload. Iron overload can damage your liver, heart, and other parts of your body.

Lung Injury

Although it's unlikely, blood transfusions can damage your lungs, making it difficult to breathe. This usually occurs within about six hours of the procedure. Most patients recover. However, 5–25 percent of patients who develop lung injuries die from the injury. These people usually were very ill before the transfusion.

Acute Immune Hemolytic Reaction

Acute immune hemolytic reaction is very serious, but also very rare. It occurs if the blood type you get during a transfusion doesn't match or work with your blood type. Your body attacks the new red blood cells, which then produce substances that harm your kidneys. The symptoms include chills, fever, nausea, pain in the chest or back, and dark urine. The doctor will stop the transfusion at the first sign of this reaction.

Delayed Hemolytic Reaction

This is a much slower version of acute immune hemolytic reaction. Your body destroys red blood cells so slowly that the problem can go unnoticed until your red blood cell level is very low. Both the acute and delayed hemolytic reactions are most common in patients who have had a previous transfusion.

Graft-Versus-Host Disease

Graft-versus-host disease (GVHD) is when white blood cells in the new blood attack your tissues. GVHD is usually fatal. People who have weakened immune systems are the most likely to get GVHD. Symptoms start within a month of the blood transfusion. They include fever, rash, and diarrhea. To protect against GVHD, patients with weakened immune systems should receive blood that has been treated so the white blood cells cannot cause GVHD.

Table 4.1. Infectious Risks of Blood Transfusion in the United States

Infectious Agent	Estimated Risk per Unit Transfused	Estimated % of Infected Units that transmit or cause clinical sequelae*
Virus		
HIV-1 and -2	1:1,400,000–1:2,400,000	90
Human T-cell lymphoma/ leukemia virus (HTLV) types I and II	1:256,000–1:2,000,000	30
Hepatitis A virus (HAV)	1:1,000,000	90
Hepatitis B virus (HBV)	1:58,000–1:140,000	70
Hepatitis C virus (HCV)	1:872,000–1:1,700,000	90
B19 parvovirus	1:3,300–1:40,000	Low
Bacteria		
Red blood cells (RBC)	1:1000	1:10,000,000 fatal
Platelets (PRP from whole blood screened with Gram stain, pH or glucose concentration)	1:2,000–1:4,000	greater than 40% result in clinical sequelae
Platelets pheresis (with early aerobic culture)	less than 1:10,000	Unknown
Parasites		
Babesia and malaria	less than 1:1,000,000	Unknown
Trypanosoma cruzi	Unknown	less than 20

* Units that were confirmed test positive for the infectious agent.

Note: West Nile Virus is not included in this table because of the regional, temporal, and testing (for example, mini-pool versus individual donation testing) variation, and decreasing rates of infection.

Excerpted from "Infectious Pathogens and Risk of Transmission by Transfusion," *AABB Technical Manual, 16th Ed.* © 2008 American Association of Blood Banks. Reprinted with permission.

Section 4.4

Contagious Disease Transmission on Airplanes and Cruise Ships

Text in this section is from "CDC Health Information for International Travel 2010 (Yellow Book): Chapter 6," Centers for Disease Control and Prevention (CDC), July 2009.

In-Flight Transmission of Communicable Diseases

Communicable diseases may be transmitted to other travelers during air travel, therefore:

- persons who are acutely ill, or still within the infectious period for a specific disease, should be discouraged from traveling; and

- travelers should be reminded to wash their hands frequently and cover their noses and mouths when coughing or sneezing.

If a passenger with a communicable disease is identified as having flown on a particular flight (or flights), passengers who may have been exposed will be contacted by public health authorities for possible screening or prophylaxis.

For certain communicable diseases, public health authorities will obtain contact information from the airline for potentially exposed travelers so they may be contacted and offered appropriate intervention. To assist in this process, travelers can provide airlines with current contact information such as a telephone number and state of residence. Travel agencies will not share passenger contact information with the airline or public health authorities.

Tuberculosis (TB)

Although the risk of transmission of *Mycobacterium tuberculosis* on board aircraft is low, international TB experts agree that contact investigations for flights longer than eight hours are warranted when the ill traveler meets World Health Organization (WHO) criteria for being infectious during flight. The concern is greatest when a person

44

may have flown with a highly resistant strain of TB. People known to have infectious TB should not travel by commercial air (or any other commercial means) until criteria for no longer being infectious is met. State health department TB controllers are valuable resources for advice (http://www.phf.org/about/links.htm).

Neisseria meningitides

Meningococcal disease is potentially rapidly fatal, thus rapid identification of close contacts and provision of prophylactic antimicrobials are critical. Antimicrobial prophylaxis should be considered for:

- household members traveling with a patient,
- travel companions with close contact, and
- passengers seated directly next to the ill traveler on flights longer than eight hours.

Measles

Most measles cases diagnosed in the United States are imported from countries where measles is endemic.

- An ill traveler is considered infectious during a flight of any duration if he or she traveled during the four days before rash onset through four days after rash onset.
- Intervention may prevent or mitigate measles in susceptible contacts if measles, mumps, rubella (MMR) vaccine is given within 72 hours of flight exposure or immunoglobulin is given within six days of flight exposure.
- International travelers should ensure they are immune to measles prior to travel.

Influenza

Transmission of the influenza virus aboard aircraft has been documented, but data are limited. Transmission is thought to be primarily due to large droplets; therefore, passengers seated closest to the source case are believed to be most at risk for exposure.

Disinsection

To reduce the accidental spread of mosquitoes and other vectors via airline cabins and luggage compartments, a number of countries require disinsection of all inbound flights. WHO and the International Civil Aviation Organization (ICAO) specify two approaches for aircraft disinsection: 1) spraying the aircraft cabin with an aerosolized insecticide while passengers are on board; and 2) treating the aircraft's interior surfaces with a residual insecticide while the aircraft is empty. Some countries use a third method, in which aircraft are sprayed with an aerosolized insecticide while passengers are not on board.

Disinsection is not routinely done on incoming flights to the United States. Although disinsection, when done appropriately, was declared safe by the WHO in 1995, there is still much debate about the safety of the agents and methods used. Guidelines for disinsection have been updated for the revised International Health Regulations (www2a.cdc .gov/phlp/docs/58assembly.pdf). Many countries, including the United States, reserve the right to increase the use of disinsection in case of increased threat of vector or disease spread. An updated list of countries that require disinsection and the types of methods used are available at the U.S. Department of Transportation website: (http://ostpxweb .ost.dot.gov/policy/safetyenergyenv/disinsection.htm).

Challenges of Cruise Ship Travel and Infectious Diseases

- Densely populated, semi-enclosed cruise ship environments may permit repeated and prolonged exposure to communicable diseases, resulting in their transmission between passengers and crew members.

- Differences in sanitation standards and disease prevalence between seaports may also lead to communicable disease exposure and spread.

- The risk of acquiring an infectious disease during cruise travel is difficult to quantify due to the diverse activities of crew and passengers, as well as the wide range of potential disease exposures.

- Senior citizens (an estimated one-third of cruise travelers) and travelers with underlying chronic health problems are at increased risk of illness from infections such as influenza, Legionella, and norovirus.

- Early detection and prevention of infectious diseases are important, not only to protect the health of cruise travelers, but also to avoid global dissemination of diseases in home communities through disembarking passengers and crew members.

Primary Health Concerns on Cruise Ships

Communicable Diseases

Communicable diseases occurring onboard cruise ships are similar to those that occur onshore. Detecting illnesses of public health significance is aided by heightened cruise line surveillance efforts in cooperation with public health authorities and passenger reporting.

- The most frequently documented cruise ship outbreaks involve respiratory infections (influenza and Legionella) and gastrointestinal infections (norovirus).

- In the past decade, clusters of illnesses due to vaccine-preventable diseases other than influenza, such as rubella and varicella (chickenpox), have also been reported.

Respiratory Illnesses

Influenza

- Outbreaks of influenza A and B can occur year-round, despite seasonality in the destination regions for cruises.

- Respiratory illness outbreaks usually result from the importation of influenza by embarking passengers and crew; the infection subsequently spreads person to person on the ship.

- Onboard control measures include isolation, infection control, and antiviral treatment of ill individuals as well as those exposed to the illness.

Legionnaires' Disease

- Legionnaires' disease has led to pneumonia outbreaks on multiple occasions, sometimes on consecutive cruises.

- Although contaminated ships' whirlpool spas and potable water supply systems are the most commonly implicated sources of Legionella outbreaks, exposure to other sources may also occur during port stops.

- Pinpointing the source of these outbreaks has proved difficult because diagnoses in returned travelers may be delayed and clinical specimens may be unavailable for culture at the time of diagnosis.

- Culture-based diagnostic tests for cruise travel-associated Legionnaires' disease are of public health importance.

• Improvements in ship design and standardization of spa and water supply disinfection have reduced the risk of Legionella growth and colonization.

Gastrointestinal (GI) Illnesses

The estimated likelihood of contracting gastroenteritis on an average seven-day cruise is less than 1%. GI illness accounts for fewer than 10% of shipboard passenger infirmary visits. In recent years, outbreaks of gastroenteritis on cruise ships have increased, despite good cruise ship environmental health standards.

Norovirus

The increase in gastroenteritis on cruise ships is primarily attributed to norovirus, also the main cause of acute viral gastroenteritis in the United States. Large, consecutive cruise ship outbreaks have resulted from Norovirus, due to their low infective dose, easy person-to-person transmissibility, and ability to survive routine cleaning procedures. Prompt implementation of disease control measures, such as the isolation of ill persons, strict application of food and water sanitation measures, and disinfection of surfaces with suitable disinfectants, are key to controlling Norovirus outbreaks.

Other Pathogens

Other known causes of GI illness clusters on cruise ships include food or water contaminated with *Salmonella spp.*, enterotoxigenic *Escherichia coli*, *Shigella spp.*, *Vibrio spp.*, *Staphylococcus aureus*, *Clostridium perfringens*, *Cyclospora sp.*, and *Trichinella spiralis*.

Vaccine-Preventable Diseases on Cruises

Other than influenza, clusters of rubella and varicella have been investigated on cruises originating in the United States, highlighting the potential global dissemination of vaccine-preventable diseases through cruise travel.

Preventive Measures for Cruise Ship Travelers

Due to multiple port visits and potential exposures, cruise ship travelers may be uncertain about which prevention medications, immunizations, and behaviors are appropriate for them and for their itineraries. Pre-travel advice for cruise ship travelers should include a complete review of the health status of the traveler, duration of travel, countries to be visited, and shore side activities.

Traveler Precautions during Travel

- Wash hands often with soap and water. If soap and water are not available, use an alcohol-based gel containing at least 60% alcohol.
- Practice respiratory hygiene by using a tissue to cover coughs and sneezes.
- Take food and water precautions by eating foods that are thoroughly cooked and of appropriate temperature.
- Prevent mosquito and other insect bites by using repellents and clothing that provides complete coverage.
- Use sun protection and drink plenty of water to avoid heat-related illness.
- Avoid excessive alcohol, get plenty of rest, avoid contact with ill persons, report illnesses to cruise staff, and practice safe sex.

After Travel

Health-care providers can contribute to healthy cruise ship environments by questioning ill travelers about recent cruise vacations and promptly reporting any suspected communicable disease to public health authorities.

Contacts for Concerns about Illnesses on Cruise Ships

Vessel Sanitation Program
National Center for Environmental Health
Centers for Disease Control and Prevention (CDC)
4770 Buford Highway, NEMS-F23
Atlanta, GA 30341
Toll-Free: 800-CDC-INFO (800-232-4636)
Website: http://www.cdc.gov/nceh/vsp
E-mail: CDCINFO@cdc.gov

For concerns about gastrointestinal (GI) illnesses. Other illnesses suggestive of a communicable disease should be reported to the nearest CDC quarantine station with jurisdiction nearest to the cruise ship's port of arrival.

Chapter 5

Screening Internationally Adopted Children for Contagious Diseases

International Adoptions

The number of internationally adopted children arriving annually to the United States has averaged 21,449 children in the past four years. These children accounted for 1.85% of all legal immigrants and approximately 10% of all legal pediatric immigrants in 2006 and 2007. The demography of international adoption is in constant flux, and the epidemiology of diseases in this population of children shifts as a consequence.

In 2007, the most common countries of origin for internationally adopted children were China, Guatemala, Russia, Ethiopia, South Korea, Vietnam, Ukraine, and Kazakhstan. In 2007, 40% of internationally adopted children were less than one year of age, 43% were 1–4 years of age, and 17% were over five years of age. Sixty-one percent were female.

International adoptees are usually not fully immunized and are at increased risk for infections such as measles and hepatitis A, due to often-crowded living conditions, malnutrition, lack of clean water, and exposure to endemic diseases that are not common in the United States. The major challenges in health care regarding international adoptees include the following:

Text in this chapter is excerpted from "CDC Health Information for International Travel 2010 (Yellow Book): Chapter 7–International Adoptions," Centers for Disease Control and Prevention (CDC), 2009; and from "Intercountry Adoption: Health Information," U.S. Department of State.

- Absence of a medical history
- Unavailability of biological family history
- Questionable reliability of immunization records
- Variation in pre-adoption living standards
- Different disease epidemiology in countries of origin
- Increased risk for developmental delays

Travel Preparation for Adoptive Parents and Their Families

Prospective adoptive parents should be encouraged to consider the following for themselves and other family members:

- A pre-travel visit is strongly recommended for prospective adoptive parents.
- Family members who remain at home, including extended family, and childcare providers should also be current on their routine immunizations, as recommended by the Advisory Committee on Immunization Practices (ACIP).
- Protection against measles, hepatitis A, and hepatitis B must be ensured for everyone who will be in the household or providing child care for the adopted child.
- Adults less than 65 years of age who are due for a tetanus booster should receive the diphtheria, tetanus and acellular pertussis (DTaP) vaccine.
- A one-time inactivated polio booster also is recommended for adults.

Overseas Medical Examination of the Adopted Child

All immigrants, including infants and children adopted internationally by U.S. citizens, and all refugees entering the United States must undergo a medical examination in their country of origin, performed by a panel physician designated by the U.S. Department of State.

- The medical examination is used primarily to detect certain serious contagious diseases that may be the basis for visa ineligibility.
- Prospective adoptive parents should be advised not to rely on this medical examination to detect all possible disabilities and illnesses. Laboratory results from the country of origin may also be unreliable.

- The medical examination consists of a brief physical examination and a medical history, a chest radiograph examination for tuberculosis, and blood tests for syphilis and human immunodeficiency virus (HIV) are required for immigrants over 15 years of age. Immigration applicants under 15 years of age are tested only if there is reason to suspect any of these diseases.

The U.S. Department of State website provides additional information about the medical examination at http://adoption.state.gov/about/how/health.html and the vaccination exemption form for internationally adopted children at http://travel.state.gov/pdf/ DS-1981.pdf (PDF).

Follow-Up Medical Examination after Arrival in the United States

The adopted child should have a medical examination within two weeks of arrival in the United States, or earlier if the child has fever, anorexia, diarrhea, or vomiting. Further evaluation will depend on:

- the country of origin,
- the age of the child,
- previous living conditions,
- the number of times a child has been moved from one residence to another (for example: home, hospital, orphanages, and adoptive families),
- nutritional status,
- developmental status,
- the adoptive family's specific questions, and
- any concerns raised during a pre-adoption medical review.

In one study, over 50% of newly arrived adopted children had an undiagnosed medical condition, and of these, more than 50% were diagnosed as an infectious disease.

Screening for Infectious and Noninfectious Diseases

Gastrointestinal Parasites

Gastrointestinal parasites have been found in up to 51% of internationally adopted children. *Giardia intestinalis* is the most common parasite identified. The highest rates of infection have been reported from Russia, Eastern Europe, and China.

Hepatitis A

Serology has proven useful in identifying the young infant or child from a hepatitis A virus-endemic area who may be asymptomatic yet is acutely infected and is shedding virus, with the potential to infect others. In 2007 and early 2008, multiple cases of hepatitis A secondary to exposure to a newly arrived internationally adopted child were reported in the United States.

Hepatitis B

Hepatitis B surface antigen has been reported in 1%–5% of newly arrived adoptees, depending on the country of origin and the year that the study was conducted. The hepatitis B virus (HBV) is highly transmissible within the household. All members of households adopting children who are HBV carriers must be immunized and should have follow-up antibody titers to determine if levels consistent with immunity have been achieved. Children found to be hepatitis B surface antigen-positive should receive additional tests and consultation with a pediatric gastroenterologist.

Hepatitis C

Hepatitis C serologic screening is recommended for children from China, Russia, Eastern Europe, and Southeast Asia. Depending on history of prevalence in the country of origin, receipt of blood products, and maternal drug use, hepatitis C screening of children from other areas may be indicated.

HIV

Clinical symptoms of malnutrition, long-term institutionalization, and acquired immunodeficiency may overlap, but positive HIV antibodies in children less than 18 months of age may reflect maternal antibody, but not infection. Assaying for the virus by HIV deoxyribonucleic acid (DNA) with polymerase chain reaction (PCR) will confirm the diagnosis of HIV in the infant or child. Some experts recommend HIV DNA PCR for any infant less than six months old on arrival. In children greater than six months of age, two negative assays for HIV DNA administered one month apart are necessary to exclude infection.

Malaria

Smears should be obtained on all children arriving from areas endemic for malaria and for any newly arrived child who has a fever. The child with fever should have three sets of malaria smears at least 12 hours apart before excluding the diagnosis.

Tuberculosis

Internationally adopted children are at four to six times the risk for tuberculosis than their U.S.-born peers.

- The tuberculin skin test (TST) of purified protein derivative is indicated for all children over three months of age, regardless of their bacille Calmette–Guérin (BCG) vaccination status.

- A chest radiograph and complete physical exam to assess for pulmonary and extrapulmonary tuberculosis are indicated for all children with positive TST results.

- Hilar lymphadenopathy is a more sensitive finding for TB in young children than are pulmonary infiltrates or cavitation.

- Some experts recommend a repeat TST 3–6 months after arrival.

- A child who has a positive TST but no evidence of active disease should be treated with isoniazid for nine months.

- If active disease is found, every effort should be made to isolate the organism and determine sensitivities, particularly if the child is from a region of the world with a high rate of multidrug-resistant TB, such as Russia, Eastern Europe, and Asia.

Eosinophilia

Children with eosinophil counts greater than 450 cells/mm^3 may warrant further evaluation. Evaluation may include testing for parasites that can migrate through tissues and filarial worms.

Immunizations

The U.S. Immigration and Nationality Act requires that any person seeking an immigrant visa for permanent residency must show proof of having received the ACIP-recommended vaccines prior to immigration. This applies to all immigrant infants and children entering the

United States, but internationally adopted children under 11 years of age have been exempted from the overseas immunization requirements. Adoptive parents are required to sign a waiver indicating their intention to comply with the immunization requirements within 30 days of the infant's or child's arrival in the United States.

Upon arrival in the United States, greater than 90% of newly arrived internationally adopted children need catch-up immunizations to meet the ACIP guidelines. Varicella, pneumococcal conjugate, rubella, mumps, and *Haemophilus influenzae* type b vaccines are not usually available in developing countries.

Reliability of Vaccine Records

- Appears to differ by and even within country.

- Either of two approaches to vaccination can be taken for internationally adopted children: 1) immunize regardless of immunization record; or 2) if the child is over six months of age, test antibody titers to the vaccines potentially administered, and immunize only for those to which the child has no protective titers.

- If the infant is over six months old and there is uncertainty regarding immunization status or validity of immunization record, immunize according to the ACIP schedule.

- Measles, mumps, rubella (MMR) vaccine is not given in most of the countries of origin. Measles vaccine is administered as a single antigen. Unless the child has had mumps and rubella, administration of the MMR vaccine is recommended over serologic testing.

- Varicella testing for children coming from tropical countries is not recommended before 12 years of age unless there is a history of disease. In the tropics, varicella is a disease of adolescents and adults.

Intercountry Adoption: Health Information

The type and quality of medical information about a child can vary greatly between countries. Your adoption agency will provide you with as much information as possible about the health of a particular child, but it will not be able to guarantee that the information is complete or up-to-date. Sometimes, the information about a child eligible for adoption will be more comprehensive from Convention countries than from non-Convention countries.

Convention Adoptions

If you are adopting a child from a Convention country, your accredited adoption service provider is responsible for providing you with an English-language translation of the child's medical records. It will provide this to you no later than two weeks before the adoption or two weeks before the date when you travel to the child's birth country to complete the adoption (whichever is earlier). Accredited adoption service providers must make reasonable efforts to obtain available information, including the following:

- The date that the Convention country or other child welfare authority assumed custody of the child and the child's condition at that time

- History of any significant illnesses, hospitalizations, special needs, and changes in the child's condition since the child came into custody

- Growth data, including prenatal and birth history

- Specific information on the known health risks in the specific region of the child's birth country

- If a medical examination of the child is arranged, the date of the examination, and the name, contact information, and credentials of the physician who examined the child

- Information detailing all tests performed on the child

- Current health data

- Information about the child's birth family, cultural, racial, ethnic, and linguistic background

- Information about the child's past placements prior to adoption

- Dates on any videotapes and photographs taken of the child

Note: Unless extenuating circumstances involving the child's best interests requires a more expedited decision, an accredited adoption service providers may not withdraw a referral until you have had two weeks to consider the medical and social needs of the child and your ability to meet those needs.

Chapter 6

Bioterrorism: Disease Used as a Weapon

Chapter Contents

Section 6.1

Bioterrorism Overview

Text in this section is from "Bioterrorism Overview,"
Centers for Disease Control and Prevention (CDC), February 2007.

A bioterrorism attack is the deliberate release of viruses, bacteria, or other germs (agents) used to cause illness or death in people, animals, or plants. These agents are typically found in nature, but it is possible that they could be changed to increase their ability to cause disease, make them resistant to current medicines, or to increase their ability to be spread into the environment. Biological agents can be spread through the air, through water, or in food. Terrorists may use biological agents because they can be extremely difficult to detect and do not cause illness for several hours to several days. Some bioterrorism agents, like the smallpox virus, can be spread from person to person and some, like anthrax, cannot.

Bioterrorism agents can be separated into three categories, depending on how easily they can be spread and the severity of illness or death they cause. Category A agents are considered the highest risk and Category C agents are those that are considered emerging threats for disease.

Category A

These high-priority agents include organisms or toxins that pose the highest risk to the public and national security because:

- they can be easily spread or transmitted from person to person;
- they result in high death rates and have the potential for major public health impact;
- they might cause public panic and social disruption; and
- they require special action for public health preparedness.

Bioterrorism: Disease Used as a Weapon

These agents are the second highest priority because:

60

- they are moderately easy to spread;
- they result in moderate illness rates and low death rates;
- they require specific enhancements of Centers for Disease Control and Prevention (CDC) laboratory capacity and enhanced disease monitoring.

Category C

These third highest priority agents include emerging pathogens that could be engineered for mass spread in the future because:

- they are easily available;
- they are easily produced and spread; and
- they have potential for high morbidity and mortality rates and major health impact.

Section 6.2

Strategic National Stockpile of Medicine

Excerpted from "Strategic National Stockpile," Centers for
Disease Control and Prevention (CDC), updated March 31, 2009.

What the Strategic National Stockpile Means to You

The Centers for Disease Control and Prevention (CDC) Strategic National Stockpile (SNS) has large quantities of medicine and medical supplies to protect the American public if there is a public health emergency (terrorist attack, flu outbreak, earthquake) severe enough to cause local supplies to run out. Once federal and local authorities agree that the SNS is needed, medicines will be delivered to any state in the U.S. within twelve hours. Each state has plans to receive and distribute SNS medicine and medical supplies to local communities as quickly as possible.

What should you know about the medicines in the SNS?

- The medicine in the SNS is free for everyone.

- The SNS has stockpiled enough medicine to protect people in several large cities at the same time.

- Federal, state, and local community planners are working together to ensure that the SNS medicines will be delivered to the affected area to protect you and your family if there is a terrorist attack.

How will you get your medicine if the SNS is delivered to your area?

- Local communities are prepared to receive SNS medicine and medical supplies from the state to provide to everyone in the community who needs them.

- Find out about how to get medicine to protect you and your family by watching television, listening to the radio, reading the newspaper, checking the community website, or learning from trusted community leaders.

A National Repository of Life-Saving Pharmaceuticals and Medical Material

The SNS is a national repository of antibiotics, chemical antidotes, antitoxins, life-support medications, intravenous (IV) administration, airway maintenance supplies, and medical/surgical items. The SNS is designed to supplement and re-supply state and local public health agencies in the event of a national emergency anywhere and at anytime within the U.S. or its territories.

The SNS is organized for flexible response. The first line of support lies within the immediate response 12-hour Push Packages. These are caches of pharmaceuticals, antidotes, and medical supplies designed to provide rapid delivery of a broad spectrum of assets for an ill-defined threat in the early hours of an event. These Push Packages are positioned in strategically located, secure warehouses ready for immediate deployment to a designated site within 12 hours of the federal decision to deploy SNS assets.

If the incident requires additional pharmaceuticals and/or medical supplies, follow-up vendor managed inventory (VMI) supplies will be shipped to arrive within 24 to 36 hours. If the agent is well defined, VMI can be tailored to provide pharmaceuticals, supplies, and/or products specific to the suspected or confirmed agent(s). In this case, the VMI could act as the first option for immediate response from the SNS Program.

Determining and Maintaining SNS Assets

To determine and review the composition of the SNS Program assets, the U.S. Department of Health and Human Services (HHS) and CDC consider many factors, such as current biological and/or chemical threats, the availability of medical material, and the ease of dissemination of pharmaceuticals. One of the most significant factors in determining SNS composition, however, is the medical vulnerability of the U.S. civilian population.

The SNS program ensures that the medical material stock is rotated and kept within potency shelf-life limits. This involves quarterly quality assurance/quality control checks (QA/QC) on all 12-hour Push Packages, annual 100% inventory of all 12-hour Push Package items, and inspections of environmental conditions, security, and overall package maintenance.

Supplementing State and Local Resources

During a national emergency, state, local, and private stocks of medical material will be depleted quickly. State and local first responders and health officials can use the SNS to bolster their response to a national emergency, with a 12-hour Push Package, VMI, or a combination of both, depending on the situation. The SNS is not a first response tool.

Rapid Coordination and Transport

The SNS Program is committed to have 12-hour Push Packages delivered anywhere in the U.S. or its territories within 12 hours of a federal decision to deploy. The 12-hour Push Packages have been configured to be immediately loaded onto either trucks or commercial cargo aircraft for the most rapid transportation. Concurrent to SNS transport, the SNS Program will deploy its Technical Advisory Response Unit (TARU). The TARU staff will coordinate with state and local officials so that the SNS assets can be efficiently received and distributed upon arrival at the site.

Section 6.3

U.S. Preparedness for Health Emergencies from Diseases, Disasters, and Bioterrorism

"Report Finds Economic Crisis Hurting U.S. Preparedness for Health Emergencies," December 9, 2008. Reprinted with permission from Trust for America's Health (www.healthyamericans.org), © 2008.

Report Finds Economic Crisis Hurting U.S. Preparedness for Health Emergencies

More Than Half of States Score Seven or Lower Out of Ten in Readiness Rankings

In December 2008, Trust for America's Health (TFAH) and the Robert Wood Johnson Foundation (RWJF) released the sixth annual *Ready or Not? Protecting the Public's Health from Diseases, Disasters, and Bioterrorism* report, which finds that progress made to better protect the country from disease outbreaks, natural disasters, and bioterrorism is now at risk, due to budget cuts and the economic crisis. In addition, the report concludes that major gaps remain in many critical areas of preparedness, including surge capacity, rapid disease detection, and food safety.

The report contains state-by-state health preparedness scores based on ten key indicators to assess health emergency preparedness capabilities. More than half of states and the District of Columbia achieved a score of seven or less out of ten key indicators. Louisiana, New Hampshire, North Carolina, Virginia, and Wisconsin scored the highest with ten out of ten. Arizona, Connecticut, Florida, Maryland, Montana, and Nebraska tied for the lowest score with five out of ten.

Over the past six years, the *Ready or Not?* report has documented steady progress toward improved public health preparedness. In 2008, the TFAH found that cuts in federal funding for state and local preparedness since 2005, coupled with the cuts states are making to their budgets in response to the economic crisis, put that progress at risk.

"The economic crisis could result in a serious rollback of the progress we've made since September 11, 2001 and Hurricane Katrina to better prepare the nation for emergencies," said Jeff Levi, PhD, Executive Director of TFAH. "The 25 percent cut in federal support to protect Americans from diseases, disasters, and bioterrorism is already hurting state response capabilities. The cuts to state budgets in the next few years could lead to a disaster for the nation's disaster preparedness."

Some serious 2008 health emergencies include a *Salmonella* outbreak in jalapeño and serrano peppers that sickened 1,442 people in 43 states, the largest beef recall in history in February, Hurricanes Gustav and Ike, severe flooding in the Midwest, major wildfires in California in June and November, and a ricin scare in Las Vegas.

Among the Key Findings

Budget cuts: Federal funding for state and local preparedness has been cut more than 25 percent from fiscal year (FY) 2005, and states are no longer receiving any supplemental funding for pandemic flu preparedness, despite increased responsibilities.

- In addition to the federal decreases, 11 states and the District of Columbia (DC) cut their public health budgets in the past year. In the coming year, according to the Center on Budget and Policy and Priorities, 33 states are facing shortfalls in their 2009 budgets and 16 states are already projecting shortfalls to their 2010 budgets.

Rapid disease detection: Since September 11, 2001, the country has made significant progress in improving disease detection capabilities, but major gaps still remain.

- Only six states do not have a disease surveillance system compatible with the U.S. Centers for Disease Control and Prevention's (CDC) National Electronic Disease Surveillance System.

- Twenty-four states and DC lack the capacity to deliver and receive lab specimens, such as suspected bioterror agents or new disease outbreak samples, on a 24 hour/7 day basis.

- Only three state public health laboratories are not able to meet the expectations of their state's pandemic flu plans.

Food safety: America's food safety system has not been fundamentally modernized in more than 100 years.

- Twenty states and DC did not meet or exceed the national average rate for being able to identify the pathogens responsible for foodborne disease outbreaks in their states.

Surge capacity: Many states do not have mechanisms in place to support and protect the community assistance that is often required during a major emergency.

- Twenty-six states do not have laws that reduce or limit liability for businesses and non-profit organizations that help during a public health emergency.

- Only eight states do not have laws that limit or reduce liability exposure for health care workers who volunteer during a public health emergency.

- Seventeen states do not have State Medical Reserve Corps Coordinators.

Vaccine and medication supplies and distribution: Ensuring the public can quickly and safely receive medications during a major health emergency is one of the most serious challenges facing public health officials.

- Sixteen states have purchased less than half of their share of federally-subsidized antivirals to use during a pandemic flu outbreak.

- Every state now has an adequate plan for distributing emergency vaccines, antidotes, and medical supplies from the Strategic National Stockpile, according to the CDC. In 2005, only seven states had adequate plans. The CDC changed to a different grading system in 2007. However, questions still remain about the contents of the federal stockpile.

"States are being asked to do more with less, jeopardizing our safety, security, and health," said Risa Lavizzo-Mourey, MD, MBA, president and chief economic officer (CEO) of the Robert Wood Johnson Foundation. "We all have a stake in strengthening America's public health system, because it is our first line of defense against health emergencies."

The report also offers a series of recommendations for improving preparedness, including:

- **Restoring full funding:** At a minimum, federal, state, and local funding for public health emergency preparedness capabilities should be restored to FY 2005 levels.

- **Strengthening leadership and accountability:** The next administration must clarify the public health emergency preparedness roles and responsibilities at the U.S. Department of Health and Human Services and U.S. Department of Homeland Security.

- **Enhancing surge capacity and the public health workforce:** Federal, state, and local governments and health care providers must better address altered standards of care, alternative care sites, legal concerns to protect community assistance, and surge workforce issues.

- **Modernizing technology and equipment:** Communications and surveillance systems and laboratories need increased resources for modernization.

- **Improving community engagement:** Additional measures must be taken to engage communities in emergency planning and to improve protections for at-risk communities.

- **Incorporating preparedness into health care reform and creating an emergency health benefit:** This is needed to contain the spread of disease by providing care to the uninsured and underinsured Americans during major disasters and disease outbreaks.

Score Summary

For the state-by-state scoring, states received one point for achieving an indicator or zero points if they did not achieve the indicator. Zero is the lowest possible overall score, ten is the highest. The data for the indicators are from publicly available sources or were provided from public officials. More information on each indicator is available in the full report on TFAH's website at www.healthyamericans.org and RWJF's website at www.rwjf.org. The report was supported by a grant from RWJF.

10 out of 10: Louisiana, New Hampshire, North Carolina, Virginia, Wisconsin

9 out of 10: Alabama, Arkansas,* Indiana, Michigan, Pennsylvania, South Carolina, Tennessee, Vermont

8 out of 10: Delaware, Georgia, Hawaii, Iowa, Minnesota, North Dakota, Ohio, South Dakota, Washington

7 out of 10: California, Colorado, D.C., Illinois, Kentucky, Missouri, New Jersey, New Mexico, New York, Oklahoma, Oregon, Rhode Island, Utah, West Virginia, Wyoming

6 out of 10: Alaska, Idaho, Kansas, Maine, Massachusetts, Mississippi, Nevada, Texas

5 out of 10: Arizona, Connecticut, Florida, Maryland, Nebraska, Montana

*Arkansas's score has been revised. The state provided information confirming they have a Medical Reserve Corps Coordinator after the original release of the report.

Chapter 7

U.S. Nationally
Notifiable Infectious Diseases:
Protecting the Public Health

A notifiable disease is one for which regular, frequent, and timely information regarding individual cases is considered necessary for the prevention and control of the disease. Notifiable disease reporting at the local level protects the public's health by ensuring the proper identification and follow-up of cases. Public health workers ensure that persons who are already ill receive appropriate treatment; trace contacts who need vaccines, treatment, quarantine, or education; investigate and halt outbreaks; eliminate environmental hazards; and close premises where spread has occurred. Surveillance of notifiable conditions helps public health authorities to monitor the impact of notifiable conditions, measure disease trends, assess the effectiveness of control and prevention measures, identify populations or geographic areas at high risk, allocate resources appropriately, formulate prevention strategies, and develop public health policies. Monitoring surveillance data enables public health authorities to detect sudden changes in disease occurrence and distribution, identify changes in agents and host factors, and detect changes in health care practices.

The list of nationally notifiable infectious diseases is revised periodically. A disease might be added to the list as a new pathogen emerges, or a disease might be deleted as its incidence declines. Public health officials at state health departments and the Centers for

Excerpted from "Summary of Notifiable Diseases: United States, 2007," *MMWR Weekly* July 9, 2009, 56(53), pp. 1–94, Centers for Disease Control and Prevention (CDC).

Table 7.1. Total Reported Cases of Some of the Notifiable Contagious Diseases,* United States, 2007 (*continued on next page*)

Disease	Total reported cases
Acquired immunodeficiency syndrome (AIDS)[A]	37,503
Chancroid	23
Chlamydia trachomatis, genital infection	1,108,374
Cryptosporidiosis	11,170
Diphtheria	0
Gonorrhea	355,991
Hansen disease (leprosy)	101
Hepatitis A	2979
Hepatitis B	4519
Hepatitis C	845
Influenza-associated pediatric mortality**	77
Measles[§]	43
Meningococcal disease, all serogroups	1,077
Mumps	800
Novel influenza A virus infections	4
Pertussis (whooping cough)	10,454
Poliomyelitis, paralytic	0
Poliovirus infection, nonparalytic	0
Rabies, animal	5,862
Rabies, human	1
Rubella[§]	4
Shigellosis	19,758
Smallpox	0
Streptococcal disease, invasive, group A	5,294
Streptococcus pneumoniae, invasive disease, drug-resistant, all ages	3,329
Streptococcus pneumonia, invasive disease, drug-resistant, under five years	563
Streptococcus pneumoniae, invasive disease, nondrug-resistant, under five years	2,032

Table 7.1. Total Reported Cases of Some of the Notifiable Contagious Diseases,* United States, 2007 (*continued*)

Disease	Total reported cases
Syphilis, all stages[§§]	40,920
Tetanus	28
Trichinellosis	5
Tuberculosis[B]	13,299
Typhoid fever	434
Vancomycin-intermediate *Staphylococcus aureus* infection (VISA)	37
Vancomycin-resistant *Staphylococcus aureus* infection (VRSA)	4
Varicella (morbidity)	40,146
Varicella (mortality)***	6

* No cases of diphtheria; neuroinvasive or non-neuroinvasive western equine encephalitis virus disease; poliomyelitis, paralytic; poliovirus infection, nonparalytic; rubella, congenital syndrome; severe acute respiratory syndrome-associated coronavirus syndrome (SARS-CoV); smallpox; and yellow fever were reported in 2007. Data on chronic hepatitis B and hepatitis C virus infection (past or present) are not included because they are undergoing data quality review. Data on human immunodeficiency virus (HIV) infections are not included because HIV infection reporting has been implemented on different dates and using different methods than for AIDS case reporting.

[A] Total number of AIDS cases reported to the Division of HIV/AIDS Prevention, National Center for HIV/AIDS, Viral Hepatitis, STD, and TB Prevention (NCHHSTP) through December 31, 2007.

[§] Totals reported to the Division of STD Prevention, NCHHSTP, as of May 9, 2008.

** Totals reported to the Influenza Division, National Center for Immunization and Respiratory Diseases (NCIRD), as of December 31, 2007.

[§§] Includes the following categories: primary, secondary, latent(including early latent, late latent, and latent syphilis of unknown duration), neurosyphilis, late (including late syphilis with clinical manifestations other than neurosyphilis), and congenital syphilis.

[B] Totals reported to the Division of TB Elimination, NCHHSTP, as of May 16, 2008.

*** Death counts provided by the Division of Viral Diseases, NCIRD, as of March 31, 2008.

Disease Control and Prevention (CDC) collaborate in determining which diseases should be nationally notifiable. The Council of State and Territorial Epidemiologists (CSTE), with input from CDC, makes recommendations annually for additions and deletions. Although disease reporting is mandated by legislation or regulation at the state and local levels, state reporting to CDC is voluntary. Reporting completeness of notifiable diseases is highly variable and related to the condition or disease being reported.

Revised International Health Regulations for Public Health Emergencies of International Concern

In May 2005, the World Health Assembly adopted revised international health regulations (IHR) that went into effect in the United States on July 18, 2007. This international legal instrument governs the role of the World Health Organization (WHO) and its member countries, including the United States, in identifying, responding to and sharing information about Public Health Emergencies of International Concern (PHEIC). A PHEIC is an extraordinary event that 1) constitutes a public health risk to other countries through international spread of disease, and 2) potentially requires a coordinated international response.

The IHR are designed to prevent and protect against the international spread of diseases while minimizing the effect on world travel and trade. Countries that have adopted these rules have a much broader responsibility to detect, respond to, and report public health emergencies that potentially require a coordinated international response in addition to taking preventive measures. The IHR will help countries work together to identify, respond to, and share information about PHEIC.

An IHR decision algorithm has been developed to help countries determine whether an event should be reported. If any two of the following four questions can be answered in the affirmative, then a determination should be made that a potential PHEIC exists and WHO should be notified:

- Is the public health impact of the event serious?

- Is the event unusual or unexpected?

- Is there a significant risk of international spread?

- Is there a significant risk of international travel or trade restrictions?

Part Two

Types of Contagious Diseases

Chapter 8

Adenovirus

About Adenoviruses

Clinical features: Adenoviruses most commonly cause respiratory illness; however, depending on the infecting serotype, they may also cause various other illnesses, such as gastroenteritis, conjunctivitis, cystitis, and rash illness. Symptoms of respiratory illness that are caused by adenovirus infection range from the common cold syndrome to pneumonia, croup, and bronchitis. Patients with compromised immune systems are especially susceptible to severe complications of adenovirus infection. Acute respiratory disease (ARD), first recognized among military recruits during World War II, can be caused by adenovirus infections during conditions of crowding and stress.

The viruses: There are 49 immunologically distinct types of adenoviruses (six subgenera: A through F) that can cause human infections. Adenoviruses are unusually stable to chemical or physical agents and adverse pH conditions, allowing for prolonged survival outside of the body.

Epidemiologic features: Although epidemiologic characteristics of the adenoviruses vary by type, all are transmitted by direct contact,

---

This chapter begins with text from "Adenoviruses," Centers for Disease Control and Prevention (CDC), January 2005, and continues with excerpts from "Key Facts and Q and As about Adenovirus 14," CDC, November 20, 2007.

fecal-oral transmission, and occasionally waterborne transmission. Some types are capable of establishing persistent asymptomatic infections in tonsils, adenoids, and intestines of infected hosts, and shedding can occur for months or years. Some adenoviruses (for example, serotypes 1, 2, 5, and 6) have been shown to be endemic in parts of the world where they have been studied, and infection is usually acquired during childhood. Other types cause sporadic infection and occasional outbreaks; for example, epidemic keratoconjunctivitis is associated with adenovirus serotypes 8, 19, and 37. Epidemics of febrile disease with conjunctivitis are associated with waterborne transmission of some adenovirus types, often centering on inadequately chlorinated swimming pools and small lakes. ARD is most often associated with adenovirus types 4 and 7 in the United States. Enteric adenoviruses 40 and 41 cause gastroenteritis, usually in children. For some adenovirus serotypes, the clinical spectrum of disease associated with infection varies depending on the site of infection; for example, infection with adenovirus 7 acquired by inhalation is associated with severe lower respiratory tract disease, whereas oral transmission of the virus typically causes no or mild disease. Outbreaks of adenovirus-associated respiratory disease have been more common in the late winter, spring, and early summer; however, adenovirus infections can occur throughout the year.

Diagnosis: Antigen detection, polymerase chain reaction assay, virus isolation, and serology can be used to identify adenovirus infections. Since adenovirus can be excreted for prolonged periods, the presence of virus does not necessarily mean it is associated with disease.

Treatment: Most infections are mild and require no therapy or only symptomatic treatment. Because there is no virus-specific therapy, serious adenovirus illness can be managed only by treating symptoms and complications of the infection.

Prevention: Vaccines were developed for adenovirus serotypes 4 and 7, but were available only for preventing ARD among military recruits. Strict attention to good infection-control practices is effective for stopping nosocomial outbreaks of adenovirus-associated disease, such as epidemic keratoconjunctivitis. Maintaining adequate levels of chlorination is necessary for preventing swimming pool-associated outbreaks of adenovirus conjunctivitis.

Key Facts and Questions and Answers about Adenovirus

A report in the November 16, 2007, issue of the *Morbidity and Mortality Weekly Report* [MMWR 56(45):1181–1184] noted an unusual number of recent cases of severe pneumonia and deaths caused by adenovirus serotype 14 (Ad14) infection among civilian and military communities. Ad14 is one of the 51 serotypes of adenoviruses.

The MMWR report was based on investigations done by state and city health authorities, the U.S. Air Force, and CDC. The study showed that Ad14 is a rarely reported but emerging serotype of adenovirus that can cause severe and sometimes fatal respiratory disease in people of all ages, including healthy young adults. However, Ad14 infections are uncommon. Most infections from Ad14 are not serious, and severe or fatal outcomes from Ad14 are rare.

Since Ad14 infections are not common and most Ad14 infections are not serious, the emergence of Ad14 should not be a concern to the general population. During the winter, many other common viral and bacterial infections, including influenza, can present with very similar symptoms. As with any illness, you should check with your health care provider if you are concerned about the seriousness of your illness. For example, you may want to consult your doctor if you have an unusually high fever or fever that lasts more than a few days, have shortness of breath, or are feeling worse over time.

Who is most at risk for complications from adenovirus infection?

Everyone is at risk of adenovirus infection, but patients with weak immune systems or with underlying respiratory or cardiac disease are most at risk for severe complications from any respiratory infection, including adenovirus infections.

How is adenovirus infection spread?

Adenoviruses are spread like the common cold. The viruses can be spread from person to person via coughing or sneezing. People may also become infected by touching something with adenovirus on it and then touching their mouth, nose, or eyes. For example, adenoviruses can be transferred to a doorknob when an infected person sneezes into his/her hands and then touches the doorknob before washing. Germs can also be spread if an infected person sneezes or coughs onto tabletops or other items that might be touched by other people. To prevent the spread of disease, it is important to practice good health habits.

What steps can health care providers and people take to protect their health?

- People can protect themselves against all respiratory diseases by washing their hands, and they can protect others by covering their mouth when coughing or sneezing.

- People should, whenever possible, take steps to prevent respiratory infections. Such steps include vaccination and good health habits. At this time, Ad14 should not be considered a concern to the general public. Other respiratory infections, such as influenza, respiratory syncytial virus, and bacterial pneumonia, are other important causes of illness.

- Physicians should be aware that Ad14 can cause severe pneumonia and consider it in the differential diagnosis if the cause of infection is unknown.

State and local health departments and health care providers should consider Ad14 as a cause of outbreaks of pneumonia of unknown etiology.

- Clinicians should contact their state health departments for guidance on testing patients with a serious illness that they suspect may be an Ad14 infection. Testing for generic adenoviruses should precede any testing for specific serotypes, including Ad14.

- Health officials should be aware that Ad14 has been detected occasionally in military bases since 2005. Adenovirus infections in the military have been a concern for many years. Vaccines for the two adenoviruses most commonly causing disease in the military, Ad4 and Ad7, were used until 1996, and new versions of the vaccines are being studied in clinical trials for future use in the military.

- Health departments should report unusual clusters of severe adenoviral respiratory disease or cases of Ad14 to CDC.

Chapter 9

Amebiasis

What is amebiasis?

Amebiasis (am-e-BI-a-sis) is a disease caused by a one-celled parasite called *Entamoeba histolytica* (ent-a-ME-ba his-to-LI-ti-ka).

Who is at risk for amebiasis?

Although anyone can have this disease, it is more common in people who live in tropical areas with poor sanitary conditions. In the United States, amebiasis is most often found in travelers to and immigrants from these areas, as well as in people who live in institutions that have poor sanitary conditions. Men who have sex with men can also become infected.

How can I become infected with E. histolytica?

- By putting anything into your mouth that has touched the stool of a person who is infected with *E. histolytica*.

- By swallowing something, such as water or food, that is contaminated with *E. histolytica*.

- By touching and bringing to your mouth *E. histolytica* cysts (eggs) picked up from surfaces that are contaminated with *E. histolytica*.

"Amebiasis," Centers for Disease Control and Prevention (CDC), September 3, 2008.

What are the symptoms of amebiasis?

Only about 10% to 20% of people who are infected with *E. histolytica* become sick from the infection. The symptoms often are quite mild and can include loose stools, stomach pain, and stomach cramping. Amebic dysentery is a severe form of amebiasis associated with stomach pain, bloody stools, and fever. Rarely, *E. histolytica* invades the liver and forms an abscess. Even less commonly, it spreads to other parts of the body, such as the lungs or brain.

If I swallowed E. histolytica, how quickly would I become sick?

Only about 10% to 20% of people who are infected with *E. histolytica* become sick from the infection. Those people who do become sick usually develop symptoms within two to four weeks, although this may range from several weeks or longer.

What should I do if I think I have amebiasis?

See your health care provider.

How is amebiasis diagnosed?

Your health care provider will ask you to submit stool samples. Because *E. histolytica* is not always found in every stool sample, you may be asked to submit several stool samples from several different days.

Diagnosis of amebiasis can be very difficult. One problem is that other parasites and cells can look very similar to *E. histolytica* when seen under a microscope. Therefore, sometimes people are told that they are infected with *E. histolytica* even though they are not. *Entamoeba histolytica* and another ameba, *Entamoeba dispar*, which is about ten times more common, look the same when seen under a microscope. Unlike infection with *E. histolytica*, which sometimes makes people sick, infection with *E. dispar* does not make people sick and therefore does not need to be treated.

If you have been told that you are infected with *E. histolytica* but you are feeling fine, you might be infected with *E. dispar* instead. Unfortunately, most laboratories do not yet have the tests that can tell whether a person is infected with *E. histolytica* or with *E. dispar*. Until these tests become more widely available, it usually is best to assume that the parasite *is E. histolytica*.

A blood test is also available but is only recommended when your health care provider thinks that your infection may have spread beyond the intestine (gut) to some other organ of your body, such as the liver. However, this blood test may not be helpful in diagnosing your current illness because the test may still be positive if you had amebiasis in the past, even if you are no longer infected now.

How is amebiasis treated?

Several antibiotics are available to treat amebiasis. Treatment must be prescribed by a physician. You will be treated with only one antibiotic if your *E. histolytica* infection has not made you sick. You probably will be treated with two antibiotics (first one and then the other) if your infection has made you sick.

I am going to travel to a country that has poor sanitary conditions. What should I eat and drink there so I will not become infected with E. histolytica *or other such germs?*

- Drink only bottled or boiled (for one minute) water or carbonated (bubbly) drinks in cans or bottles. Do not drink fountain drinks or any drinks with ice cubes. Another way to make water safe is by filtering it through an "absolute one micron or less" filter and dissolving chlorine, chlorine dioxide, or iodine tablets in the filtered water. "Absolute one micron" filters can be found in camping/outdoor supply stores.

- Do not eat fresh fruit or vegetables that you did not peel yourself.

- Do not eat or drink milk, cheese, or dairy products that may not have been pasteurized.

- Do not eat or drink anything sold by street vendors.

Should I be concerned about spreading infection to the rest of my household?

Yes. However, the risk of spreading infection is low if the infected person is treated with antibiotics and practices good personal hygiene. This includes thorough hand washing with soap and water after using the toilet, after changing diapers, and before handling food.

Note: This information is not meant to be used for self-diagnosis or as a substitute for consultation with a health care provider. If you have any questions about the disease described or think that you may have a parasitic infection, consult a health care provider.

Chapter 10

Chancroid

What is chancroid?

Chancroid is a highly contagious sexually transmitted disease (or STD), but it is curable. It is caused by bacteria called *Haemophilus ducreyi* (or *H. ducreyi*). Chancroid causes ulcers or sores, usually of the genitals. Swollen, painful lymph glands in the groin area are often associated with chancroid. Left untreated, chancroid may make the transmission of human immunodeficiency virus (HIV) easier.

How common is it?

Chancroid is very common in Africa and parts of Asia, and it is becoming more common in the United States.

How is it transmitted?

Chancroid is transmitted in two ways:

- sexual transmission through skin-to-skin contact with an open sore, and

- non-sexual transmission by means of autoinoculation when contact is made with the pus-like fluid from the ulcer.

A person is considered to be infectious (able to pass the bacteria to others) when ulcers or sores are present. This means what as long as there are chancroid sores on the body, the person can spread the infection. There has been no reported disease in infants born to women with active chancroid at time of delivery.

Symptoms

- Symptoms usually occur within ten days from exposure. They rarely develop earlier than three days or later than ten days.

- The ulcer or sore begins as a tender, elevated bump, or papule that becomes a pus-filled, open sore with eroded or ragged edges.

- It is soft to the touch (unlike a syphilis chancre that is hard or rubbery). The term soft chancre is frequently used to describe the chancroid sore.

- The ulcers can be very painful in men, but women are often unaware of them.

- Because chancroid is often asymptomatic in women, they are often unaware that they are infected.

- Painful lymph glands (or lymph nodes) may occur in the groin, usually only on one side of the body. However, they can sometimes occur on both the left and right sides.

Testing and Diagnosis

Diagnosis is made by isolating the bacteria *Haemophilus ducreyi* in a culture from a genital ulcer or sore. The chancre is often confused with symptoms of other sexually transmitted diseases (STDs) like syphilis or herpes. Therefore, it is important that a health care provider rule these diseases out.

A gram stain to identify *H. ducreyi* is possible but can be misleading because of other organisms found in most genital ulcers.

Treatment

Chancroid can be treated with antibiotics. Successful treatment does two things:

- It resolves symptoms (or causes them to disappear).

- It prevents transmission.

A follow-up examination should be conducted three to seven days after treatment begins. If treatment is successful, ulcers usually improve within three to seven days. The time required for complete healing is related to the size of the ulcer. Large ulcers may require two weeks or longer to heal. In severe cases, scarring may result.

Partners should be examined and treated regardless of whether symptoms are present.

What does it mean for my health?

Chancroid has been well established as a cofactor for HIV transmission. In other words, someone infected with chancroid may be more easily infected with HIV. Also, someone infected with both chancroid and HIV may transmit HIV more easily to a partner who is not infected. Moreover, persons with HIV may experience slower healing of chancroid, even with treatment, and may need to take medications for a longer period of time.

In addition there may be complications from chancroid. Complications include the following:

- In 50% of cases, the lymph node glands in the groin become infected within five to eight days of appearance of initial sores.

- Glands on one side become enlarged, hard, painful, and fuse together to form a bubo, an inflammation and swelling of one or more lymph nodes with overlying red skin. Surgical drainage of the bubo may be necessary to relieve pain.

- Ruptured buboes are susceptible to secondary bacterial infections.

- In uncircumcised males, new scar tissue may result in phimosis (constriction so the foreskin cannot be retracted over the glans or head of the penis). Circumcision may be required to correct this.

Reduce Your Risk

As with other sexually transmitted diseases (STDs) there are things people can do to reduce or eliminate the risk of infection with chancroid. These include the following:

- Abstinence (not having sex) is a sure way to avoid infection.

- Mutual monogamy (having sex with only one uninfected partner) is another way to avoid infection.

- Latex condoms for vaginal, oral, and anal sex reduce risk. Using latex condoms may protect the penis or vagina from infection but does not protect other areas such as the scrotum or anal area.

- Water-based spermicides can be used along with latex condoms for additional protection during vaginal intercourse. Use of spermicide is not recommended nor found to be effective for oral or anal intercourse.

If a person does get chancroid, it is important for the infected person to avoid touching the infected area to prevent chance of autoinoculation.

Talk to Your Partner

You should talk to your partner as soon as you learn you have chancroid. Telling a partner can be hard, but it's important that you talk to your partner as soon as possible so she or he can get treatment.

Chapter 11

Chickenpox (Varicella) and Shingles

Chickenpox Vaccine: What You Need to Know

Why get vaccinated?

Chickenpox (also called varicella) is a common childhood disease. It is usually mild, but it can be serious, especially in young infants and adults.

- It causes a rash, itching, fever, and tiredness.

- It can lead to severe skin infection, scars, pneumonia, brain damage, or death.

- The chickenpox virus can be spread from person to person through the air, or by contact with fluid from chickenpox blisters.

- A person who has had chickenpox can get a painful rash called shingles years later.

- Before the vaccine, about 11,000 people were hospitalized for chickenpox each year in the United States.

This chapter includes text from "Chickenpox Vaccine: What You Need to Know," Centers for Disease Control and Prevention (CDC), March 13, 2008; "Varicella Disease Questions and Answers," CDC, reviewed June 2009; "Varicella Treatment Questions and Answers," CDC, June 2009; and "NINDS Shingles Information Page," National Institute of Neurological Disorders and Stroke (NINDS), updated April 24, 2009.

- Before the vaccine, about 100 people died each year as a result of chickenpox in the United States.

Chickenpox vaccine can prevent chickenpox. Most people who get chickenpox vaccine will not get chickenpox. But if someone who has been vaccinated does get chickenpox, it is usually very mild. They will have fewer blisters, are less likely to have a fever, and will recover faster.

Who should get chickenpox vaccine and when?

Routine: Children who have never had chickenpox should get two doses of chickenpox vaccine at these ages:

- First dose: 12–15 months of age
- Second dose: 4–6 years of age (may be given earlier, if at least three months after the first dose)

People 13 years of age and older (who have never had chickenpox or received chickenpox vaccine) should get two doses at least 28 days apart.

Catch-Up: Anyone who is not fully vaccinated, and never had chickenpox, should receive one or two doses of chickenpox vaccine. The timing of these doses depends on the person's age. Ask your provider. Chickenpox vaccine may be given at the same time as other vaccines.

Note: A combination vaccine called measles, mumps, rubella, varicella (MMRV), which contains both chickenpox and MMR vaccines, may be given instead of the two individual vaccines to people 12 years of age and younger.

Are there some people who should not get chickenpox vaccine or who should wait?

- People should not get chickenpox vaccine if they have ever had a life-threatening allergic reaction to a previous dose of chickenpox vaccine or to gelatin or the antibiotic neomycin.
- People who are moderately or severely ill at the time the shot is scheduled should usually wait until they recover before getting chickenpox vaccine.
- Pregnant women should wait to get chickenpox vaccine until

after they have given birth. Women should not get pregnant for one month after getting chickenpox vaccine.

- Some people should check with their doctor about whether they should get chickenpox vaccine, including anyone who:
  - has human immunodeficiency virus (HIV), acquired immunodeficiency syndrome (AIDS), or another disease that affects the immune system;
  - is being treated with drugs that affect the immune system, such as steroids, for two weeks or longer;
  - has any kind of cancer; or
  - is getting cancer treatment with radiation or drugs.
- People who recently had a transfusion or were given other blood products should ask their doctor when they may get chickenpox vaccine.

What are the risks from chickenpox vaccine?

A vaccine, like any medicine, is capable of causing serious problems, such as severe allergic reactions. The risk of chickenpox vaccine causing serious harm, or death, is extremely small. Getting chickenpox vaccine is much safer than getting chickenpox disease. Most people who get chickenpox vaccine do not have any problems with it. Reactions are usually more likely after the first dose than after the second.

Note: The first dose of MMRV vaccine has been associated with rash and higher rates of fever than MMR and varicella vaccines given separately. Rash has been reported in about one person in 20 and fever in about one person in five. Seizures caused by a fever are also reported more often after MMRV. These usually occur 5–12 days after the first dose.

What should I do if there is a reaction?

- Call a doctor, or get the person to a doctor right away if there is any unusual condition, such as a high fever, weakness, or behavior changes. Signs of a serious allergic reaction can include difficulty breathing, hoarseness or wheezing, hives, paleness, weakness, a fast heart beat or dizziness.
- Tell your doctor what happened, the date and time it happened, and when the vaccination was given.

89

Varicella Disease Questions and Answers

How do you get chickenpox?

Chickenpox is highly infectious and spreads from person to person by direct contact or through the air from an infected person's coughing or sneezing or from aerosolization of virus from skin lesions. A person with chickenpox is contagious 1–2 days before the rash appears and until all blisters have formed scabs. It takes from 10–21 days after exposure for someone to develop chickenpox.

Can you get chickenpox if you've been vaccinated?

Yes. About 15%–20% of people who have received one dose of chickenpox vaccine do still get chickenpox if they are exposed, but their disease is usually mild. Vaccinated persons who get chickenpox generally have fewer than 50 spots or bumps, which may resemble bug bites more than typical, fluid-filled chickenpox blisters. In 2006, the Advisory Committee on Immunization Practices (ACIP) voted to recommend routine two-dose varicella vaccination for children. In one study, children who received two doses of the chickenpox vaccine were three times less likely to get chickenpox than individuals who have had only one dose.

Varicella Treatment Questions and Answers

What home treatments are available for chickenpox?

Parents can do several things at home to help relieve their child's chickenpox symptoms. Because scratching the blisters may cause them to become infected, keep your child's fingernails trimmed short. Calamine lotion and Aveeno® (oatmeal) baths may help relieve some of the itching. Do not use aspirin or aspirin-containing products to relieve your child's fever. The use of aspirin in children with chickenpox has been associated with development of Reye syndrome (a severe disease affecting all organs, but most seriously affecting the liver and brain, and may cause death). Use non-aspirin medications such as acetaminophen (Tylenol®).

Are there any treatments that my doctor can prescribe for chickenpox?

Your health care provider will advise you on treatment options. Acyclovir, famciclovir, or valacyclovir (medicines that work against herpes viruses) are recommended for persons who are more likely to develop serious disease, including persons with chronic skin or lung disease, otherwise healthy individuals 13 years of age or older, and persons receiving steroid therapy. However, only acyclovir is currently licensed for use in treating varicella.

Persons whose immune systems have been weakened from disease or medication should contact their doctor immediately if they are exposed to or develop chickenpox. If you are pregnant and are either exposed to or develop chickenpox, you should immediately discuss prevention and treatment options with your doctor.

Is there any preventive treatment available after exposure to chickenpox for susceptible persons who are not eligible to receive chickenpox vaccine?

Yes, varicella zoster immune globulin (VZIG) can prevent or modify disease after exposure to someone with chickenpox. However, because it is costly and only provides temporary protection, VZIG is only recommended for persons at high risk of developing severe disease who are not eligible to receive chickenpox vaccine.

VZIG should be administered as soon as possible, but no later than 96 hours, after exposure to chickenpox. If you have had a varicella exposure and you fit into one of these groups, contact your doctor.

The only U.S. licensed manufacturer of VZIG discontinued production of VZIG in 2006. However, a similar product, VariZIG™ (Cangene Corporation, Winnipeg, Canada), became available under an investigational new drug (IND) application submitted to the Food and Drug Administration (FDA) in February 2006. Doctors in the U.S. can now request VariZIG from the sole authorized U.S. distributor, FFF Enterprises (Temecula, California), for their patients who have been exposed to varicella and who are at increased risk for severe disease and complications.

Shingles Information

Shingles (herpes zoster) is an outbreak of rash or blisters on the skin that is caused by the same virus that causes chickenpox—the varicella-zoster virus (VZV). The first sign of shingles is often burning or tingling pain, or sometimes numbness or itch, in one particular location on only one side of the body. After several days or a week, a rash of fluid-filled blisters, similar to chickenpox, appears in one area on one side of the body. Shingles pain can be mild or intense. Some people have mostly itching; some feel pain from the gentlest touch or breeze. The most common location for shingles is a band, called a dermatome, spanning one side of the trunk around the waistline. Anyone who has had chickenpox is at risk for shingles. Scientists think that in the original battle with the varicella-zoster virus, some of the virus particles leave the skin blisters and move into the nervous system. When the varicella-zoster virus reactivates, the virus moves back down the long nerve fibers that extend from the sensory cell bodies to the skin. The viruses multiply, the tell-tale rash erupts, and the person now has shingles.

Is there any treatment?

The severity and duration of an attack of shingles can be significantly reduced by immediate treatment with antiviral drugs, which include acyclovir, valacyclovir, or famciclovir. Antiviral drugs may also help stave off the painful aftereffects of shingles known as postherpetic neuralgia. Other treatments for postherpetic neuralgia include steroids, antidepressants, anticonvulsants, and topical agents.

In 2006, the Food and Drug Administration approved a VZV vaccine (Zostavax) for use in people 60 and older who have had chickenpox. When the vaccine becomes more widely available, many older adults will for the first time have a means of preventing shingles. Researchers found that giving older adults the vaccine reduced the expected number of later cases of shingles by half. And in people who still got the disease despite immunization, the severity and complications of shingles were dramatically reduced. The shingles vaccine is only a preventive therapy and is not a treatment for those who already have shingles or postherpetic neuralgia.

What is the prognosis?

For most healthy people who receive treatment soon after the outbreak of blisters, the lesions heal, the pain subsides within 3–5 weeks, and the blisters often leave no scars. However, shingles is a serious threat in immunosuppressed individuals.

A person with a shingles rash can pass the virus to someone, usually a child, who has never had chickenpox, but the child will develop chickenpox, not shingles. A person with chickenpox cannot communicate shingles to someone else. Shingles comes from the virus hiding inside the person's body, not from an outside source.

Chapter 12

Chlamydia and
Lymphogranuloma Venereum
(LGV)

What is chlamydia?

Chlamydia is a common sexually transmitted disease (STD) caused by the bacterium, *Chlamydia trachomatis*, which can damage a woman's reproductive organs. Even though symptoms of chlamydia are usually mild or absent, serious complications that cause irreversible damage, including infertility, can occur silently before a woman ever recognizes a problem. Chlamydia also can cause discharge from the penis of an infected man.

How common is chlamydia?

Chlamydia is the most frequently reported bacterial sexually transmitted disease in the United States. In 2006, 1,030,911 chlamydial infections were reported to the Centers for Disease Control and Prevention (CDC) from 50 states and the District of Columbia. Underreporting is substantial because most people with chlamydia are not aware of their infections and do not seek testing. Also, testing is not often done if patients are treated for their symptoms. An estimated 2,291,000 non-institutionalized U.S. civilians ages 14–39 are infected with chlamydia based on the U.S. National Health and Nutrition

Text in this chapter is from "STD Facts: Chlamydia," Centers for Disease Control and Prevention (CDC), December 20, 2007; and "STD Facts: LGV," CDC, January 4, 2008.

Examination Survey. Women are frequently re-infected if their sex partners are not treated.

How do people get chlamydia?

Chlamydia can be transmitted during vaginal, anal, or oral sex. Chlamydia can also be passed from an infected mother to her baby during vaginal childbirth. Any sexually active person can be infected with chlamydia. The greater the number of sex partners, the greater the risk of infection. Because the cervix of teenage girls and young women is not fully matured and is probably more susceptible to infection, they are at particularly high risk for infection if sexually active. Since chlamydia can be transmitted by oral or anal sex, men who have sex with men are also at risk for chlamydial infection.

What are the symptoms of chlamydia?

Chlamydia is known as a silent disease because about three-quarters of infected women and about half of infected men have no symptoms. If symptoms do occur, they usually appear within one to three weeks after exposure.

In women, the bacteria initially infect the cervix and the urethra. Women who have symptoms might have an abnormal vaginal discharge or a burning sensation when urinating. When the infection spreads from the cervix to the fallopian tubes, some women still have no signs or symptoms; others have lower abdominal pain, low back pain, nausea, fever, pain during intercourse, or bleeding between menstrual periods. Chlamydial infection of the cervix can spread to the rectum.

Men with signs or symptoms might have a discharge from their penis or a burning sensation when urinating. Men might also have burning and itching around the opening of the penis. Pain and swelling in the testicles are uncommon.

Men or women who have receptive anal intercourse may acquire chlamydial infection in the rectum, which can cause rectal pain, discharge, or bleeding. Chlamydia can also be found in the throats of women and men having oral sex with an infected partner.

What complications can result from untreated chlamydia?

If untreated, chlamydial infections can progress to serious reproductive and other health problems with both short-term and long-term consequences. Like the disease itself, the damage that chlamydia causes is often silent.

In women, untreated infection can spread into the uterus or fallopian tubes and cause pelvic inflammatory disease (PID). This happens in up to 40 percent of women with untreated chlamydia. PID can cause permanent damage to the fallopian tubes, uterus, and surrounding tissues. The damage can lead to chronic pelvic pain, infertility, and potentially fatal ectopic pregnancy. Women infected with chlamydia are up to five times more likely to become infected with human immunodeficiency virus (HIV), if exposed.

To help prevent the serious consequences of chlamydia, screening at least annually for chlamydia is recommended for all sexually active women age 25 years and younger. An annual screening test also is recommended for older women with risk factors for chlamydia (a new sex partner or multiple sex partners). All pregnant women should have a screening test for chlamydia.

Complications among men are rare. Infection sometimes spreads to the epididymis, causing pain, fever, and, rarely, sterility. Rarely, genital chlamydial infection can cause arthritis that can be accompanied by skin lesions and inflammation of the eye and urethra (Reiter syndrome).

How does chlamydia affect a pregnant woman and her baby?

In pregnant women, there is some evidence that untreated chlamydial infections can lead to premature delivery. Babies who are born to infected mothers can get chlamydial infections in their eyes and respiratory tracts. Chlamydia is a leading cause of early infant pneumonia and conjunctivitis (pink eye) in newborns.

How is chlamydia diagnosed?

There are laboratory tests to diagnose chlamydia. Some can be performed on urine, other tests require that a specimen be collected from a site such as the penis or cervix.

What is the treatment for chlamydia?

Chlamydia can be easily treated and cured with antibiotics. A single dose of azithromycin or a week of doxycycline (twice daily) are the most commonly used treatments. HIV-positive persons with chlamydia should receive the same treatment as those who are HIV negative.

All sex partners should be evaluated, tested, and treated. Persons with chlamydia should abstain from sexual intercourse until they and their sex partners have completed treatment, otherwise re-infection is possible.

Women whose sex partners have not been appropriately treated are at high risk for re-infection. Having multiple infections increases a woman's risk of serious reproductive health complications, including infertility. Retesting should be encouraged for women three to four months after treatment. This is especially true if a woman does not know if her sex partner received treatment.

How can chlamydia be prevented?

- The surest way to avoid transmission of STD is to abstain from sexual contact, or to be in a long-term mutually monogamous relationship with a partner who has been tested and is known to be uninfected.

- Latex male condoms, when used consistently and correctly, can reduce the risk of transmission of chlamydia.

- CDC recommends yearly chlamydia testing of all sexually active women age 25 or younger, older women with risk factors for chlamydial infections (those who have a new sex partner or multiple sex partners), and all pregnant women.

- If a woman has any symptoms, she should stop having sex and consult a health care provider immediately. Sexual activity should not resume until all sex partners have been examined and, if necessary, treated.

Lymphogranuloma Venereum *(LGV)*

What is LGV?

Lymphogranuloma venereum (LGV) is a sexually transmitted disease (STD) caused by three strains of the bacterium *Chlamydia trachomatis*. The visual signs include genital papule(s) (raised surface or bumps) and or ulcers, and swelling of the lymph glands in the genital area. LGV may also produce rectal ulcers, bleeding, pain, and discharge, especially among those who practice receptive anal intercourse. Genital lesions caused by LGV can be mistaken for other ulcerative STD such as syphilis, genital herpes, and chancroid. Complications of untreated LGV may include enlargement and ulcerations of the external genitalia and lymphatic obstruction, which may lead to elephantiasis of the genitalia.

How common is LGV?

Signs and symptoms associated with rectal infection can be mistakenly thought to be caused by ulcerative colitis. While the frequency of LGV infection is thought to be rare in industrialized countries, its identification is not always obvious, so the number of cases of LGV in the United States is unknown. However, outbreaks in the Netherlands and other European countries among men who have sex with men (MSM) have raised concerns about cases of LGV in the U.S.

How do people get LGV?

LGV is passed from person to person through direct contact with lesions, ulcers, or other area where the bacteria is located. Transmission of the organism occurs during sexual penetration (vaginal, oral, or anal) and may also occur via skin to skin contact. The likelihood of LGV infection following an exposure is unknown, but it is considered less infectious than some other STD. A person who has had sexual contact with a LGV-infected partner within 60 days of symptom onset should be examined, tested for urethral or cervical chlamydial infection, and treated with doxycycline, twice daily for seven days.

What are the signs and symptoms?

LGV can be difficult to diagnose. Typically, the primary lesion produced by LGV is a small genital or rectal lesion, which can ulcerate at the site of transmission after an incubation period of 3–30 days. These ulcers may remain undetected within the urethra, vagina, or rectum. As with other STD that causes ulcers, LGV may facilitate transmission and acquisition of HIV.

How is LGV diagnosed?

Because of limitations in a commercially available test, diagnosis is primarily based on clinical findings. Direct identification of the bacteria from a lesion or site of the infection may be possible through testing for chlamydia but, this would not indicate if the chlamydia infection is LGV. However, the usual chlamydia tests that are available have not been FDA approved for testing rectal specimens. In a patient with rectal signs or symptoms suspicious for LGV, a health care provider can collect a specimen and send the sample to his/her state health department for referral to CDC, which is working with state and local health departments to test specimens and validate diagnostic methods for LGV.

What is the treatment for LGV?

There is no vaccine against the bacteria. LGV can be treated with three weeks of antibiotics. CDC STD Treatment Guidelines recommend the use of doxycycline, twice a day for 21 days. An alternative treatment is erythromycin base or azithromycin. The health care provider will determine which is best.

If you have been treated for LGV, you should notify any sex partners you had sex with within 60 days of the symptom onset so they can be evaluated and treated. This will reduce the risk that your partners will develop symptoms and/or serious complications of LGV. It will reduce your risk of becoming re-infected as well as reduce the risk of ongoing transmission in the community. You and all of your sex partners should avoid sex until you have completed treatment for the infection and your symptoms and your partners' symptoms have disappeared.

Persons with both LGV and HIV infection should receive the same LGV treatment as those who are HIV-negative. Prolonged therapy may be required, and delay in resolution of symptoms may occur among persons with HIV.

How can LGV be prevented?

The surest way to avoid transmission of sexually transmitted diseases is to abstain from sexual contact, or to be in a long-term mutually monogamous relationship with a partner who has been tested and is asymptomatic and uninfected.

Male latex condoms, when used consistently and correctly, may reduce the risk of LGV transmission. Genital ulcer diseases can occur in male or female genital areas that may or may not be covered (protected by the condom).

Having had LGV and completing treatment does not prevent re-infection. Effective treatment is available and it is important that persons suspected of having LGV be treated as if they have it. Persons who are treated for LGV treatment should abstain from sexual contact until the infection is cleared.

Chapter 13

Clostridium Difficile *Infection*

Potentially Deadly Infection Doubles among Hospital Patients over the Last Five Years

The number of hospital patients stricken by an infection that can lead to diarrhea, blood poisoning, and even death increased by 200 percent between 2000 and 2005, according to the latest *News and Numbers* from the Agency for Healthcare Research and Quality (AHRQ). The sharp upturn follows a 74 percent increase in the number of cases between 1993 and 2000.

The infection—*Clostridium difficile*, or *C. difficile*-associated disease—results after previous antibiotic therapy suppresses the normal bacteria of the colon. This allows growth of *Clostridium difficile* following exposure by unwashed hands or infected surfaces such as bedpans, toilet seats, or floors. Symptoms can range from mild diarrhea to severe, life-threatening illness that, in its most severe form, can be treated only by completely removing the colon.

This chapter includes text from "Potentially Deadly Infection Doubles among Hospital Patients Over Last 5 Years," Agency for Healthcare Research and Quality (AHRQ), April 23, 2008; "General Information about *Clostridium Difficile* Infections," Centers for Disease Control and Prevention (CDC), June 6, 2007; and "*Clostridium Difficile* Toxin: The Test and Common Questions," © 2009 American Association for Clinical Chemistry. Reprinted with permission. For additional information about clinical lab testing, visit the Lab Tests Online website at www.labtestsonline.org.

AHRQ's analysis also found:

- There were over two million cases of *C. difficile* in U.S. hospitals between 1993 and 2005.

- Two out of three infected hospital patients in 2005 were elderly.

- On average, patients with *C. difficile* were hospitalized almost three times longer than uninfected patients. The in-hospital death rate for patients with *C. difficile* was 9.5 percent compared with 2.1 percent overall.

- The highest rate of *C. difficile* infection in hospital patients was in the Northeast (144 stays per 100,000 population) and the lowest (67 stays per 100,000 population) was in the West.

General Information about Clostridium Difficile Infections

Clostridium difficile is a bacterium that causes diarrhea and more serious intestinal conditions such as colitis. The diseases that result from *C. difficile* infections include colitis, more serious intestinal conditions, sepsis, and rarely death.

Symptoms include:

- watery diarrhea (at least three bowel movements per day for two or more days),

- fever,

- loss of appetite,

- nausea,

- abdominal pain/tenderness.

How is C. difficile disease treated?

C. difficile is generally treated for ten days with antibiotics prescribed by a health care provider. The drugs are effective and appear to have few side-effects. Do the following to reduce the chance of spread to others:

- wash hands with soap and water, especially after using the restroom and before eating; and

- clean surfaces in bathrooms, kitchens, and other areas on a regular basis with household detergent or disinfectants.

Clostridium Difficile *Toxin Test and Common Questions*

The *Clostridium difficile* toxin test is used to diagnose antibiotic-associated diarrhea and pseudomembranous colitis that is caused by *C. difficile.* It may also be ordered to detect recurrent disease.

If the patient has a positive toxin test, the doctor will typically discontinue any antibiotics that the patient may be taking and prescribe an appropriate treatment of oral antibiotic, such as metronidazole or vancomycin, to eliminate the *C. difficile* bacteria.

When is it ordered?

A *C. difficile* toxin test may be ordered when a hospitalized patient has frequent loose stools, abdominal pain, fever, and/or nausea during or following a course of antibiotics or following a recent gastrointestinal surgery. It may be ordered when an outpatient develops these symptoms within 6–8 weeks after taking antibiotics, several days after chemotherapy, or when a patient has a chronic gastrointestinal disorder that the doctor suspects is being worsened by a *C. difficile* infection. The *C. difficile* toxin test may be ordered to help diagnose the cause of frequent diarrhea when no other discernible cause (such as parasites or pathogenic bacteria) has been detected.

If a patient treated for antibiotic-associated diarrhea or colitis relapses and symptoms re-emerge, *C. difficile* toxin testing may be ordered to confirm the presence of the toxin.

What does the test result mean?

If the *C. difficile* toxin test is positive, it is likely that the patient's diarrhea and related symptoms are due to an overgrowth of toxin-producing *C. difficile.* Occasionally, false positives may be seen with grossly (visibly) bloody stool samples.

If the test is negative but the diarrhea continues, another sample needs to be tested. The rapid *C. difficile* toxin tests detect less than 85% of cases, so the toxin may have been missed the first time. Since the toxin breaks down at room temperature, a negative result may also indicate that the sample was not transported, stored, or processed promptly. A negative test result may also mean that the diarrhea and other symptoms are being caused by something other than *C. difficile.*

101

Is there anything else I should know?

There is a rapid test to detect a common antigen expressed by all strains of *C. difficile*, but it does not tell the doctor if the bacteria are producing the harmful toxins. An additional test to detect toxin A and B must be performed to confirm *C. difficile*-associated disease. The usual method to detect *C. difficile* toxin A and B is by a rapid enzyme immunoassay. Results are available after one to four hours, depending on the test. A cytotoxin test that looks for the toxic effects of stool on human cells grown in culture is a more sensitive method to detect toxin, but it requires 24 to 48 hours to get the result.

Clostridium difficile can be grown and isolated on a stool culture, but its presence does not indicate whether the strain present is a toxin producer. It also does not distinguish between *C. difficile* colonization and overgrowth/infection.

An endoscopic procedure can be used to diagnose *C. difficile* colitis. A specialist (gastroenterologist) can observe and biopsy any characteristic pseudomembranous lesions that may be present.

Molecular testing methods are being investigated for use in the detection of the presence of *C. difficile* toxin A and B. However, these tests are not able to distinguish between an active infection and a prior infection since the toxin can be detected long after the patient has recovered.

What else can cause diarrhea?

Diarrhea can be due to a pathogenic bacterial infection, a viral infection, a parasite, food intolerance, certain medications, chronic bowel disorders such as irritable bowel syndrome (IBS), or malabsorption disorders (such as celiac disease). Diarrhea may also be caused or exacerbated by psychological stresses.

Why must the stool sample be fresh?

For *C. difficile* toxin testing, the sample must be fresh because the toxin will break down in one to two hours and may result in a false negative test.

Why shouldn't I take an over-the-counter antidiarrhea medicine when I have diarrhea caused by C. difficile?

Antidiarrhea medicine can slow down the passage of stool through the gastrointestinal tract, increasing the length of time that the colon is exposed to the toxin and increasing tissue damage and inflammation.

Once I've had a C. difficile *infection, can I be re-infected?*

Yes, but in the short-term it is generally a case of recurrence of overgrowth and toxin production rather than re-infection; this happens because the normal flora has not reestablished itself fully yet. A patient who has had *C. difficile* diarrhea may also be at an increased risk of developing a new case of it with future courses of antibiotics.

Are some antibiotics more likely to cause antibiotic-related diarrhea?

Almost any antibiotic may lead to diarrhea since the drugs alter the normal population of good bacteria in the bowel. Broad-spectrum antibiotics, which kill many different types of bacteria, are more likely to wipe out normal bowel flora and allow *C. difficile* to overgrow and produce toxin.

Chapter 14

Common Cold: Rhinoviruses, Coronaviruses, and Others

Sneezing, scratchy throat, runny nose—everyone knows the first signs of a cold, probably the most common illness known. Although the common cold is usually mild, with symptoms lasting 1–2 weeks, it is a leading cause of doctor visits and missed days from school and work. People in the United States suffer one billion colds each year, according to some estimates. According to the Centers for Disease Control and Prevention (CDC), 22 million school days are lost annually in the United States due to the common cold.

Children have about 6–10 colds a year. One important reason why colds are so common in children is because they are often in close contact with each other in daycare centers and schools. In families with children in school, the number of colds per child can be as high as 12 a year. Adults average about two to four colds a year, although the range varies widely. Women, especially those aged 20–30 years, have more colds than men, possibly because of their closer contact with children. On average, people older than 60 have fewer than one cold a year.

The cold season: In the United States, most colds occur during the fall and winter. Beginning in late August or early September, the rate of colds increases slowly for a few weeks and remains high until March or April, when it declines. The seasonal variation may relate to the

"Common Cold: Overview, Cause, Transmission, Symptoms, Treatment, Prevention, and Complications," National Institute of Allergy and Infectious Diseases (NIAID), December 7, 2007.

opening of schools and to cold weather, which prompt people to spend more time indoors and increase the chances that viruses will spread to you from someone else.

Seasonal changes in relative humidity also may affect the prevalence of colds. The most common cold-causing viruses survive better when humidity is low—the colder months of the year. Cold weather also may make the inside lining of your nose drier and more vulnerable to viral infection.

Cause of the Common Cold

The viruses: More than 200 different viruses are known to cause the symptoms of the common cold. Some, such as the rhinoviruses, seldom produce serious illnesses. Others, such as parainfluenza and respiratory syncytial virus, produce mild infections in adults but can lead to severe lower respiratory tract infections in young children.

Rhinoviruses (from the Greek *rhin*, meaning nose) cause an estimated 30–35 percent of all adult colds, and are most active in early fall, spring, and summer. Scientists have identified than 110 distinct rhinovirus types. These agents grow best at temperatures of about 91 degrees Fahrenheit, the temperature inside the human nose.

Scientists think coronaviruses cause a large percentage of all adult colds. They bring on colds primarily in the winter and early spring. Of the more than 30 kinds, three or four infect humans. The importance of coronaviruses as a cause of colds is hard to assess because, unlike rhinoviruses, they are difficult to grow in the laboratory.

Approximately 10–15 percent of adult colds are caused by viruses also responsible for other, more severe illnesses: adenoviruses, coxsackievirus, echoviruses, orthomyxoviruses (including influenza A and B viruses, which cause flu), paramyxoviruses (including several parainfluenza viruses), respiratory syncytial virus, and enterovirus.

The causes of 30–50 percent of adult colds, presumed to be viral, remain unidentified. The same viruses that produce colds in adults appear to cause colds in children. The relative importance of various viruses in pediatric colds, however, is unclear because it's difficult to isolate the precise cause of symptoms in research studies of children with colds.

The weather: There is no evidence that you can get a cold from exposure to cold weather or from getting chilled or overheated.

Other factors: There is also no evidence that your chances of getting a cold are related to factors such as exercise, diet, or enlarged tonsils or adenoids. On the other hand, research suggests that psychological stress and allergic diseases affecting your nose or throat may have an impact on your chances of getting infected by cold viruses.

Transmission

You can get infected by cold viruses by either of these methods:

- Touching your skin or environmental surfaces, such as telephones and stair rails, that have cold germs on them and then touching your eyes or nose
- Inhaling drops of mucus full of cold germs from the air

Symptoms

Symptoms of the common cold usually begin 2–3 days after infection and often include the following: mucus buildup in your nose, difficulty breathing through your nose, swelling of your sinuses, sneezing, sore throat, cough, and headache.

Fever is usually slight but can climb to 102 degrees Fahrenheit in infants and young children. Cold symptoms can last from 2–14 days, but like most people, you'll probably recover in a week. If symptoms recur often or last much longer than two weeks, you might have an allergy rather than a cold.

Colds occasionally can lead to bacterial infections of your middle ear or sinuses, requiring treatment with antibiotics. High fever, significantly swollen glands, severe sinus pain, and a cough that produces mucus may indicate a complication or more serious illness requiring a visit to your health care provider.

Treatment

There is no cure for the common cold, but you can get relief from your cold symptoms by doing the following:

- Resting in bed
- Drinking plenty of fluids
- Gargling with warm salt water or using throat sprays or lozenges for a scratchy or sore throat
- Using petroleum jelly for a raw nose
- Taking aspirin or acetaminophen—Tylenol, for example—for headache or fever

A word of caution: Several studies have linked aspirin use to the development of Reye syndrome in children recovering from flu or chickenpox. Reye syndrome is a rare but serious illness that usually occurs in children between the ages of 3–12 years. It can affect all organs of the body but most often the brain and liver. While most children who survive an episode of Reye syndrome do not suffer any lasting consequences, the illness can lead to permanent brain damage or death. The American Academy of Pediatrics recommends children and teenagers not be given aspirin or medicine containing aspirin when they have any viral illness such as the common cold.

Over-the-counter cold medicines: Nonprescription cold remedies, including decongestants and cough suppressants, may relieve some of your cold symptoms but will not prevent or even shorten the length of your cold. Moreover, because most of these medicines have some side effects, such as drowsiness, dizziness, insomnia, or upset stomach, you should take them with care.

Questions have been raised about the safety of nonprescription cold medicines in children and whether the benefits justify any potential risks from the use of these products in children, especially in those under two years of age. Recently, a Food and Drug Administration panel recommended that nonprescription cold medicines not be given to children under the age of six, because cold medicines do not appear to be effective for these children and may not be safe.

Over-the-counter antihistamines: Nonprescription antihistamines may give you some relief from symptoms such as runny nose and watery eyes, which are symptoms commonly associated with colds.

Antibiotics: Never take antibiotics to treat a cold because antibiotics do not kill viruses. You should use these prescription medicines only if you have a rare bacterial complication, such as sinusitis or ear infection. In addition, you should not use antibiotics just in case, because they will not prevent bacterial infections.

Steam: Although inhaling steam may temporarily relieve symptoms of congestion, health experts have found that this approach is not an effective treatment.

Prevention

There are several ways you can keep yourself from getting a cold or passing one on to others:

- Because cold germs on your hands can easily enter through your eyes and nose, keep your hands away from those areas of your body.

- If possible, avoid being close to people who have colds.

- If you have a cold, avoid being close to people.

- If you sneeze or cough, cover your nose or mouth, and sneeze or cough into your elbow rather than your hand.

Handwashing: Handwashing with soap and water is the simplest and one of the most effective ways to keep from getting colds or giving them to others. During cold season, you should wash your hands often and teach your children to do the same. When water isn't available, Centers for Disease Control and Prevention (CDC) recommends using alcohol-based products made for disinfecting your hands.

Disinfecting: Rhinoviruses can live up to three hours on your skin. They also can survive up to three hours on objects such as telephones and stair railings. Cleaning environmental surfaces with a virus-killing disinfectant might help prevent spread of infection.

Vaccine: Because so many different viruses can cause the common cold, the outlook for developing a vaccine that will prevent transmission of all of them is dim. Scientists, however, continue to search for a solution to this problem.

Unproven Prevention Methods

Echinacea: Echinacea is a dietary herbal supplement that some people use to treat their colds. Researchers, however, have found that while the herb may help treat your colds if taken in the early stages, it will not help prevent them.

One research study funded by the National Center for Complementary and Alternative Medicine, a part of the National Institutes of Health, found that echinacea is not effective at all in treating children aged 2–11.

Vitamin C: Many people are convinced that taking large quantities of vitamin C will prevent colds or relieve symptoms. To test this theory, several large-scale, controlled studies involving children and adults have been conducted. To date, no conclusive data has shown that large doses of vitamin C prevent colds. The vitamin may reduce the severity or duration of symptoms, but there is no clear evidence of this effect. Taking vitamin C over long periods of time in large amounts may be harmful. Too much vitamin C can cause severe diarrhea, a particular danger for elderly people and small children.

Honey: Honey has been considered to be a treatment for coughs and to soothe a sore throat. A recent study conducted at the Penn State College of Medicine compared the effectiveness of a little bit of buckwheat honey before bedtime versus either no treatment or dextromethorphan (DM), the cough suppressant found in many over-the-counter cold medicines. The results of this study suggest that honey may be useful to relieve coughing, but researchers need to do additional studies.

You should never give honey to children under the age of one because of the risk of infantile botulism, a serious disease.

Zinc: Zinc lozenges and zinc lollipops are available over the counter as a treatment for the common cold; however, results from studies designed to test the efficacy of zinc are inconclusive. Although several studies have shown zinc to be effective for reducing the symptoms of the common cold, an equal number of studies have shown zinc is not effective. This may be due to flaws in the way these studies were conducted, or the particular form of zinc used in each case. Therefore, additional studies are needed.

Complications

Colds occasionally can lead to bacterial infections of your middle ear or sinuses, requiring treatment with antibiotics. High fever, significantly swollen glands, severe sinus pain, and a cough that produces mucus, may indicate a complication or more serious illness requiring a visit to your health care provider.

Chapter 15

Conjunctivitis (Pinkeye)

About Pinkeye

Conjunctivitis, commonly known as pinkeye, is an inflammation of the conjunctiva, the clear membrane that covers the white part of the eye and the inner surface of the eyelids.

While pinkeye can be alarming because it may make the eyes extremely red and can spread rapidly, it's a fairly common condition and usually causes no long-term eye or vision damage. But if your child shows symptoms of pinkeye, it's important to see a doctor. Some kinds of pinkeye go away on their own, but other types require treatment.

Causes

Pinkeye can be caused by many of the bacteria and viruses responsible for colds and other infections,—including ear infections, sinus infections, and sore throats—and by the same types of bacteria that cause the sexually transmitted diseases (STDs) chlamydia and gonorrhea.

Pinkeye also can be caused by allergies. These cases tend to happen more frequently among kids who also have other allergic conditions, such as hay fever. Triggers of allergic conjunctivitis include grass, ragweed pollen, animal dander, and dust mites.

Sometimes a substance in the environment can irritate the eyes and cause pinkeye; for example, chemicals (such as chlorine and soaps) and air pollutants (such as smoke and fumes).

Pinkeye in Newborns

Newborns are particularly susceptible to pinkeye and can be more prone to serious health complications if it goes untreated.

If a baby is born to a mother who has an STD, during delivery the bacteria or virus can pass from the birth canal into the baby's eyes, causing pinkeye. To prevent this, doctors give antibiotic ointment or eye drops to all babies immediately after birth. Occasionally, this preventive treatment causes a mild chemical conjunctivitis, which typically clears up on its own. Doctors also can screen pregnant women for STDs and treat them during pregnancy to prevent transmission of the infection to the baby.

Many babies are born with a narrow or blocked tear duct, a condition which usually clears up on its own. Sometimes, though, it can lead to conjunctivitis.

Symptoms

The different types of pinkeye can have different symptoms. And symptoms can vary from child to child.

One of the most common symptoms is discomfort in the eye. A child may say that it feels like there's sand in the eye. Many kids have redness of the eye and inner eyelid, which is why conjunctivitis is often called pinkeye. It can also cause discharge from the eyes, which may cause the eyelids to stick together when the child awakens in the morning. Some kids have swollen eyelids or sensitivity to bright light.

In cases of allergic conjunctivitis, itchiness and tearing are common symptoms.

Contagiousness

Cases of pinkeye that are caused by bacteria and viruses are contagious; cases caused by allergies or environmental irritants are not.

A child can get pinkeye by touching an infected person or something an infected person has touched, such as a used tissue. In the summertime, pinkeye can spread when kids swim in contaminated water or share contaminated towels. It also can be spread through coughing and sneezing.

Doctors usually recommend keeping kids diagnosed with contagious conjunctivitis out of school, day care, or summer camp for a short time.

Someone who has pinkeye in one eye can also inadvertently spread it to the other eye by touching the infected eye, then touching the other eye.

Preventing Pinkeye

To prevent pinkeye caused by infections, teach kids to wash their hands often with warm water and soap. They also should not share eye drops, tissues, eye makeup, washcloths, towels, or pillowcases with other people.

Be sure to wash your own hands thoroughly after touching an infected child's eyes, and throw away items like gauze or cotton balls after they've been used. Wash towels and other linens that the child has used in hot water separately from the rest of the family's laundry to avoid contamination.

If you know your child is prone to allergic conjunctivitis, keep windows and doors closed on days when the pollen is heavy, and dust and vacuum frequently to limit allergy triggers in the home. Irritant conjunctivitis can only be prevented by avoiding the irritating causes.

Many cases of pinkeye in newborns can be prevented by screening and treating pregnant women for STDs. A pregnant woman may have bacteria in her birth canal even if she shows no symptoms, which is why prenatal screening is important.

Treatment

Pinkeye caused by a virus usually goes away on its own without any treatment. If a doctor suspects that the pinkeye has been caused by a bacterial infection, antibiotic eye drops or ointment will be prescribed.

Sometimes it can be a challenge to get kids to tolerate eye drops several times a day. If you're having trouble, put the drops on the inner corner of your child's closed eye—when the child opens the eye, the medicine will flow into it. If you continue to have trouble with drops, ask the doctor about antibiotic ointment. It can be applied in a thin layer where the eyelids meet, and will melt and enter the eye.

If your child has allergic conjunctivitis, your doctor may prescribe antiallergy medication, which comes in the form of pills, liquid, or eye drops.

Cool or warm compresses and acetaminophen or ibuprofen may make a child with pinkeye feel more comfortable. You can clean the edges of the infected eye carefully with warm water and gauze or cotton balls. This can also remove the crusts of dried discharge that may cause the eyelids to stick together first thing in the morning.

When to Call the Doctor

If you think your child has pinkeye, it's important to contact your doctor to learn what's causing it and how to treat it. Other serious eye conditions can mimic conjunctivitis, so a child who complains of severe pain, changes in eyesight, or sensitivity to light should be examined. If the pinkeye does not improve after two to three days of treatment, or after a week when left untreated, call your doctor.

If your child has pinkeye and starts to develop increased swelling, redness, and tenderness in the eyelids and around the eye, along with a fever, call your doctor. Those symptoms may mean the infection has started to spread beyond the conjunctiva and will require additional treatment.

Chapter 16

Coxsackievirus Infections

Coxsackieviruses are part of the enterovirus family of viruses (which also includes polioviruses and hepatitis A virus) that live in the human digestive tract. They can spread from person to person, usually on unwashed hands and surfaces contaminated by feces, where they can live for several days.

In cooler climates, outbreaks of coxsackievirus infections most often occur in the summer and fall, though they cause infections year-round in tropical parts of the world.

In most cases, coxsackieviruses cause mild flu-like symptoms and go away without treatment. But in some cases, they can lead to more serious infections.

Signs and Symptoms

Coxsackievirus can produce a wide variety of symptoms. About half of all kids infected with coxsackievirus have no symptoms. Others suddenly develop high fever, headache, and muscle aches, and some also develop a sore throat, abdominal discomfort, or nausea. A child with a coxsackievirus infection may simply feel hot but have no other symptoms. In most kids, the fever lasts about three days, then disappears.

Coxsackieviruses can also cause several different symptoms that affect different body parts, including:

- **Hand, foot, and mouth disease**, a type of coxsackievirus syndrome, causes painful red blisters in the throat and on the tongue, gums, hard palate, inside of the cheeks, and the palms of hands and soles of the feet.

- **Herpangina**, an infection of the throat which causes red-ringed blisters and ulcers on the tonsils and soft palate, the fleshy back portion of the roof of the mouth.

- **Hemorrhagic conjunctivitis**, an infection that affects the whites of the eyes. Hemorrhagic conjunctivitis usually begins as eye pain, followed quickly by red, watery eyes with swelling, light sensitivity, and blurred vision.

Occasionally, coxsackieviruses can cause more serious infections that may need to be treated in a hospital, including:

- viral meningitis, an infection of the meninges (the three membranes that envelop the brain and spinal cord);

- encephalitis, a brain infection;

- myocarditis, an infection of the heart muscle.

Newborns can be infected from their mothers during or shortly after birth and are more at risk for developing serious infection, including myocarditis, hepatitis, and meningoencephalitis (an inflammation of the brain and meninges). In newborns, symptoms can develop within two weeks after birth.

Contagiousness

Coxsackieviruses are very contagious. They can be passed from person to person on unwashed hands and surfaces contaminated by feces. They can also be spread through droplets of fluid sprayed into the air when someone sneezes or coughs.

When an outbreak affects a community, risk for coxsackievirus infection is highest among infants and children younger than five. The virus spreads easily in group settings like schools, childcare centers, or summer camps. People who are infected with a coxsackievirus are most contagious the first week they're sick.

Prevention

There is no vaccine to prevent coxsackievirus infection. Hand washing is the best protection. Remind everyone in your family to wash their hands frequently, particularly after using the toilet (especially those in public places), after changing a diaper, before meals, and before preparing food. Shared toys in child care centers should be routinely cleaned with a disinfectant because the virus can live on these objects for days.

Kids who are sick with a coxsackievirus infection should be kept out of school or child care for a few days to avoid spreading the infection.

The duration of an infection varies widely. For coxsackie fever without other symptoms, a child's temperature may return to normal within 24 hours, although the average fever lasts three to four days. Hand, foot, and mouth disease usually lasts for two or three days, while viral meningitis can take three to seven days to clear up.

Treating Coxsackievirus Infections

Depending on the type of infection and symptoms, the doctor may prescribe medications to make your child feel more comfortable. However, because antibiotics only work against bacteria, they can't be used to fight a coxsackievirus infection.

Acetaminophen may be given to relieve any minor aches and pains. If the fever lasts for more than 24 hours or if your child has any symptoms of a more serious coxsackievirus infection, call your doctor.

Most children with a simple coxsackievirus infection recover completely after a few days without needing any treatment. A child who has a fever without any other symptoms should rest in bed or play quietly indoors. Offer plenty of fluids to prevent dehydration.

When to Call the Doctor

Call the doctor immediately if your child develops any of the following symptoms:

- fever higher than 100.4° Fahrenheit (38° Celsius) for infants younger than six months and higher than 102° Fahrenheit (38.8° Celsius) for older kids
- poor appetite
- trouble feeding

- vomiting
- diarrhea
- difficulty breathing
- convulsions
- unusual sleepiness
- pain in the chest or abdomen
- sores on the skin or inside the mouth
- severe sore throat
- severe headache, especially with vomiting, confusion, unusual sleepiness, or convulsions
- neck stiffness
- red, swollen, and watery eyes
- pain in one or both testicles

Chapter 17

Cryptosporidiosis

Cryptosporidiosis is a diarrheal disease caused by microscopic parasites, *Cryptosporidium*, that can live in the intestine of humans and animals and is passed in the stool of an infected person or animal. Both the disease and the parasite are commonly known as "crypto." The parasite is protected by an outer shell that allows it to survive outside the body for long periods of time and makes it very resistant to chlorine-based disinfectants. During the past two decades, crypto has become recognized as one of the most common causes of waterborne disease (recreational water and drinking water) in humans in the United States. The parasite is found in every region of the United States and throughout the world.

How is cryptosporidiosis spread?

Cryptosporidium lives in the intestine of infected humans or animals. An infected person or animal sheds crypto parasites in the stool. Millions of crypto germs can be released in a bowel movement from an infected human or animal. Shedding of crypto in the stool begins when the symptoms begin and can last for weeks after the symptoms (for example, diarrhea) stop. You can become infected after accidentally swallowing the parasite. *Cryptosporidium* may be found in soil, food, water, or surfaces that have been contaminated

"Cryptosporidiosis: Fact Sheets: Infection–General Public," Centers for Disease Control and Prevention (CDC), April 16, 2008.

with the feces from infected humans or animals. Crypto is not spread by contact with blood. Crypto can be spread in the following situations:

- By putting something in your mouth or accidentally swallowing something that has come into contact with stool of a person or animal infected with crypto. **Note:** You may not be able to tell by looking whether something has been in contact with stool.

- By swallowing recreational water contaminated with crypto. Recreational water is water in swimming pools, hot tubs, Jacuzzis, fountains, lakes, rivers, springs, ponds, or streams. Recreational water can be contaminated with sewage or feces from humans or animals.

- By swallowing water or beverages contaminated with stool from infected humans or animals.

- By eating uncooked food contaminated with crypto. Thoroughly wash with uncontaminated water all vegetables and fruits you plan to eat raw.

- By touching your mouth with contaminated hands. Hands can become contaminated through a variety of activities, such as touching surfaces (toys, bathroom fixtures, changing tables, diaper pails) that have been contaminated by stool from an infected person, changing diapers, caring for an infected person, changing diapers, caring for an infected person, and handling an infected cow or calf.

- By exposure to human feces through sexual contact.

What are the symptoms of cryptosporidiosis?

The most common symptom of cryptosporidiosis is watery diarrhea. Other symptoms include the following:

- Stomach cramps or pain
- Dehydration
- Nausea
- Vomiting
- Fever
- Weight loss

Some people with crypto will have no symptoms at all. While the small intestine is the site most commonly affected, crypto infections could possibly affect other areas of the digestive tract or the respiratory tract.

Symptoms of cryptosporidiosis generally begin 2–10 days (average seven days) after becoming infected with the parasite.

In persons with healthy immune systems, symptoms usually last about 1–2 weeks. The symptoms may go in cycles in which you may seem to get better for a few days, then feel worse again before the illness ends.

Who is most at risk for cryptosporidiosis?

People who are most likely to become infected with *Cryptosporidium* include the following:

- Children who attend day care centers, including diaper-aged children
- Child care workers
- Parents of infected children
- People who take care of other people with cryptosporidiosis
- International travelers
- Backpackers, hikers, and campers who drink unfiltered, untreated water
- People who drink from untreated shallow, unprotected wells
- People, including swimmers, who swallow water from contaminated sources
- People who handle infected cattle
- People exposed to human feces through sexual contact

Contaminated water may include water that has not been boiled or filtered, as well as contaminated recreational water sources. Several community-wide outbreaks of cryptosporidiosis have been linked to drinking municipal water or recreational water contaminated with *Cryptosporidium*.

Although crypto can infect all people, some groups are likely to develop more serious illness. If you have a severely weakened immune system, talk to your health care provider for additional guidance.

If you suspect that you have cryptosporidiosis, see your health care provider.

How is a cryptosporidiosis diagnosed?

Your health care provider will ask you to submit stool samples to see if you are infected. Because testing for crypto can be difficult, you may be asked to submit several stool specimens over several days. Tests for crypto are not routinely done in most laboratories. Therefore, your health care provider should specifically request testing for the parasite.

What is the treatment for cryptosporidiosis?

Nitazoxanide has been Food and Drug Administration (FDA)-approved for treatment of diarrhea caused by *Cryptosporidium* in people with healthy immune systems and is available by prescription. Consult with your health care provider for more information. Most people who have healthy immune systems will recover without treatment. Diarrhea can be managed by drinking plenty of fluids to prevent dehydration. Young children and pregnant women may be more susceptible to dehydration. Rapid loss of fluids from diarrhea may be especially life threatening to babies. Therefore, parents should talk to their health care provider about fluid replacement therapy options for infants. Antidiarrheal medicine may help slow down diarrhea, but a health care provider should be consulted before such medicine is taken.

People who are in poor health or who have weakened immune systems are at higher risk for more severe and more prolonged illness. The effectiveness of nitazoxanide in immunosuppressed individuals is unclear. Human immunodeficiency virus (HIV)-positive individuals who suspect they have crypto should contact their health care provider. For persons with acquired immunodeficiency syndrome (AIDS), anti-retroviral therapy that improves immune status will also decrease or eliminate symptoms of crypto. However, even if symptoms disappear, cryptosporidiosis is often not curable and the symptoms may return if the immune status worsens.

Cryptosporidium can be very contagious. Infected individuals should follow these guidelines to avoid spreading the disease to others:

1. Wash your hands frequently with soap and water, especially after using the toilet, after changing diapers, and before eating or preparing food.

2. Do not swim in recreational water (pools, hot tubs, lakes, rivers, oceans, etc.) if you have cryptosporidiosis and for at least

two weeks after the diarrhea stops. You can pass crypto in your stool and contaminate water for several weeks after your symptoms have ended. You do not even need to have a fecal accident in the water. Immersion in the water may be enough for contamination to occur. Water contaminated in this manner has resulted in outbreaks of cryptosporidiosis among recreational water users. **Note:** You may not be protected in a chlorinated recreational water venue (such as a swimming pool, water park, splash pad, spray park) because *Cryptosporidium* is chlorine-resistant and can live for days in chlorine-treated water.

3. Avoid sexual practices that might result in oral exposure to stool (for example, oral-anal contact).

4. Avoid close contact with anyone who has a weakened immune system.

5. Children with diarrhea should be excluded from childcare settings until the diarrhea has stopped.

Chapter 18

Diphtheria

About Diphtheria

Diphtheria is a bacterial infection that spreads easily and occurs quickly. It mainly affects the nose and throat. Children under five and adults over 60 years old are particularly at risk for contracting the infection. People living in crowded or unclean conditions, those who aren't well nourished, and children and adults who don't have up-to-date immunizations are also at risk.

Diphtheria is rare in the United States and Europe, where health officials have been immunizing children against it for decades. However, it's still common in developing countries where immunizations aren't given routinely. In 1993 and 1994, more than 50,000 cases were reported during a serious outbreak of diphtheria in countries of the former Soviet Union.

Signs and Symptoms

In its early stages, diphtheria can be mistaken for a bad sore throat. A low-grade fever and swollen neck glands are the other early symptoms.

"Diphtheria," October 2008, reprinted with permission from www.kidshealth .org. Copyright © 2008 The Nemours Foundation. This information was provided by KidsHealth, one of the largest resources online for medically reviewed health information written for parents, kids, and teens. For more articles like this one, visit www.KidsHealth.org, or www.TeensHealth.org.

The toxin, or poison, caused by the bacteria can lead to a thick coating in the nose, throat, or airway. This coating is usually fuzzy gray or black and can cause breathing problems and difficulty in swallowing. The formation of this coating (or membrane) in the nose, throat, or airway makes a diphtheria infection different from other more common infections (such as strep throat) that cause sore throat.

As the infection progresses, the person may:

• have difficulty breathing or swallowing,

• complain of double vision,

• have slurred speech,

• even show signs of going into shock (skin that's pale and cold, rapid heartbeat, sweating, and an anxious appearance).

In cases that progress beyond a throat infection, diphtheria toxin spreads through the bloodstream and can lead to potentially life-threatening complications that affect other organs of the body, such as the heart and kidneys. The toxin can cause damage to the heart that affects its ability to pump blood or the kidneys' ability to clear wastes. It can also cause nerve damage, eventually leading to paralysis. Up to 40% to 50% of those who don't get treated can die.

Prevention

Preventing diphtheria depends almost completely on immunizing children with the diphtheria/tetanus/pertussis (DTP or DTaP) vaccine and non-immunized adults with the diphtheria/tetanus vaccine (DT). Most cases of diphtheria occur in people who haven't received the vaccine at all or haven't received the entire course.

The immunization schedule calls for:

• DTaP vaccines at two, four, and six months of age;

• booster dose given at twelve to eighteen months;

• booster dose given again at four to six years;

• booster shots given every ten years after that to maintain protection.

Although most children tolerate it well, the vaccine sometimes causes mild side effects such as redness or tenderness at the injection site, a low-grade fever, or general fussiness or crankiness. Severe complications, such as an allergic reaction, are rare.

Contagiousness

Diphtheria is highly contagious. It's easily passed from the infected person to others through sneezing, coughing, or even laughing. It can also be spread to others who pick up tissues or drinking glasses that have been used by the infected person.

People who have been infected by the diphtheria bacteria can infect others for up to four weeks, even if they don't have any symptoms. The incubation period (the time it takes for a person to become infected after being exposed) for diphtheria is two to four days, although it can range from one to six days.

Treatment

Children and adults with diphtheria are treated in a hospital. After a doctor confirms the diagnosis through a throat culture, the infected person receives a special anti-toxin, given through injections or through an intravenous (IV), to neutralize the diphtheria toxin already circulating in the body, as well as antibiotics to kill the remaining diphtheria bacteria.

If the infection is advanced, people with diphtheria may need a ventilator to help them breathe. In cases in which the toxins may have spread to the heart, kidneys, or central nervous system, patients may need intravenous fluids, oxygen, or heart medications.

A person with diphtheria must also be isolated. Family members (as well as others who spend a lot of time with the person with diphtheria) who haven't been immunized, or who are very young or elderly, must be protected from contact with the patient.

When someone is diagnosed with diphtheria, the doctor will notify the local health department and will take steps to treat everyone in the household who may have been exposed to the bacteria. This will include assessment of immune status, throat cultures, and booster doses of the diphtheria vaccine. They will also receive antibiotics as a precaution.

Immediate hospitalization and early intervention allow most patients to recover from diphtheria. After the antibiotics and anti-toxin have taken effect, someone with diphtheria will need bed rest for a while (four to six weeks, or until full recovery). Bed rest is particularly important if the person's heart has been affected by the disease. Myocarditis, or inflammation of the heart muscle, can be a complication of diphtheria.

Those who have recovered should still receive a full course of the diphtheria vaccine to prevent a recurrence because contracting the disease doesn't guarantee lifetime immunity.

When to Call the Doctor

Call your doctor immediately if you or your child has symptoms of diphtheria, if you observe symptoms in someone else, if anyone in your family is exposed to diphtheria, or if you think that you or a family member is at risk. It's important to remember, though, that most throat infections are not diphtheria, especially in countries that have routine immunizations against it.

If you're not sure if your child has been vaccinated against diphtheria, make an appointment. Also make sure your own booster immunizations are current. International studies have shown that a significant percentage of adults over 40 years of age aren't adequately protected against diphtheria and tetanus.

Chapter 19

Epstein-Barr Virus and Infectious Mononucleosis

Epstein-Barr virus, frequently referred to as EBV, is a member of the herpesvirus family and one of the most common human viruses. The virus occurs worldwide, and most people become infected with EBV sometime during their lives. In the United States, as many as 95% of adults between 35 and 40 years of age have been infected. Infants become susceptible to EBV as soon as maternal antibody protection (present at birth) disappears. Many children become infected with EBV, and these infections usually cause no symptoms or are indistinguishable from the other mild, brief illnesses of childhood. In the United States and in other developed countries, many persons are not infected with EBV in their childhood years. When infection with EBV occurs during adolescence or young adulthood, it causes infectious mononucleosis 35% to 50% of the time.

Symptoms of infectious mononucleosis are fever, sore throat, and swollen lymph glands. Sometimes, a swollen spleen or liver involvement may develop. Heart problems or involvement of the central nervous system occurs only rarely, and infectious mononucleosis is almost never fatal. There are no known associations between active EBV infection and problems during pregnancy, such as miscarriages or birth defects. Although the symptoms of infectious mononucleosis usually resolve in one or two months, EBV remains dormant or latent in a few cells in the throat and blood for the rest of the person's

---

Text in this chapter is excerpted from "Epstein-Barr Virus and Infectious Mononucleosis," Centers for Disease Control and Prevention (CDC), May 16, 2006.

life. Periodically, the virus can reactivate and is commonly found in the saliva of infected persons. This reactivation usually occurs without symptoms of illness.

EBV also establishes a lifelong dormant infection in some cells of the body's immune system. A late event in a very few carriers of this virus is the emergence of Burkitt lymphoma and nasopharyngeal carcinoma, two rare cancers that are not normally found in the United States. EBV appears to play an important role in these malignancies, but is probably not the sole cause of disease.

Most individuals exposed to people with infectious mononucleosis have previously been infected with EBV and are not at risk for infectious mononucleosis. In addition, transmission of EBV requires intimate contact with the saliva (found in the mouth) of an infected person. Transmission of this virus through the air or blood does not normally occur. The incubation period, or the time from infection to appearance of symptoms, ranges from 4–6 weeks. Persons with infectious mononucleosis may be able to spread the infection to others for a period of weeks. However, no special precautions or isolation procedures are recommended, since the virus is also found frequently in the saliva of healthy people. In fact, many healthy people can carry and spread the virus intermittently for life. These people are usually the primary reservoir for person-to-person transmission. For this reason, transmission of the virus is almost impossible to prevent.

The clinical diagnosis of infectious mononucleosis is suggested on the basis of the symptoms of fever, sore throat, swollen lymph glands, and the age of the patient. Usually, laboratory tests are needed for confirmation. Serologic results for persons with infectious mononucleosis include an elevated white blood cell count, an increased percentage of certain atypical white blood cells, and a positive reaction to a mono spot test.

There is no specific treatment for infectious mononucleosis, other than treating the symptoms. No antiviral drugs or vaccines are available. Some physicians have prescribed a five-day course of steroids to control the swelling of the throat and tonsils. The use of steroids has also been reported to decrease the overall length and severity of illness, but these reports have not been published.

It is important to note that symptoms related to infectious mononucleosis caused by EBV infection seldom last for more than four months. When such an illness lasts more than six months, it is frequently called chronic EBV infection. However, valid laboratory evidence for continued active EBV infection is seldom found in these patients. The illness should be investigated further to determine if it meets the criteria for chronic fatigue syndrome (CFS). This process includes ruling out other causes of chronic illness or fatigue.

Diagnosis of EBV Infections

In most cases of infectious mononucleosis, the clinical diagnosis can be made from the characteristic triad of fever, pharyngitis, and lymphadenopathy lasting for 1–4 weeks. Serologic test results include a normal to moderately elevated white blood cell count, an increased total number of lymphocytes, greater than 10% atypical lymphocytes, and a positive reaction to a mono spot test. In patients with symptoms compatible with infectious mononucleosis, a positive Paul-Bunnell heterophile antibody test result is diagnostic, and no further testing is necessary. Moderate-to-high levels of heterophile antibodies are seen during the first month of illness and decrease rapidly after week four. False-positive results may be found in a small number of patients, and false-negative results may be obtained in 10% to 15% of patients, primarily in children younger than ten years of age. True outbreaks of infectious mononucleosis are extremely rare. A substantial number of pseudo-outbreaks have been linked to laboratory error, as reported in CDC's *Morbidity and Mortality Weekly Report*, vol. 40, no. 32, on August 16, 1991.

When mono spot or heterophile test results are negative, additional laboratory testing may be needed to differentiate EBV infections from a mononucleosis-like illness induced by cytomegalovirus, adenovirus, or *Toxoplasma gondii*. Direct detection of EBV in blood or lymphoid tissues is a research tool and is not available for routine diagnosis. Instead, serologic testing is the method of choice for diagnosing primary infection.

Summary of Interpretation

The diagnosis of EBV infection is summarized as follows:

Susceptibility

If antibodies to the viral capsid antigen are not detected, the patient is susceptible to EBV infection.

Primary Infection

Primary EBV infection is indicated if immunoglobulin (Ig) M antibody to the viral capsid antigen is present and antibody to EBV nuclear antigen, or EBV nuclear antigen (EBNA), is absent. A rising or high IgG antibody to the viral capsid antigen and negative antibody to EBNA after at least four weeks of illness is also strongly suggestive of primary infection. In addition, 80% of patients with active EBV infection produce antibody to early antigen.

Past Infection

If antibodies to both the viral capsid antigen and EBNA are present, then past infection (from 4–6 months to years earlier) is indicated. Since 95% of adults have been infected with EBV, most adults will show antibodies to EBV from infection years earlier. High or elevated antibody levels may be present for years and are not diagnostic of recent infection.

Reactivation

In the presence of antibodies to EBNA, an elevation of antibodies to early antigen suggests reactivation. However, when EBV antibody to the early antigen test is present, this result does not automatically indicate that a patient's current medical condition is caused by EBV. A number of healthy people with no symptoms have antibodies to the EBV early antigen for years after their initial EBV infection. Many times reactivation occurs subclinically.

Chronic EBV Infection

Reliable laboratory evidence for continued active EBV infection is very seldom found in patients who have been ill for more than four months. When the illness lasts more than six months, it should be investigated to see if other causes of chronic illness or CFS are present.

Chapter 20

Fifth Disease (Parvovirus B19)

What's Fifth Disease?

Especially common in kids between the ages of five and fifteen, fifth disease typically produces a distinctive red rash on the face that makes the child appear to have a "slapped cheek." The rash then spreads to the trunk, arms, and legs. Fifth disease is actually just a viral illness that most kids recover from quickly and without complications.

Fifth disease (also called erythema infectiosum) is caused by parvovirus B19. A human virus, parvovirus B19 is not the same parvovirus that veterinarians may be concerned about in pets, especially dogs, and it cannot be passed from humans to animals or vice versa.

Studies show that although 40% to 60% of adults worldwide have laboratory evidence of a past parvovirus B19 infection, most of these adults can't remember having had symptoms of fifth disease. This leads medical experts to believe that most people with a B19 infection have either very mild symptoms or no symptoms at all.

Fifth disease occurs everywhere in the world. Outbreaks of parvovirus tend to happen in the late winter and early spring, but there may also be sporadic cases of the disease any time throughout the year.

"Fifth Disease," November 2007, reprinted with permission from www .kidshealth.org. Copyright © 2007 The Nemours Foundation. This information was provided by KidsHealth, one of the largest resources online for medically reviewed health information written for parents, kids, and teens. For more articles like this one, visit www.KidsHealth.org. or www.TeensHealth.org.

Signs and Symptoms

Fifth disease begins with a low-grade fever, headache, and mild cold-like symptoms (a stuffy or runny nose). These symptoms pass, and the illness seems to be gone until a rash appears a few days later. The bright red rash typically begins on the face. Several days later, the rash spreads and red blotches (usually lighter in color) extend down to the trunk, arms, and legs. The rash usually spares the palms of the hands and soles of the feet. As the centers of the blotches begin to clear, the rash takes on a lacy, net-like appearance. Kids younger than ten years old are most likely to get the rash.

Older kids and adults sometimes complain that the rash itches, but most children with a rash caused by fifth disease do not look sick and no longer have fever. It may take one to three weeks for the rash to completely clear, and during that time it may seem to worsen until it finally fades away entirely.

Certain stimuli (including sunlight, heat, exercise, and stress) may reactivate the rash until it completely fades. Other symptoms that sometimes occur with fifth disease include swollen glands, red eyes, sore throat, diarrhea, and rarely, rashes that look like blisters or bruises.

In some cases, especially in adults and older teens, an attack of fifth disease may be followed by joint swelling or pain, often in the hands, wrists, knees, or ankles.

Contagiousness

A person with parvovirus infection is most contagious before the rash appears—either during the incubation period (the time between infection and the onset of symptoms) or during the time when he or she has only mild respiratory symptoms. Because the rash of fifth disease is due to an immune reaction (a defense response launched by the body against foreign substances like viruses) that occurs after the infection has passed, a child is usually not contagious once the rash appears.

Parvovirus B19 spreads easily from person to person in fluids from the nose, mouth, and throat of someone with the infection, especially through large droplets from coughs and sneezes.

In households where a child has fifth disease, another family member who hasn't previously had parvovirus B19 has about a 50% chance of also getting the infection. Children with fifth disease may attend childcare or school, since they are no longer contagious. Once infected with parvovirus B19, a person develops immunity to it and won't usually become infected again.

Parvovirus B19 infection during pregnancy may cause problems for the fetus. Some fetuses may develop severe anemia if the mother is infected while pregnant—especially if the infection occurs during the first half of the pregnancy. In some cases, this anemia is so severe that the fetus doesn't survive. Fortunately, about half of all pregnant women are immune from having had a previous infection with parvovirus. Serious problems occur in less than 5% of women who become infected during pregnancy.

Prevention

There is no vaccine for fifth disease, and no real way to prevent spreading the virus. Isolating someone with a fifth disease rash won't prevent spread of the infection because the person usually isn't contagious by that time.

Practicing good hygiene, especially frequent hand washing, is always a good idea since it can help prevent the spread of many infections.

Incubation

The incubation period (the time between infection and the onset of symptoms) for fifth disease ranges from four to 28 days, with the average being 16 to 17 days.

Duration

The rash of fifth disease usually lasts one to three weeks. In a few cases in older kids and adults, joint swelling and pain because of fifth disease have lasted from a few months up to a few years.

Diagnosis

Doctors can usually diagnose fifth disease by the distinctive rash on the face and body. If a child or adult has no telltale rash but has been sick for a while, a doctor may perform blood tests to see if the illness could be caused by parvovirus B19.

Treatment

Fifth disease is caused by a virus, and it cannot be treated with antibiotics used to treat bacterial infections. Although antiviral medicines do exist, there are currently none available that will treat fifth disease. In most cases, this is such a mild illness that no medicine is necessary.

Usually, kids with fifth disease feel fairly well and need little home treatment other than rest. After the fever and mild cold symptoms have passed, there may be little to treat except any discomfort from the rash itself. If your child has itching from the rash of fifth disease, ask the doctor for advice about relieving discomfort. The doctor may also recommend acetaminophen for fever or joint pain.

Complications

The majority of kids with fifth disease recover with no complications. By the time the rash appears and while it's present, they usually feel well and are back to their normal activities.

However, some children with weakened immune systems (such as those with acquired immunodeficiency syndrome [AIDS] or leukemia) or with certain blood disorders (like sickle cell anemia or hemolytic anemia) may become significantly ill when infected with parvovirus B19. Parvovirus B19 can temporarily slow down or stop the body's production of the oxygen-carrying red blood cells (RBCs), causing anemia.

When a child is healthy, this slowdown of red blood cell production usually goes unnoticed because it doesn't affect overall health. But some kids who are already anemic can become sick if their RBC production is further affected by the virus. The RBC levels may drop dangerously low, affecting the supply of oxygen to the body's tissues.

When to Call the Doctor

Call the doctor if your child develops a rash, especially if the rash is widespread over the body or accompanied by other symptoms.

If you're pregnant and develop a rash or if you've been exposed to someone with fifth disease (or to anyone with an unusual rash), call your obstetrician.

Chapter 21

Genital Herpes

What is genital herpes?

Genital herpes is a sexually transmitted disease (STD) caused by the herpes simplex viruses type 1 (HSV-1) or type 2 (HSV-2). Most genital herpes is caused by HSV-2. Most individuals have no or only minimal signs or symptoms from HSV-1 or HSV-2 infection. When signs do occur, they typically appear as one or more blisters on or around the genitals or rectum. The blisters break, leaving tender ulcers (sores) that may take two to four weeks to heal the first time they occur. Typically, another outbreak can appear weeks or months after the first, but it almost always is less severe and shorter than the first outbreak. Although the infection can stay in the body indefinitely, the number of outbreaks tends to decrease over a period of years.

How common is genital herpes?

Results of a nationally representative study show that genital herpes infection is common in the United States. Nationwide, at least 45 million people ages 12 and older, or one out of five adolescents and adults, have had genital HSV infection. Over the past decade, the percent of Americans with genital herpes infection in the U.S. has decreased.

This chapter includes text from "STD Facts: Genital Herpes," Centers for Disease Control and Prevention (CDC) January 4, 2008; and text from "Shutting Down the Genital Herpes Virus," National Institute of Allergy and Infectious Diseases (NIAID), May 4, 2007.

Genital HSV-2 infection is more common in women (approximately one out of four women) than in men (almost one out of eight). This may be due to male-to-female transmission being more likely than female-to-male transmission.

How do people get genital herpes?

HSV-1 and HSV-2 can be found in and released from the sores that the viruses cause, but they also are released between outbreaks from skin that does not appear to have a sore. Generally, a person can only get HSV-2 infection during sexual contact with someone who has a genital HSV-2 infection. Transmission can occur from an infected partner who does not have a visible sore and may not know that he or she is infected.

HSV-1 can cause genital herpes, but it more commonly causes infections of the mouth and lips, so-called fever blisters. HSV-1 infection of the genitals can be caused by oral-genital or genital-genital contact with a person who has HSV-1 infection. Genital HSV-1 outbreaks recur less regularly than genital HSV-2 outbreaks.

What are the signs and symptoms of genital herpes?

Most people infected with HSV-2 are not aware of their infection. However, if signs and symptoms occur during the first outbreak, they can be quite pronounced. The first outbreak usually occurs within two weeks after the virus is transmitted, and the sores typically heal within two to four weeks. Other signs and symptoms during the primary episode may include a second crop of sores, and flu-like symptoms, including fever and swollen glands. However, most individuals with HSV-2 infection never have sores, or they have very mild signs that they do not even notice or that they mistake for insect bites or another skin condition.

People diagnosed with a first episode of genital herpes can expect to have several (typically four or five) outbreaks (symptomatic recurrences) within a year. Over time these recurrences usually decrease in frequency. It is possible that a person becomes aware of the first episode years after the infection is acquired.

What are the complications of genital herpes?

Genital herpes can cause recurrent painful genital sores in many adults, and herpes infection can be severe in people with suppressed immune systems. Regardless of severity of symptoms, genital herpes frequently causes psychological distress in people who know they are infected.

In addition, genital HSV can lead to potentially fatal infections in babies. It is important that women avoid contracting herpes during pregnancy because a newly acquired infection during late pregnancy poses a greater risk of transmission to the baby. If a woman has active genital herpes at delivery, a cesarean delivery is usually performed. Fortunately, infection of a baby from a woman with herpes infection is rare.

Herpes may play a role in the spread of human immunodeficiency virus (HIV), the virus that causes acquired immunodeficiency syndrome (AIDS). Herpes can make people more susceptible to HIV infection, and it can make HIV-infected individuals more infectious.

How is genital herpes diagnosed?

The signs and symptoms associated with HSV-2 can vary greatly. Health care providers can diagnose genital herpes by visual inspection if the outbreak is typical, and by taking a sample from the sore(s) and testing it in a laboratory. HSV infections can be diagnosed between outbreaks by the use of a blood test. Blood tests, which detect antibodies to HSV-1 or HSV-2 infection, can be helpful, although the results are not always clear-cut.

Is there a treatment for herpes?

There is no treatment that can cure herpes, but antiviral medications can shorten and prevent outbreaks during the period of time the person takes the medication. In addition, daily suppressive therapy for symptomatic herpes can reduce transmission to partners.

How can herpes be prevented?

The surest way to avoid transmission of sexually transmitted diseases, including genital herpes, is to abstain from sexual contact, or to be in a long-term mutually monogamous relationship with a partner who has been tested and is known to be uninfected.

Genital ulcer diseases can occur in both male and female genital areas that are covered or protected by a latex condom, as well as in areas that are not covered. Correct and consistent use of latex condoms can reduce the risk of genital herpes.

Persons with herpes should abstain from sexual activity with uninfected partners when lesions or other symptoms of herpes are present. It is important to know that even if a person does not have any symptoms he or she can still infect sex partners. Sex partners of infected persons should be advised that they may become infected and they should use condoms to reduce the risk. Sex partners can seek testing to determine if they are infected with HSV. A positive HSV-2 blood test most likely indicates a genital herpes infection.

Shutting Down the Genital Herpes Virus

Once acquired, herpes simplex virus (HSV) 2—a common, sexually transmitted infection that can cause painful, recurring sores around the genitals—never goes away. Although genital herpes symptoms can be controlled with antiviral drugs, preventing HSV-2 infection altogether is an important public health goal because HSV-2 infection increases a person's risk of acquiring HIV, the virus that causes AIDS.

NIAID grantee Judy Lieberman, MD, PhD, and her colleagues at Harvard Medical School in Boston made headway toward this goal by creating a fatty liquid that effectively silenced the expression of HSV-2 genes and protected mice from an otherwise lethal dose of the virus. Significantly, the liquid's power seemed long-lasting.

The liquid the Boston group is developing is one of a class of experimental substances called microbicides. Several dozen microbicides are being tested in labs, animal studies, and human clinical trials. Whether formulated as a gel, cream, or foam, microbicides would be applied to the vagina prior to intercourse, giving women a discreet way to protect themselves from sexually transmitted infections. An ideal microbicide would not only be safe, easy to use, and inexpensive, it would be effective even if applied many hours or days before intercourse.

RNA Interference

Since its discovery—first in plants and insects and later in higher animals—the naturally occurring viral defense process called ribonucleic acid (RNA) interference (RNAi) has generated great excitement throughout the scientific world. Researchers hope to harness the gene-silencing effects of RNAi with lab-created small interfering (si) RNAs that can target the genetic machinery of viruses while sparing host tissue.

Chapter 22

Gonorrhea

What is gonorrhea?

Gonorrhea is a sexually transmitted disease (STD). Gonorrhea is caused by *Neisseria gonorrhoeae,* a bacterium that can grow and multiply easily in the warm, moist areas of the reproductive tract, including the cervix (opening to the womb), uterus (womb), and fallopian tubes (egg canals) in women, and in the urethra (urine canal) in women and men. The bacterium can also grow in the mouth, throat, eyes, and anus.

How common is gonorrhea?

Gonorrhea is a very common infectious disease. The Centers for Disease Control and Prevention (CDC) estimates that more than 700,000 persons in the U.S. get new gonorrheal infections each year. Only about half of these infections are reported to CDC. In 2006, 358,366 cases of gonorrhea were reported to CDC. In the period from 1975 to 1997, the national gonorrhea rate declined, following the implementation of the national gonorrhea control program in the mid-1970s. After several years of stable gonorrhea rates, however, the national gonorrhea rate increased for the second consecutive year. In 2006, the rate of reported gonorrheal infections was 120.9 per 100,000 persons.

Excerpted from "CDC Fact Sheet: Gonorrhea," Centers for Disease Control and Prevention (CDC), reviewed February 28, 2008.

How do people get gonorrhea?

Gonorrhea is spread through contact with the penis, vagina, mouth, or anus. Ejaculation does not have to occur for gonorrhea to be transmitted or acquired. Gonorrhea can also be spread from mother to baby during delivery. People who have had gonorrhea and received treatment may get infected again if they have sexual contact with a person infected with gonorrhea.

Who is at risk for gonorrhea?

Any sexually active person can be infected with gonorrhea. In the United States, the highest reported rates of infection are among sexually active teenagers, young adults, and African Americans.

What are the signs and symptoms of gonorrhea?

Some men with gonorrhea may have no symptoms at all. However, some men have signs or symptoms that appear two to five days after infection; symptoms can take as long as 30 days to appear. Symptoms and signs include a burning sensation when urinating, or a white, yellow, or green discharge from the penis. Sometimes men with gonorrhea get painful or swollen testicles.

In women, the symptoms of gonorrhea are often mild, but most women who are infected have no symptoms. Even when a woman has symptoms, they can be so non-specific as to be mistaken for a bladder or vaginal infection. The initial symptoms and signs in women include a painful or burning sensation when urinating, increased vaginal discharge, or vaginal bleeding between periods. Women with gonorrhea are at risk of developing serious complications from the infection, regardless of the presence or severity of symptoms.

Symptoms of rectal infection in both men and women may include discharge, anal itching, soreness, bleeding, or painful bowel movements. Rectal infection also may cause no symptoms. Infections in the throat may cause a sore throat but usually causes no symptoms.

What are the complications of gonorrhea?

Untreated gonorrhea can cause serious and permanent health problems in both women and men.

In women, gonorrhea is a common cause of pelvic inflammatory disease (PID). About one million women each year in the United States develop PID. The symptoms may be quite mild or can be very severe and can include abdominal pain and fever. PID can lead to internal abscesses (pus-filled pockets that are hard to cure) and long-lasting, chronic pelvic pain. PID can damage the fallopian tubes enough to cause infertility or increase the risk of ectopic pregnancy. Ectopic pregnancy is a life-threatening condition in which a fertilized egg grows outside the uterus, usually in a fallopian tube.

In men, gonorrhea can cause epididymitis, a painful condition of the ducts attached to the testicles that may lead to infertility if left untreated.

Gonorrhea can spread to the blood or joints. This condition can be life threatening. In addition, people with gonorrhea can more easily contract human immunodeficiency virus (HIV), the virus that causes acquired immunodeficiency syndrome (AIDS). HIV-infected people with gonorrhea can transmit HIV more easily to someone else than if they did not have gonorrhea.

How does gonorrhea affect a pregnant woman and her baby?

If a pregnant woman has gonorrhea, she may give the infection to her baby as the baby passes through the birth canal during delivery. This can cause blindness, joint infection, or a life-threatening blood infection in the baby. Treatment of gonorrhea as soon as it is detected in pregnant women will reduce the risk of these complications. Pregnant women should consult a health care provider for appropriate examination, testing, and treatment, as necessary.

How is gonorrhea diagnosed?

Several laboratory tests are available to diagnose gonorrhea. A doctor or nurse can obtain a sample for testing from the parts of the body likely to be infected (cervix, urethra, rectum, or throat) and send the sample to a laboratory for analysis. Gonorrhea that is present in the cervix or urethra can be diagnosed in a laboratory by testing a urine sample. A quick laboratory test for gonorrhea that can be done in some clinics or doctor's offices is a Gram stain. A Gram stain of a sample from a urethra or a cervix allows the doctor to see the gonorrhea bacterium under a microscope. This test works better for men than for women.

What is the treatment for gonorrhea?

Several antibiotics can successfully cure gonorrhea in adolescents and adults. However, drug-resistant strains of gonorrhea are increasing in many areas of the world, including the United States, and successful treatment of gonorrhea is becoming more difficult. Because many people with gonorrhea also have chlamydia, another STD, antibiotics for both infections are usually given together. Persons with gonorrhea should be tested for other STDs.

It is important to take all of the medication prescribed to cure gonorrhea. Although medication will stop the infection, it will not repair any permanent damage done by the disease. People who have had gonorrhea and have been treated can get the disease again if they have sexual contact with persons infected with gonorrhea. If a person's symptoms continue even after receiving treatment, he or she should return to a doctor to be reevaluated.

How can gonorrhea be prevented?

The surest way to avoid transmission of STDs is to abstain from sexual intercourse, or to be in a long-term mutually monogamous relationship with a partner who has been tested and is known to be uninfected.

Latex condoms, when used consistently and correctly, can reduce the risk of transmission of gonorrhea.

Any genital symptoms such as discharge or burning during urination or unusual sore or rash should be a signal to stop having sex and to see a doctor immediately. If a person has been diagnosed and treated for gonorrhea, he or she should notify all recent sex partners so they can see a health care provider and be treated. This will reduce the risk that the sex partners will develop serious complications from gonorrhea and will also reduce the person's risk of becoming reinfected. The person and all of his or her sex partners must avoid sex until they have completed their treatment for gonorrhea.

Chapter 23

Hand, Foot, and Mouth Disease

Hand, foot, and mouth disease (HFMD) is a common viral illness of infants and children. The disease causes fever and blister-like eruptions in the mouth and/or a skin rash. HFMD is often confused with foot-and-mouth (also called hoof-and-mouth) disease, a disease of cattle, sheep, and swine; however, the two diseases are not related—they are caused by different viruses. Humans do not get the animal disease, and animals do not get the human disease.

Illness

* The disease usually begins with a fever, poor appetite, malaise (feeling vaguely unwell), and often with a sore throat.

* One or two days after fever onset, painful sores usually develop in the mouth. They begin as small red spots that blister and then often become ulcers. The sores are usually located on the tongue, gums, and inside of the cheeks.

* A non-itchy skin rash develops over 1–2 days. The rash has flat or raised red spots, sometimes with blisters. The rash is usually located on the palms of the hands and soles of the feet; it may also appear on the buttocks and/or genitalia.

This chapter includes text from "Hand, Foot, and Mouth Disease," Centers for Disease Control and Prevention (CDC), June 5, 2008; and excerpts from "Hand, Foot, and Mouth Disease: Q and A," CDC, June 5, 2008.

- A person with HFMD may have only the rash or only the mouth sores.

Cause

- HFMD is caused by viruses that belong to the enterovirus genus (group). This group of viruses includes polioviruses, coxsackieviruses, echoviruses, and enteroviruses.
- Coxsackievirus A16 is the most common cause of HFMD, but other coxsackieviruses have been associated with the illness.
- Enteroviruses, including enterovirus 71, have also been associated with HFMD and with outbreaks of the disease.

How HFMD Is Spread

- Infection is spread from person to person by direct contact with infectious virus. Infectious virus is found in the nose and throat secretions, saliva, blister fluid, and stool of infected persons. The virus is most often spread by persons with unwashed, virus-contaminated hands and by contact with virus-contaminated surfaces.
- Infected persons are most contagious during the first week of the illness.
- The viruses that cause HFMD can remain in the body for weeks after a patient's symptoms have gone away. This means that the infected person can still pass the infection to other people even though he/she appears well. Also, some persons who are infected and excreting the virus, including most adults, may have no symptoms.
- HFMD is not transmitted to or from pets or other animals.

Factors That Increase the Chance for Infection or Disease

- Everyone who has not already been infected with an enterovirus that causes HFMD is at risk of infection, but not everyone who is infected with an enterovirus becomes ill with HFMD.
- HFMD occurs mainly in children under ten years old but can also occur in adults. Children are more likely to be at risk for infection and illness because they are less likely than adults to have antibodies to protect them. Such antibodies develop in the

body during a person's first exposure to the enteroviruses that cause HFMD.

- Infection results in immunity to (protection against) the specific virus that caused HFMD. A second case of HFMD may occur following infection with a different member of the enterovirus group.

Diagnosis

- HFMD is one of many infections that result in mouth sores. However, health care providers can usually tell the difference between HFMD and other causes of mouth sores by considering the patient's age, the symptoms reported by the patient or parent, and the appearance of the rash and sores.

- Samples from the throat or stool may be sent to a laboratory to test for virus and to find out which enterovirus caused the illness. However, it can take 2–4 weeks to obtain test results, so health care providers usually do not order tests.

Treatment and Medical Management

- There is no specific treatment for HFMD.
- Symptoms can be treated to provide relief from pain from mouth sores and from fever and aches:
  - Fever can be treated with antipyretics (drugs that reduce fevers).
  - Pain can be treated with acetaminophen, ibuprofen, or other over-the-counter pain relievers.
  - Mouthwashes or sprays that numb pain can be used to lessen mouth pain.
- Fluid intake should be enough to prevent dehydration (lack of body fluids). If moderate-to-severe dehydration develops, it can be treated medically by giving fluids through the veins.

Prevention

- A specific preventive for HFMD is not available, but the risk of infection can be lowered by following good hygiene practices.
- Good hygiene practices that can lower the risk of infection include the following:

- Washing hands frequently and correctly and especially after changing diapers and after using the toilet

- Cleaning dirty surfaces and soiled items, including toys, first with soap and water and then disinfecting them by cleansing with a solution of chlorine bleach (made by adding one tablespoon of bleach to four cups of water)

- Avoiding close contact (kissing, hugging, sharing eating utensils or cups, etc.) with persons with HFMD

Vaccination Recommendations

- No vaccine is available to protect against the enteroviruses that cause HFMD.

Complications

- Complications from the virus infections that cause HFMD are not common, but if they do occur, medical care should be sought.

- Viral or aseptic meningitis can rarely occur with HFMD. Viral meningitis causes fever, headache, stiff neck, or back pain. The condition is usually mild and clears without treatment; however, some patients may need to be hospitalized for a short time.

- Other more serious diseases, such as encephalitis (swelling of the brain) or a polio-like paralysis, result even more rarely. Encephalitis can be fatal.

- There have been reports of fingernail and toenail loss occurring mostly in children within four weeks of their having hand, foot, and mouth disease (HFMD). At this time, it is not known whether the reported nail loss is or is not a result of the infection. However, in the reports reviewed, the nail loss has been temporary and nail growth resumed without medical treatment.

Trends and Statistics

- Individual cases and outbreaks of HFMD occur worldwide. In temperate climates, cases occur more often in summer and early autumn.

- Since 1997, outbreaks of HFMD caused by enterovirus 71 have been reported in Asia and Australia.

- HFMD caused by coxsackievirus A16 infection is a mild disease. Nearly all patients recover in 7 to 10 days without medical treatment.

- HFMD caused by enterovirus 71 has shown a higher incidence of neurologic (nervous system) involvement.

- Fatal cases of encephalitis (swelling of the brain) caused by enterovirus 71 have occurred during outbreaks.

Questions and Answers about Hand, Foot and Mouth Disease

Who is at risk for hand, foot, and mouth disease?

HFMD occurs mainly in children under 10 years old, but it can occur in adults too. Everyone is at risk of infection with viruses that cause HFMD, but not everyone who is infected becomes ill. Infants, children, and adolescents are more likely to be susceptible to infection and illness from these viruses because they are less likely than adults to be immune to them. Many adults have developed protective antibodies due to previous exposures to the viruses. Infection results in immunity to the specific virus, but a second episode of HFMD may occur following infection with a different member of the enterovirus group of viruses.

What are the risks to pregnant women exposed to children with hand, foot, and mouth disease?

Because enterovirus, including those that cause HFMD, are very common, pregnant women are frequently exposed to them, especially during summer and fall months. For all adults, including pregnant women, the risk of infection is higher among those who do not have antibodies from earlier exposures to these viruses and for those who are exposed to young children—the primary spreaders of enterovirus.

Most enterovirus infections during pregnancy cause mild or no illness in the mother. Although the available information is limited, currently there is no clear evidence that maternal enterovirus infection causes adverse outcomes of pregnancy, such as abortion, stillbirth, or congenital defects. However, mothers infected shortly before delivery may pass the virus to the newborn. Babies born to mothers who have symptoms of enteroviral illness around the time of delivery are more likely to be infected. Most newborns infected with an enterovirus have mild illness, but, in rare cases, they may develop an overwhelming infection of many organs, including liver and heart, and die from the infection. The risk of this severe illness in newborns is higher during the first two weeks of life.

Strict adherence to generally recommended good hygiene practices by pregnant women may help to decrease the risk of infection during pregnancy and around the time of delivery.

How should hand, foot, and mouth disease in the child care setting be handled?

In the United States, HFMD outbreaks in child care facilities occur most often in the summer and fall months and usually coincide with an increased number of cases in the community.

CDC has no specific recommendations regarding the exclusion of children with HFMD from child care programs, schools, or other group settings. Children are often excluded from group settings during the first few days of the illness, which may reduce the spread of infection, but will not completely interrupt it. Exclusion of ill persons may not prevent additional cases since the viruses that cause HFMD can remain in the body for weeks after the patient's symptoms have gone away. This means that the infected person can still pass the infection to other people even though they appear well. Also, some persons who are infected and excreting the virus, including most adults, may have no symptoms. Some benefit may be gained, however, by excluding children who have blisters in their mouths and drool or who have weeping lesions on their hands.

If an outbreak occurs in the child care setting follow these procedures:

- Make sure that all children and adults wash their hands frequently and thoroughly, especially after changing diapers or using the toilet.

- Thoroughly wash and disinfect contaminated items and surfaces, using a diluted solution of chlorine-containing bleach.

Chapter 24

Hansen Disease (Leprosy)

What Is Leprosy?

Leprosy (Hansen disease), is a chronic infectious disease that primarily affects the peripheral nerves, skin, upper respiratory tract, eyes, and nasal mucosa. The disease is caused by a bacillus (rod-shaped) bacterium known as *Mycobacterium leprae* (*M. leprae*).

The Bacterium: **Mycobacterium leprae**

M. leprae, discovered by G.A. Hansen in Norway in 1873, is a slow growing, intracellular pathogen, incapable of living outside its host. The organism has never been grown in a laboratory, making it more difficult to study than other bacteria; at this point it can only be grown in animals. Armadillos and immunocompromised mice are the only two sources for growing the bacteria for research purposes.

Another factor complicating studies of leprosy is that *M. leprae* multiplies slowly, with an average doubling time of 12–14 days, and only in a select group of animals. Armadillos and three species of monkeys—chimpanzees, sooty mangabeys, and cynomolgus macaques—are the only animals other than humans that have been found to become naturally infected with *M. leprae*. Symptoms can take as long as 20 years to appear.

"Leprosy," National Institute of Allergy and Infectious Diseases (NIAID), updated June 2, 2008.

The Disease

The mode of transmission of leprosy is still unclear and has been assumed to be via the respiratory system mainly through nasal droplets; broken skin also remains a possibility. The primary tissues that are affected by *M. leprae* are the superficial sites of the skin and peripheral nerves because the bacteria survive best at low temperatures.

Leprosy has been described by Ridley and Joplin as a continuous spectrum of disease. The course of human leprosy depends on the immunity of infected persons. Some people in a family may have the infection, but other close family members will not develop it, depending on their personal ability to fight off the bacteria.

Leprosy usually affects the skin, peripheral nerves, and upper airways but has a wide range of clinical manifestations. Clinical forms of leprosy represent a spectrum reflecting the cellular immune response to *M. leprae*. Patients with good T-cell immunity (Th1 type) exhibit tuberculoid (TT) leprosy which is also known as paucibacillary leprosy, a milder form of the disease, characterized by skin discoloration. Those with poor T-cell immunity typically exhibit lepromatous (LL) leprosy or multibacillary leprosy which is associated with symmetric skin lesions, nodules, plaques, thickened dermis, and frequent involvement of the nasal mucosa resulting in congestion and nose bleeds. In between these forms of leprosy are the borderline tuberculoid (BT), borderline-borderline (BB) and borderline lepromatous (BL) forms.

LL leprosy is also characterized by large numbers of organisms in the skin, many skin lesions with slight hypopigmentation, and less sensory loss in the lesions. While individuals with LL have high titer antibodies to *M. leprae*, they also have an impaired cellular immune response to the bacillus. Changes in immunity of the host as well as treatment can result in worsening of the clinical course of the disease.

All forms of leprosy may cause some degree of peripheral neurological damage (nerve damage in the arms and legs) which causes sensory loss in the skin as well as muscle weakness. People with long-term leprosy may lose the use of their hands or feet due to repeated traumatic injury resulting from lack of sensation. If left untreated, it can cause progressive and permanent damage to the skin, nerves, eyes, and limbs.

Diagnosis and Treatment

In the United States, most physicians do not have experience identifying leprosy because it is extremely rare (about 100–200 new cases per year, mostly occurring in the Gulf Coast, Hawaii, Massachusetts, and New York and among individuals who have lived in areas of the world where the disease is more widespread). It is important that people who have unusual rashes that do not respond to treatment seek out skilled dermatologists who can make an accurate diagnosis.

Diagnosis of leprosy is typically based on clinical symptoms, especially localized skin lesions that show sensory loss (loss of sensation to stimuli such as touch and heat). Thickened, enlarged peripheral nerves are also a hallmark of the disease. Skin and blood samples can also be tested in order to reach a conclusive diagnosis.

With early diagnosis, leprosy can be treated. People who are getting treatment for leprosy are not contagious, and they can lead a normal lifestyle.

In 1981, the World Health Organization (WHO) recommended multidrug therapy (MDT) with dapsone, rifampicin, and clofazimine. The regimen for multibacillary is monthly for a period of one year and for paucibacillary it is monthly doses of rifampicin and daily doses of dapsone for a period of six months. Although several groups are now advocating uniform treatment for all forms of leprosy; this is being debated in the scientific community.

Leprosy Today

At the beginning of 2007, the registered prevalence of leprosy in the world was 224,717 cases, while the number of new cases detected during 2006 was 259,017, as reported by 109 countries (World Health Organization). The global number of new cases detected during the past five years has decreased at an average rate of nearly 20 percent per year largely due to the success of early diagnosis and treatment with MDT.

Since the 1980s, when the World Health Organization (WHO) initiated its Leprosy Elimination Project, more than 14 million cases have been cured. However, the number of new cases being detected annually is raising the unanswered questions about the source of infection, transmission, and incubation period of leprosy. In other words, what is the basis of this steady stream of new cases detected in the midst of such a dramatic drop in the numbers of people living with the disease? This may be attributed to a number of factors including intensified efforts in case detection, and/or high transmission of the disease in certain areas.

Today, leprosy is found mainly in Angola, Brazil, Central African Republic, Democratic Republic of Congo, India, Madagascar, Mozambique,

Nepal, and the United Republic of Tanzania. These countries account for a remarkable 75 percent of the global leprosy burden and they are taking steps to control the disease through information campaigns and by providing diagnostic and treatment services to all communities, including the poor and underserved, and by incorporating leprosy diagnosis and treatment into general health services.

Chapter 25

Hepatitis:
A through E and Beyond

Viral hepatitis is inflammation of the liver caused by a virus. Several different viruses, named the hepatitis A, B, C, D, and E viruses, cause viral hepatitis. All of these viruses cause acute, or short-term, viral hepatitis. The hepatitis B, C, and D viruses can also cause chronic hepatitis, in which the infection is prolonged, sometimes lifelong. Chronic hepatitis can lead to cirrhosis, liver failure, and liver cancer.

Researchers are looking for other viruses that may cause hepatitis, but none have been identified with certainty. Other viruses that less often affect the liver include cytomegalovirus; Epstein-Barr virus, also called infectious mononucleosis; herpes virus; parvovirus; and adenovirus.

What are the symptoms of viral hepatitis?

Symptoms include the following:

- jaundice, which causes a yellowing of the skin and eyes

- fatigue

- abdominal pain

- loss of appetite

Text in this chapter is from "Viral Hepatitis: A through E and Beyond," National Institute of Diabetes and Digestive and Kidney Diseases (NIDDK), February 2008.

- nausea

- vomiting

- diarrhea

- low grade fever

- headache

However, some people do not have symptoms.

Hepatitis A

Hepatitis A is spread primarily through food or water contaminated by feces from an infected person. Rarely, it spreads through contact with infected blood.

People most likely to get hepatitis A are:

- international travelers, particularly those traveling to developing countries;

- people who live with or have sex with an infected person;

- people living in areas where children are not routinely vaccinated against hepatitis A, where outbreaks are more likely;

- daycare children and employees, during outbreaks;

- men who have sex with men; and

- users of illicit drugs.

How can hepatitis A be prevented?

The hepatitis A vaccine offers immunity to adults and children older than one year. The Centers for Disease Control and Prevention (CDC) recommends routine hepatitis A vaccination for children aged 12 to 23 months and for adults who are at high risk for infection. Treatment with immune globulin can provide short-term immunity to hepatitis A when given before exposure or within two weeks of exposure to the virus. Avoiding tap water when traveling internationally and practicing good hygiene and sanitation also help prevent hepatitis A.

What is the treatment for hepatitis A?

Hepatitis A usually resolves on its own over several weeks.

Hepatitis B

Hepatitis B is spread through contact with infected blood, through sex with an infected person, and from mother to child during childbirth, whether the delivery is vaginal or via cesarean section.

People most likely to get hepatitis B are:

- people who live with or have sexual contact with an infected person;
- men who have sex with men;
- people who have multiple sex partners;
- injection drug users;
- immigrants and children of immigrants from areas with high rates of hepatitis B;
- infants born to infected mothers;
- health care workers;
- hemodialysis patients;
- people who received a transfusion of blood or blood products before 1987, when better tests to screen blood donors were developed; and
- international travelers.

How can hepatitis B be prevented?

The hepatitis B vaccine offers the best protection. All infants and unvaccinated children, adolescents, and at-risk adults should be vaccinated. For people who have not been vaccinated, reducing exposure to the virus can help prevent hepatitis B. Reducing exposure means using latex condoms, which may lower the risk of transmission; not sharing drug needles; and not sharing personal items such as toothbrushes, razors, and nail clippers with an infected person.

What is the treatment for hepatitis B?

Drugs approved for the treatment of chronic hepatitis B include alpha interferon and peginterferon, which slow the replication of the virus in the body and also boost the immune system, and the antiviral drugs lamivudine, adefovir dipivoxil, entecavir, and telbivudine. Other drugs are also being evaluated. Infants born to infected mothers should receive hepatitis B immune globulin and the hepatitis B vaccine within 12 hours of birth to help prevent infection.

People who develop acute hepatitis B are generally not treated with antiviral drugs because, depending on their age at infection, the disease often resolves on its own. Infected newborns are most likely to progress to chronic hepatitis B, but by young adulthood, most people with acute infection recover spontaneously. Severe acute hepatitis B can be treated with an antiviral drug such as lamivudine.

Hepatitis C

Hepatitis C is spread primarily through contact with infected blood. Less commonly, it can spread through sexual contact and childbirth.

People most likely to be exposed to the hepatitis C virus are:

- injection drug users;
- people who have sex with an infected person;
- people who have multiple sex partners;
- health care workers;
- infants born to infected women;
- hemodialysis patients;
- people who received a transfusion of blood or blood products before July 1992, when sensitive tests to screen blood donors for hepatitis C were introduced; and
- people who received clotting factors made before 1987, when methods to manufacture these products were improved.

How can hepatitis C be prevented?

There is no vaccine for hepatitis C. The only way to prevent the disease is to reduce the risk of exposure to the virus. Reducing exposure means avoiding behaviors like sharing drug needles or personal items such as toothbrushes, razors, and nail clippers with an infected person.

What is the treatment for hepatitis C?

Chronic hepatitis C is treated with peginterferon together with the antiviral drug ribavirin. If acute hepatitis C does not resolve on its own within two to three months, drug treatment is recommended.

Hepatitis D

Hepatitis D is spread through contact with infected blood. This disease only occurs at the same time as infection with hepatitis B or in people who are already infected with hepatitis B.

Anyone infected with hepatitis B is at risk for hepatitis D. Injection drug users have the highest risk. Others at risk include people who live with or have sex with a person infected with hepatitis D and people who received a transfusion of blood or blood products before 1987.

How can hepatitis D be prevented?

People not already infected with hepatitis B should receive the hepatitis B vaccine. Other preventive measures include avoiding exposure to infected blood, contaminated needles, and an infected person's personal items such as toothbrushes, razors, and nail clippers.

What is the treatment for hepatitis D?

Chronic hepatitis D is usually treated with pegylated interferon, although other potential treatments are under study.

Hepatitis E

Hepatitis E is spread through food or water contaminated by feces from an infected person. This disease is uncommon in the United States.

People most likely to be exposed to the hepatitis E virus are:

- international travelers, particularly those traveling to developing countries;
- people living in areas where hepatitis E outbreaks are common; and
- people who live with or have sex with an infected person.

How can hepatitis E be prevented?

There is no U.S. Food and Drug Administration (FDA)-approved vaccine for hepatitis E. The only way to prevent the disease is to reduce the risk of exposure to the virus. Reducing risk of exposure means avoiding tap water when traveling internationally and practicing good hygiene and sanitation.

What is the treatment for hepatitis E?

Hepatitis E usually resolves on its own over several weeks to months.

Points to Remember

- Viral hepatitis is inflammation of the liver caused by the hepatitis A, B, C, D, or E viruses.

- Depending on the type of virus, viral hepatitis is spread through contaminated food or water, contact with infected blood, sexual contact with an infected person, or from mother to child during childbirth.

- Vaccines offer protection from hepatitis A and hepatitis B.

- No vaccines are available for hepatitis C, D, and E. Reducing exposure to the viruses offers the best protection.

- Hepatitis A and E usually resolve on their own. Hepatitis B, C, and D can be chronic and serious. Drugs are available to treat chronic hepatitis.

What else causes viral hepatitis?

Some cases of viral hepatitis cannot be attributed to the hepatitis A, B, C, D, or E viruses, or even the less common viruses that can infect the liver, such as cytomegalovirus, Epstein-Barr virus, herpes virus, parvovirus, and adenovirus. These cases are called non-A–E hepatitis. Scientists continue to study the causes of non-A–E hepatitis.

Chapter 26

Human Immunodeficiency Virus (HIV) and Acquired Immunodeficiency Syndrome (AIDS)

HIV and AIDS: Are You at Risk?

Human immunodeficiency virus (HIV): A virus that kills your body's CD4 cells. CD4 cells (also called T-helper cells) help your body fight off infection and disease. HIV can be passed from person to person.

Acquired immunodeficiency syndrome (AIDS): A disease you get when HIV destroys your body's immune system. Normally, your immune system helps you fight off illness. When your immune system fails you can become very sick and can die.

Transmission of HIV

Anyone can get HIV. You can get HIV:

- by having unprotected sex—sex without a condom—with someone who has HIV. The virus can be in an infected person's blood, semen, or vaginal secretions and can enter your body through tiny cuts or sores in your skin, or in the lining of your vagina, penis, rectum, or mouth;

This chapter includes text from "HIV and AIDS: Are You at Risk?" Centers for Disease Control and Prevention (CDC), August 2007; and excerpts from "HIV and AIDS in the United States: CDC HIV/AIDS Facts," CDC, August 2008.

- by sharing a needle and syringe to inject drugs or sharing drug equipment used to prepare drugs for injection with someone who has HIV;

- from a blood transfusion or blood clotting factor that you got before 1985. (All blood in the United States has been tested for HIV since 1985.)

Babies born to women with HIV also can become infected during pregnancy, birth, or breast feeding.
   You cannot get HIV:

- by working with or being around someone who has HIV;

- from sweat, spit, tears, clothes, drinking fountains, phones, toilet seats, or through everyday things like sharing a meal;

- from insect bites or stings;

- from donating blood; or

- from a closed-mouth kiss (but there is a very small chance of getting it from open-mouthed or French kissing with an infected person because of possible blood contact).

How can I protect myself?

- Don't share needles and syringes used to inject drugs, steroids, vitamins, or for tattooing or body piercing. Also, do not share equipment (works) used to prepare drugs to be injected. Many people have been infected with HIV, hepatitis, and other germs this way. Germs from an infected person can stay in a needle and then be injected directly into the next person who uses the needle.

- The surest way to avoid transmission of sexually transmitted diseases (STDs) is to abstain from sexual intercourse, or to be in a long-term mutually monogamous relationship with a partner who has been tested and you know is uninfected.

- For persons whose sexual behaviors place them at risk for STDs, correct and consistent use of the male latex condom can reduce the risk of STD transmission. However, no protective method is 100 percent effective, and condom use cannot guarantee absolute protection against any STD. The more sex partners you have, the greater your chances are of getting HIV or other diseases passed through sex.

- Condoms used with a lubricant are less likely to break. However, condoms with the spermicide nonoxynol-9 are not recommended for STD/HIV prevention. Condoms must be used correctly and consistently to be effective and protective.

- Don't share razors or toothbrushes because of they may have the blood of another person on them.

- If you are pregnant or think you might be soon, talk to a doctor or your local health department about being tested for HIV. If you share HIV, drug treatments are available to help you and they can reduce the chance of passing HIV to your baby.

How do I know if I have HIV or AIDS?

You might have HIV and still feel perfectly healthy. The only way to know for sure if you are infected or not is to be tested. Talk with a knowledgeable health care provider or counselor both before and after you are tested. You can go to your doctor or health department for testing. To find out where to go in your area for HIV counseling and testing, call your local health department or the Centers for Disease Control and Prevention (CDC) at 800-CDC-INFO (232-4636).

Your doctor or health care provider can give you a confidential HIV test. The information on your HIV test and test results are confidential, as is your other medical information. This means it can be shared only with people authorized to see your medical records.

CDC recommends that everyone know their HIV status. How often you should an HIV test depends on your circumstances. If you have never been tested for HIV, you should be tested. CDC recommends being tested at least once a year if you do things that can transmit HIV infection.

In many states, you can be tested anonymously. These tests are usually given at special places known as anonymous testing sites. When you get an anonymous HIV test, the testing site records only a number or code with the test result, not your name. A counselor gives you this number at the time your blood, saliva, or urine is taken for the test, then you return to the testing site (or perhaps call the testing site, for example with home collection kits) and give them your number or code to learn the results of your test.

If you have been tested for HIV and the result is negative and you never do things that might transmit HIV infection, then you and your health care provider can decide whether you need to get tested again.

What can I do if the test shows I have HIV?

Although HIV is a very serious infection, many people with HIV and AIDS are living longer, healthier lives today, thanks to new and effective treatments. It is very important to make sure you have a doctor who knows how to treat HIV. If you don't know which doctor to use, talk with a health care professional or trained HIV counselor. If you are pregnant or are planning to become pregnant, this is especially important.

There also are other things you can do for yourself to stay healthy:

- Follow your doctor's instructions. Keep your appointments. Your doctor may prescribe medicine for you. Take the medicine just the way he or she tells you to because taking only some of your medicine gives your HIV infection more chance to grow.

- Get immunizations (shots) to prevent infections such as pneumonia and flu. Your doctor will tell you when to get these shots.

- If you smoke or if you use drugs not prescribed by your doctor, quit.

- Eat healthy foods. This will help keep you strong, keep your energy and weight up, and help your body protect itself.

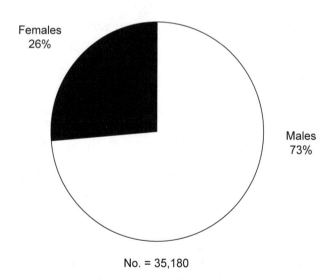

No. = 35,180

Based on data from 33 states with long-term, confidential name-based HIV reporting.

Figure 26.1. *Sex of adults and adolescents with HIV/AIDS diagnosed during 2006 (Based on data from 33 states with long-term, confidential name-based HIV reporting.)*

• Exercise regularly to stay strong and fit.

• Get enough sleep and rest.

HIV/AIDS in the United States

By Sex

In 2006, almost three quarters of HIV/AIDS diagnoses among adolescents and adults were for males.

By Transmission Category

In 2006, the largest estimated proportion of HIV/AIDS diagnoses among adults and adolescents were for men who have sex with men (MSM), followed by persons infected through high-risk heterosexual contact.

Trends in AIDS Diagnoses and Deaths

During the mid-to-late 1990s, advances in HIV treatments slowed the progression of HIV infection to AIDS and led to dramatic decreases in deaths among persons with AIDS living in the 50 states and the District of Columbia. In general, the trend in the estimated numbers of AIDS cases and deaths remained stable from 2002 through 2005. Estimates for 2006 suggest that the number of AIDS cases remained stable and that the number of deaths decreased; however, it is too early to determine whether this trend will hold. Better treatments have also led to an increase in the number of persons who are living with AIDS.

Table 26.1. Estimated numbers of AIDS diagnoses, deaths, and persons living with AIDS, 2002–2006

	2002	2003	2004	2005	2006	Cumulative (1981–2006)
AIDS diagnoses	38,132	38,538	37,726	36,552	36,828	982,498
Deaths of persons with AIDS	16,948	16,690	16,395	16,268	14,016	545,805
Persons living with AIDS	350,419	372,267	393,598	413,882	436,693	NA*

*NA, not applicable (the values given for each year are cumulative).

Based on data for the 50 states and the District of Columbia.

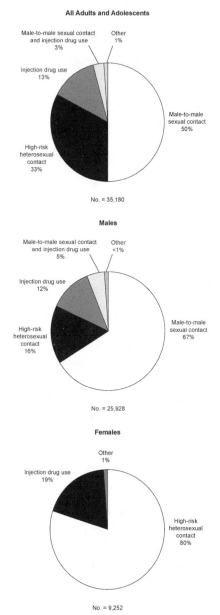

All Adults and Adolescents

Male-to-male sexual contact
and injection drug use
3%

Other
1%

Injection drug use
13%

Male-to-male
sexual contact
50%

High-risk
heterosexual
contact
33%

No. = 35,180

Males

Male-to-male sexual contact
and injection drug use
5%

Other
<1%

Injection drug use
12%

High-risk
heterosexual
contact
16%

Male-to-male
sexual contact
67%

No. = 25,928

Females

Other
1%

Injection drug use
19%

High-risk
heterosexual
contact
80%

No. = 9,252

Based on data from 33 states with long-term, confidential name-based HIV reporting.

Figure 26.2. *All Adults and Adolescents with HIV/AIDS Diagnosed during 2006 (Based on data from 33 states with long-term, confidential name-based HIV reporting.)*

Chapter 27

Human Papillomavirus (HPV)

What is genital HPV infection?

Genital human papillomavirus (HPV) is the most common sexually transmitted infection (STI). The virus infects the skin and mucous membranes. There are more than 40 HPV types that can infect the genital areas of men and women, including the skin of the penis, vulva (area outside the vagina), and anus, and the linings of the vagina, cervix, and rectum. You cannot see HPV. Most people who become infected with HPV do not even know they have it.

What are the symptoms and potential health consequences of HPV?

Most people with HPV do not develop symptoms or health problems. But sometimes, certain types of HPV can cause genital warts in men and women. Other HPV types can cause cervical cancer and other less common cancers, such as cancers of the vulva, vagina, anus, and penis. The types of HPV that can cause genital warts are not the same as the types that can cause cancer.

HPV types are often referred to as low-risk (wart-causing) or high-risk (cancer-causing), based on whether they put a person at risk for cancer. In 90% of cases, the body's immune system clears the HPV infection naturally within two years. This is true of both high-risk and low-risk types.

Text in this chapter is from "STD Facts: Human Papillomavirus (HPV)," Centers for Disease Control and Prevention (CDC), April 10, 2008.

Genital warts usually appear as small bumps or groups of bumps, usually in the genital area. They can be raised or flat, single or multiple, small or large, and sometimes cauliflower shaped. They can appear on the vulva, in or around the vagina or anus, on the cervix, and on the penis, scrotum, groin, or thigh. Warts may appear within weeks or months after sexual contact with an infected person. Or, they may not appear at all. If left untreated, genital warts may go away, remain unchanged, or increase in size or number. They will not turn into cancer.

Cervical cancer does not have symptoms until it is quite advanced. For this reason, it is important for women to get screened regularly for cervical cancer.

Other less common HPV-related cancers, such as cancers of the vulva, vagina, anus, and penis, also may not have signs or symptoms until they are advanced.

How do people get genital HPV infections?

Genital HPV is passed on through genital contact, most often during vaginal and anal sex. A person can have HPV even if years have passed since he or she had sex. Most infected persons do not realize they are infected or that they are passing the virus to a sex partner.

Very rarely, a pregnant woman with genital HPV can pass HPV to her baby during vaginal delivery. In these cases, the child may develop warts in the throat or voice box—a condition called recurrent respiratory papillomatosis (RRP).

How does HPV cause genital warts and cancer?

HPV can cause normal cells on infected skin or mucous membranes to turn abnormal. Most of the time, you cannot see or feel these cell changes. In most cases, the body fights off HPV naturally and the infected cells then go back to normal.

- Sometimes, low-risk types of HPV can cause visible changes that take the form of genital warts.

- If a high-risk HPV infection is not cleared by the immune system, it can linger for many years and turn abnormal cells into cancer over time. About 10% of women with high-risk HPV on their cervix will develop long-lasting HPV infections that put them at risk for cervical cancer. Similarly, when high-risk HPV lingers and infects the cells of the penis, anus, vulva, or vagina, it can cause cancer in those areas. But these cancers are much less common than cervical cancer.

How common are HPV and related diseases?

HPV infection: Approximately 20 million Americans are currently infected with HPV, and another 6.2 million people become newly infected each year. At least 50% of sexually active men and women acquire genital HPV infection at some point in their lives.

Genital warts: About 1% of sexually active adults in the U.S. have genital warts at any one time.

Cervical cancer: The American Cancer Society estimates that in 2008, 11,070 women would be diagnosed with cervical cancer in the U.S.

Other HPV-related cancers are much less common than cervical cancer. The American Cancer Society estimated that in 2008, there would be:

- 3,460 women diagnosed with vulvar cancer;
- 2,210 women diagnosed with vaginal and other female genital cancers;
- 1,250 men diagnosed with penile and other male genital cancers; and
- 3,050 women and 2,020 men diagnosed with anal cancer.

Certain populations may be at higher risk for HPV-related cancers, such as gay and bisexual men, and individuals with weak immune systems (including those who have HIV/AIDS). Recurrent respiratory papillomatosis (RRP) is very rare. It is estimated that less than 2,000 children get RRP every year.

How can people prevent HPV?

A vaccine can now protect females from the four types of HPV that cause most cervical cancers and genital warts. The vaccine is recommended for 11 and 12 year-old girls. It is also recommended for girls and women age 13 through 26 who have not yet been vaccinated or completed the vaccine series.

For those who choose to be sexually active, condoms may lower the risk of HPV, if used all the time and the right way. Condoms may also lower the risk of developing HPV-related diseases, such as genital warts and cervical cancer. But HPV can infect areas that are not covered by a condom—so condoms may not fully protect against HPV. So, the only sure way to prevent HPV is to avoid all sexual activity.

Individuals can also lower their chances of getting HPV by being in a mutually faithful relationship with someone who has had no or few sex partners. However, even people with only one lifetime sex partner can get HPV, if their partner was infected with HPV. For those who are not in long-term mutually monogamous relationships, limiting the number of sex partners and choosing a partner less likely to be infected may lower the risk of HPV. Partners less likely to be infected include those who have had no or few prior sex partners. But it may not be possible to determine if a partner who has been sexually active in the past is currently infected.

How can people prevent HPV-related diseases?

There are important steps girls and women can take to prevent cervical cancer. The HPV vaccine can protect against most cervical cancers. Cervical cancer can also be prevented with routine cervical cancer screening and follow-up of abnormal results. The Pap test can identify abnormal or pre-cancerous changes in the cervix so that they can be removed before cancer develops. An HPV deoxyribonucleic acid (DNA) test, which can find high-risk HPV on a woman's cervix, may also be used with a Pap test in certain cases. The HPV test can help health care professionals decide if more tests or treatment are needed. Even women who got the vaccine when they were younger need regular cervical cancer screening because the vaccine does not protect against all cervical cancers.

There is currently no vaccine licensed to prevent HPV-related diseases in men. Studies are now being done to find out if the vaccine is also safe in men, and if it can protect them against HPV and related conditions. There is also no approved screening test to find early signs of penile or anal cancer. Some experts recommend yearly anal Pap tests for gay and bisexual men and for HIV-positive persons because anal cancer is more common in these populations. Scientists are still studying how best to screen for penile and anal cancers in those who may be at highest risk for those diseases.

Generally, cesarean delivery is not recommended for women with genital warts to prevent RRP in their babies. This is because it is unclear whether cesarean delivery actually prevents RRP in infants and children.

Is there a test for HPV?

The HPV test on the market is only used as part of cervical cancer screening. There is no general test for men or women to check one's overall HPV status. HPV usually goes away on its own, without causing health problems. So an HPV infection that is found today will most likely not be there a year or two from now. For this reason, there is no need to be tested just to find out if you have HPV now. However, you should get tested for signs of disease that HPV can cause, such as cervical cancer.

- Genital warts are diagnosed by visual inspection. Some health care providers may use acetic acid, a vinegar solution, to help identify flat warts. But this is not a sensitive test so it may wrongly identify normal skin as a wart.

- Cervical cell changes (early signs of cervical cancer) can be identified by routine Pap tests. The HPV test can identify high-risk HPV types on a woman's cervix, which can cause cervical cell changes and cancer.

Is there a treatment for HPV?

There is no treatment for the virus itself, but a healthy immune system can usually fight off HPV naturally. There are treatments for the diseases that HPV can cause:

Visible genital warts can be removed by patient-applied medications, or by treatments performed by a health care provider. Some individuals choose to forego treatment to see if the warts will disappear on their own. No one treatment is better than another.

Cervical cancer is most treatable when it is diagnosed and treated early. There are new forms of surgery, radiation therapy, and chemotherapy available for patients. But women who get routine Pap testing and follow up as needed can identify problems before cancer develops. Prevention is always better than treatment.

Other HPV-related cancers are also more treatable when diagnosed and treated early. There are new forms of surgery, radiation therapy, and chemotherapy available for patients.

For More Information

American Cancer Society (ACS)
13599 Clifton Rd., NE
Atlanta, GA 30329
Toll-Free 24 Hr. Hotline: 800-ACS (227)-2345
Toll-Free TTY: 866-228-4327
Website: http://www.cancer.org

CDC National Prevention Information Network (NPIN)
P.O. Box 6003
Rockville, MD 20849
Toll-Free: 800-458-5231
Phone: 404-679-3860
Toll-Free Fax: 888-282-7681
Toll-Free TTY: 800-243-7012
Website: http://www.cdcnpin.org
E-mail: info@cdcnpin.org

National HPV and Cervical Cancer Prevention Resource Center
American Social Health Association
P.O. Box 13827
Research Triangle Park, NC 27709
Toll-Free Hotline: 800-227-8922
Phone: 919-361-8400
Fax: 919-361-8425
Website: http://www.ashastd.org/hpv/hpv_overview.cfm

Chapter 28

Impetigo

Impetigo, a contagious skin infection that usually produces blisters or sores on the face, neck, hands, and diaper area, is one of the most common skin infections among kids.

It is generally caused by one of two bacteria: *Staphylococcus aureus* or group A *Streptococcus*. Impetigo usually affects preschool and school-age children. A child may be more likely to develop impetigo if the skin has already been irritated by other skin problems, such as eczema, poison ivy, and insect bites.

Good hygiene can help prevent impetigo, which often develops when there is a sore or a rash that has been scratched repetitively (for example, poison ivy can get infected and turn into impetigo). Impetigo is typically treated with either an antibiotic cream or medication taken by mouth.

Signs and Symptoms

Impetigo may affect skin anywhere on the body but commonly occurs around the nose and mouth, hands, and forearms, and diaper area in young children.

There are two types of impetigo: bullous impetigo (large blisters) and non-bullous impetigo (crusted) impetigo. The non-bullous or crusted

"Impetigo," November 2008, reprinted with permission from www.kidshealth .org. Copyright © 2008 The Nemours Foundation. This information was provided by KidsHealth, one of the largest resources online for medically reviewed health information written for parents, kids, and teens. For more articles like this one, visit www.KidsHelath.org, or www.TeensHealth.org.

form is most common. This is usually caused by *Staphylococcus aureus* but can also be caused by infection with group A *Streptococcus*. Nonbullous begins as tiny blisters. These blisters eventually burst and leave small wet patches of red skin that may weep fluid. Gradually, a tan or yellowish-brown crust covers the affected area, making it look like it has been coated with honey or brown sugar.

Bullous impetigo is nearly always caused by *Staphylococcus aureus*, which triggers larger fluid-containing blisters that appear clear, then cloudy. These blisters are more likely to stay intact longer on the skin without bursting.

Contagiousness

Impetigo may itch and kids can spread the infection by scratching it and then touching other parts of the body.

Impetigo is contagious and can spread to anyone who comes into contact with infected skin or other items, such as clothing, towels, and bed linens, that have been touched by infected skin.

Treatment

When it just affects a small area of the skin, impetigo can usually be treated with antibiotic ointment. But if the infection has spread to other areas of the body, or the ointment isn't working, the doctor may prescribe an antibiotic pill or liquid.

Once antibiotic treatment begins, healing should start within a few days. It's important to make sure that your child takes the medication as the doctor has prescribed. If that doesn't happen, a deeper and more serious skin infection could develop.

While the infection is healing, gently wash the areas of infected skin with clean gauze and antiseptic soap every day. Soak any areas of crusted skin in warm soapy water to help remove the layers of crust (it is not necessary to completely remove all of it).

To keep your child from spreading impetigo to other parts of the body, the doctor or nurse will probably recommend covering infected areas of skin with gauze and tape or a loose plastic bandage. Keep your child's fingernails short and clean.

Prevention

Good hygiene practices, such as regular hand washing, can help prevent impetigo. Have kids use soap and water to clean their skin and be sure they take baths or showers regularly. Pay special attention to areas of the skin that have been injured, such as cuts, scrapes, bug bites, areas of eczema, and rashes such as poison ivy. Keep these areas clean and covered.

Anyone in your family with impetigo should keep fingernails cut short and the impetigo sores covered with gauze and tape.

Prevent impetigo infection from spreading among family members by using antibacterial soap and making sure that each family member uses a separate towel. If necessary, substitute paper towels for cloth ones until the impetigo is gone. Separate the infected person's bed linens, towels, and clothing from those of other family members, and wash these items in hot water.

When to Call the Doctor

Call the doctor if your child has signs of impetigo, especially if he or she has been exposed to a family member or classmate with the infection. If your child is already being treated for impetigo, keep an eye on the sores and call the doctor if the skin doesn't begin to heal after three days of treatment or if a fever develops. If the area around the rash becomes red, warm, or tender to the touch, notify the doctor as soon as possible.

Chapter 29

Influenza

Chapter Contents

Section 29.1

Seasonal Flu

This section includes "Key Facts about Seasonal Influenza (Flu),"
Centers for Disease Control and Prevention (CDC), March 12, 2009;
and "Types of Influenza Viruses," CDC, December 20, 2007.

Key Facts about Seasonal Influenza

What is influenza (also called flu)?

The flu is a contagious respiratory illness caused by influenza viruses. It can cause mild to severe illness, and at times can lead to death. The best way to prevent the flu is by getting a flu vaccination each year.

Every year in the United States, on average:

- 5% to 20% of the population gets the flu;
- more than 200,000 people are hospitalized from flu-related complications; and
- about 36,000 people die from flu-related causes.

Some people, such as older people, young children, and people with certain health conditions (such as asthma, diabetes, or heart disease), are at high risk for serious flu complications.

Symptoms of Flu

Symptoms of flu include the following:

- fever (usually high)
- headache
- extreme tiredness
- dry cough
- sore throat
- runny or stuffy nose
- muscle aches

Stomach symptoms, such as nausea, vomiting, and diarrhea, also can occur but are more common in children than adults.

Complications of Flu

Complications of flu can include bacterial pneumonia, ear infections, sinus infections, dehydration, and worsening of chronic medical conditions, such as congestive heart failure, asthma, or diabetes.

How Flu Spreads

Flu viruses are thought to spread mainly from person to person through coughing or sneezing of people with influenza. Sometimes people may become infected by touching something with flu viruses on it and then touching their mouth or nose. Most healthy adults may be able to infect others beginning one day before symptoms develop and up to five days after becoming sick. That means that you may be able to pass on the flu to someone else before you know you are sick, as well as while you are sick.

Preventing Seasonal Flu: Get Vaccinated

The single best way to prevent the flu is to get a flu vaccination each year. There are two types of vaccines:

- The flu shot—an inactivated vaccine (containing killed virus) that is given with a needle. The flu shot is approved for use in people six months of age and older, including healthy people and people with chronic medical conditions.

- The nasal-spray flu vaccine—a vaccine made with live, weakened flu viruses that do not cause the flu (live attenuated influenza vaccine [LAIV]). LAIV is approved for use in healthy people 2–49 years of age who are not pregnant. Healthy indicates persons who do not have an underlying medical condition that predisposes them to influenza complications.

About two weeks after vaccination, antibodies develop that protect against influenza virus infection. Flu vaccines will not protect against flu-like illnesses caused by non-influenza viruses.

When to Get Vaccinated

Yearly flu vaccination should begin in September or as soon as vaccine is available and continue throughout the influenza season, into

December, January, and beyond. This is because the timing and duration of influenza seasons vary. While influenza outbreaks can happen as early as October, most of the time influenza activity peaks in January or later.

Who should get vaccinated?

In general, anyone who wants to reduce their chances of getting the flu can get vaccinated. However, certain people should get vaccinated each year either because they are at high risk of having serious flu-related complications or because they live with or care for high risk persons. During flu seasons when vaccine supplies are limited or delayed, the Advisory Committee on Immunization Practices (ACIP) makes recommendations regarding priority groups for vaccination.

People who should get vaccinated each year include the following:

- Children aged six months up to their 19th birthday
- Pregnant women
- People 50 years of age and older
- People of any age with certain chronic medical conditions
- People who live in nursing homes and other long-term care facilities
- People who live with or care for those at high risk for complications from flu, including:
  - health care workers,
  - household contacts of persons at high risk for complications from the flu,
  - household contacts and out of home caregivers of children less than six months of age (these children are too young to be vaccinated).

Use of the Nasal Spray Flu Vaccine

Vaccination with the nasal-spray flu vaccine is an option for healthy people 2–49 years of age who are not pregnant, even healthy persons who live with or care for those in a high-risk group. The one exception is healthy persons who care for persons with severely weakened immune systems who require a protected environment; these healthy persons should get the inactivated vaccine.

Who should not be vaccinated?

Some people should not be vaccinated without first consulting a physician. They include the following:

- People who have a severe allergy to chicken eggs
- People who have had a severe reaction to an influenza vaccination in the past
- People who developed Guillain-Barré syndrome (GBS) within six weeks of getting an influenza vaccine previously
- Children less than six months of age (influenza vaccine is not approved for use in this age group)
- People who have a moderate or severe illness with a fever should wait to get vaccinated until their symptoms lessen

If you have questions about whether you should get a flu vaccine, consult your health care provider.

Types of Influenza Viruses

There are three types of influenza viruses: A, B, and C. Influenza A and B viruses cause seasonal epidemics of disease almost every winter in the United States. Influenza type C infections cause a mild respiratory illness and are not thought to cause epidemics.

Influenza A viruses are divided into subtypes based on two proteins on the surface of the virus: the hemagglutinin (H) and the neuraminidase (N). There are 16 different hemagglutinin subtypes and nine different neuraminidase subtypes, Influenza A viruses can be further broken down into different strains. The current subtypes of influenza A viruses found in people are A (H1N1) and A (H3N2).

Influenza B viruses are not divided into subtypes. Influenza B viruses also can be further broken down into different strains.

Influenza A (H1N1), A (H3N2), and influenza B strains are included in each year's influenza vaccine. Getting a flu vaccine can protect against influenza A and B viruses. The flu vaccine does not protect against influenza C viruses.

Section 29.2

Pandemic Flu

This section includes text from the following Centers for Disease Control and Prevention (CDC) documents: "What Is an Influenza Pandemic?" "How Does Seasonal Flu Differ from Pandemic Flu?" and "Avian Influenza (Bird Flu)," 2009. These documents are available online at http://www.PandemicFlu.gov.

What is an influenza pandemic?

A pandemic is a global disease outbreak. An influenza pandemic occurs when a new influenza A virus emerges for which there is little or no immunity in the human population, begins to cause serious illness and then spreads easily person-to-person worldwide.

Historically, the 20th century saw three pandemics of influenza:

- 1918 influenza pandemic caused at least 675,000 U.S. deaths and up to 50 million deaths worldwide;

- 1957 influenza pandemic caused at least 70,000 U.S. deaths and 1–2 million deaths worldwide; and

- 1968 influenza pandemic caused about 34,000 U.S. deaths and 700,000 deaths worldwide.

Characteristics and Challenges of a Pandemic

Rapid Worldwide Spread

- When a pandemic influenza virus emerges, its global spread is considered inevitable.

- Preparedness activities should assume that the entire world population would be susceptible.

- Countries might, through measures such as border closures and travel restrictions, delay arrival of the virus, but cannot stop it.

Health Care Systems Overloaded

- Most people have little or no immunity to a pandemic virus. Infection and illness rates soar. A substantial percentage of the world's population will require some form of medical care.

- Nations are unlikely to have the staff, facilities, equipment, and hospital beds needed to cope with large numbers of people who suddenly fall ill.

- Death rates are high, largely determined by four factors: the number of people who become infected, the virulence of the virus, the underlying characteristics and vulnerability of affected populations, and the effectiveness of preventive measures.

- Past pandemics have spread globally in two and sometimes three waves.

Medical Supplies Inadequate

- The need for vaccine is likely to outstrip supply.

- The need for antiviral drugs is also likely to be inadequate early in a pandemic.

- A pandemic can create a shortage of hospital beds, ventilators, and other supplies. Surge capacity at non-traditional sites such as schools may be created to cope with demand.

- Difficult decisions will need to be made regarding who gets antiviral drugs and vaccines.

Economic and Social Disruption

- Travel bans, closings of schools and businesses, and cancellations of events could have major impact on communities and citizens.

- Care for sick family members and fear of exposure can result in significant worker absenteeism.

Communications and Information Are Critical Components of Pandemic Response

Education and outreach are critical to preparing for a pandemic. Understanding what a pandemic is, what needs to be done at all levels to prepare for pandemic influenza, and what could happen during a pandemic helps us make informed decisions both as individuals and as a nation. Should a pandemic occur the public must be able to depend on its government to provide scientifically sound public health information quickly, openly, and dependably.

Table 29.1. Differences between Seasonal Flu and Pandemic Flu

Seasonal Flu	Pandemic Flu
Outbreaks follow predictable seasonal patterns; occurs annually, usually in winter, in temperate climates	Occurs rarely (three times in 20th century—last in 1968)
Usually some immunity built up from previous exposure	No previous exposure; little or no pre-existing immunity
Healthy adults usually not at risk for serious complications; the very young, the elderly and those with certain underlying health conditions at increased risk for serious complications	Healthy people may be at increased risk for serious complications
Health systems can usually meet public and patient needs	Health systems may be overwhelmed
Vaccine developed based on known flu strains and available for annual flu season	Vaccine probably would not be available in the early stages of a pandemic
Adequate supplies of antivirals are usually available	Effective antivirals may be in limited supply
Average U.S. deaths approximately 36,000/year	Number of deaths could be quite high (for example, U.S. 1918 death toll approximately 675,000)
Symptoms: fever, cough, runny nose, muscle pain. Deaths often caused by complications, such as pneumonia.	Symptoms may be more severe and complications more frequent
Generally causes modest impact on society (for example, some school closing, encouragement of people who are sick to stay home)	May cause major impact on society (for example, widespread restrictions on travel, closings of schools and businesses, cancellation of large public gatherings)
Manageable impact on domestic and world economy	Potential for severe impact on domestic and world economy

Avian Influenza (Bird Flu)

Avian Flu in Birds Is Spreading in Asia and Other Countries

- Avian influenza—commonly called bird flu—is an infection caused by influenza viruses that occur naturally in birds.

- Wild birds can carry the viruses, but usually do not get sick from them. However, some domesticated birds, including chickens, ducks, and turkeys, can become infected, often fatally.

- One strain of avian influenza, the H5N1 virus, is endemic in much of Asia and has spread into parts of Europe and Africa. Avian H5N1 infections have recently killed poultry and other birds in a number of countries.

- Strains of avian H5N1 influenza may infect various types of animals, including wild birds, pigs, and tigers.

- Symptoms in birds and other animals vary, but virulent strains can cause death within a few days.

Avian H5N1 Flu in Humans Is Currently Very Limited and Not a Pandemic

- Human H5N1 influenza infection was first recognized in 1997 when this virus infected 18 people in Hong Kong, causing six deaths.

- The World Health Organization is tracking the number of human cases of the H5N1 virus.

- Currently, close contact with infected poultry has been the primary source for human infection. Though rare, there have been isolated reports of human-to-human transmission of the virus.

- Genetic studies confirm that the influenza A virus H5N1 mutates rapidly. Should it adapt to allow easy human-to-human transmission, a pandemic could ensue—it has not done so to date.

- At this time, it is uncertain whether the currently circulating H5N1 virus will lead to a global disease outbreak in humans—a pandemic.

- The reported symptoms of avian influenza in humans have ranged from typical influenza-like symptoms (fever, cough, sore throat, and muscle aches) to eye infections (conjunctivitis), acute respiratory distress, viral pneumonia, and other severe, life-threatening complications.

Preventing and Treating Avian Flu in Humans

- Vaccines to protect humans against H5N1 viruses currently are under development. In addition, research is underway on methods to make large quantities of vaccine more quickly.

• So far, research suggests that two antiviral medicines, osel-tamivir (Tamiflu®) and zanamivir (Relenza®), may be useful treatments for H5N1 avian influenza. Some adverse reactions have been reported in children. However, H5N1 viruses are generally resistant to two other available antiviral medications, amantadine and rimantadine, so they cannot be used to treat avian flu.

Section 29.3

H1N1 Flu (Swine Flu)

This section includes text from "Novel H1N1 Flu (Swine Flu) and You," Centers for Disease Control and Prevention (CDC), updated June 30, 2009; "Outbreak Notice Novel H1N1 Flu: Global Situation," CDC, July 30, 2009; "What to Do if You Get Flu-Like Symptoms," CDC, July 8, 2009; and "CDC Advisors Make Recommendations for Use of Vaccine Against Novel H1N1," CDC Press Release, July 29, 2009.

Novel H1N1 Flu

Novel H1N1 (referred to as swine flu) is a new influenza virus causing illness in people. This new virus was first detected in people in the United States in April 2009. Other countries, including Mexico and Canada, have reported people sick with this new virus. This virus is spreading from person-to-person, probably in much the same way that regular seasonal influenza viruses spread.

Why is novel H1N1 virus sometimes called swine flu?

This virus was originally referred to as swine flu because laboratory testing showed that many of the genes in this new virus were very similar to influenza viruses that normally occur in pigs in North America. But further study has shown that this new virus is very different from what normally circulates in North American pigs. It has two genes from flu viruses that normally circulate in pigs in Europe and Asia and avian genes and human genes.

Are there human infections with novel H1N1 virus in the U.S.?

Yes. Cases of human infection with novel H1N1 influenza virus were first confirmed in the U.S. in Southern California and near Guadalupe County, Texas. The outbreak intensified rapidly from that time and more and more states have been reporting cases of illness from this virus. An updated case count of confirmed novel H1N1 flu infections in the United States is kept at http://www.cdc.gov/h1n1flu/update.htm.

Is novel H1N1 virus contagious?

The Centers for Disease Control and Prevention (CDC) has determined that novel H1N1 virus is contagious and is spreading from human to human. However, at this time, it is not known how easily the virus spreads between people.

What are the signs and symptoms of this virus in people?

The symptoms of novel H1N1 flu virus in people are similar to the symptoms of seasonal flu and include fever, cough, sore throat, runny or stuffy nose, body aches, headache, chills, and fatigue. A significant number of people who have been infected with this virus also have reported diarrhea and vomiting. Also, like seasonal flu, severe illnesses and death have occurred as a result of illness associated with this virus.

How severe is illness associated with novel H1N1 flu virus?

It's not known at this time how severe novel H1N1 flu virus will be in the general population. In seasonal flu, there are certain people that are at higher risk of serious flu-related complications. This includes people 65 years and older, children younger than five years old, pregnant women, and people of any age with certain chronic medical conditions. Early indications are that pregnancy and other previously recognized medical conditions that increase the risk of influenza-related complications, like asthma and diabetes, also appear to be associated with increased risk of complications from novel H1N1 virus infection as well.

One thing that appears to be different from seasonal influenza is that adults older than 64 years do not yet appear to be at increased risk of novel H1N1-related complications thus far in the outbreak. CDC is conducting laboratory studies to see if certain people might have natural immunity to this virus, depending on their age. Early reports indicate that no children and few adults younger than 60 years old have existing antibody to novel H1N1 flu virus; however, about one-third of adults older than 60 may have antibodies against this virus. It is unknown how much, if any, protection may be afforded against novel H1N1 flu by any existing antibody.

So far, with novel H1N1 flu, the largest number of novel H1N1 flu confirmed and probable cases have occurred in people between the ages of 5–24 years. At this time, there are few cases and no deaths reported in people older than 64 years old, which is unusual when compared with seasonal flu. However, pregnancy and other previously recognized high-risk medical conditions from seasonal influenza appear to be associated with increased risk of complications from this novel H1N1.

How does novel H1N1 virus spread?

Spread of novel H1N1 virus is thought to be happening in the same way that seasonal flu spreads. Flu viruses are spread mainly from person to person through coughing or sneezing by people with influenza. Sometimes people may become infected by touching something with flu viruses on it and then touching their mouth or nose.

How long can an infected person spread this virus to others?

At the current time, CDC believes that this virus has the same properties in terms of spread as seasonal flu viruses. With seasonal flu, studies have shown that people may be contagious from one day before they develop symptoms to up to seven days after they get sick. Children, especially younger children, might potentially be contagious for longer periods.

Are there medicines to treat novel H1N1 infection?

Yes. CDC recommends the use of oseltamivir or zanamivir for the treatment and/or prevention of infection with novel H1N1 flu virus. Antiviral drugs are prescription medicines (pills, liquid, or an inhaled powder) that fight against the flu by keeping flu viruses from reproducing in your body. If you get sick, antiviral drugs can make your illness milder and make you feel better faster. They may also prevent serious flu complications. During the current outbreak, the priority use for influenza antiviral drugs during is to treat severe influenza illness.

How long can influenza virus remain viable on objects (such as books and doorknobs)?

Studies have shown that influenza virus can survive on environmental surfaces and can infect a person for up to 2–8 hours after being deposited on the surface.

What kills influenza virus?

Influenza virus is destroyed by heat (167–212° Fahrenheit [75–100° Celsius]). In addition, several chemical germicides, including chlorine, hydrogen peroxide, detergents (soap), iodophors (iodine-based antiseptics), and alcohols are effective against human influenza viruses if used in proper concentration for a sufficient length of time. For example, wipes or gels with alcohol in them can be used to clean hands. The gels should be rubbed into hands until they are dry.

What is CDC doing in response to the outbreak?

The agency's goals are to reduce transmission and illness severity, and provide information to help health care providers, public health officials, and the public address the challenges posed by the new virus. CDC is working with state and local health departments to enhance surveillance in the United States and to collect and analyze data to assess the impact of the virus and determine the groups at increased risk of complications. In addition, CDC continues to issue new and updated interim guidance for clinicians, public health professionals and the public for the prevention and treatment of this new virus.

To expand the national and international laboratory capacity for detecting novel H1N1 influenza, CDC has developed and distributed new influenza diagnostic kits and reagents to more than 350 laboratories, including laboratories in 131 countries. CDC's Division of the Strategic National Stockpile (SNS) continues to send antiviral drugs, personal protective equipment, and respiratory protection devices to all 50 states and U.S. territories to help them respond to the outbreak.

The U.S. government also is aggressively taking early steps in the process to manufacture a novel H1N1 influenza vaccine, working closely with manufacturing. CDC has isolated the new H1N1 virus, made a candidate vaccine virus that can be used to create vaccine, and has provided this virus to industry so they can begin scaling up for production of a vaccine, if necessary.

What to Do If You Get Flu-Like Symptoms

The symptoms of novel H1N1 flu virus in people are similar to the symptoms of seasonal flu and include fever, cough, sore throat, runny or stuffy nose, body aches, headache, chills, and fatigue. A significant number of people who have been infected with novel H1N1 flu virus also have reported diarrhea and vomiting.

Avoid Contact with Others

If you are sick, you may be ill for a week or longer. Unless necessary for medical care, you should stay home and minimize contact with others, including avoiding travel and not going to work or school, for seven days after your symptoms begin or until you have been symptom-free for 24 hours, whichever is longer. If you leave the house to seek medical care, wear a face mask, if available and tolerable, and cover your coughs and sneezes with a tissue. In general, you should avoid contact with other people as much as possible to keep from spreading your illness, especially people at increased risk of severe illness from influenza. With seasonal flu, people may be contagious from one day before they develop symptoms to up to seven days after they get sick. Children, especially younger children, might potentially be contagious for longer periods. People infected with the novel H1N1 are likely to have similar patterns of infectiousness as with seasonal flu.

Treatment Is Available for Those Who Are Seriously Ill

It is expected that most people will recover without needing medical care. If you have severe illness or you are at high risk for flu complications, contact your health care provider or seek medical care. Your health care provider will determine whether flu testing or treatment is needed. Be aware that if the flu becomes widespread, less testing will be needed, so your health care provider may decide not to test for the flu virus.

Antiviral drugs can be given to treat those who become severely ill with influenza. These antiviral drugs are prescription medicines (pills, liquid, or an inhaler) with activity against influenza viruses, including novel H1N1 flu virus. These medications must be prescribed by a health care professional.

There are two influenza antiviral medications that are recommended for use against novel H1N1 flu. The drugs that are used for treating novel H1N1 flu are called oseltamivir (trade name Tamiflu®) and zanamivir (Relenza®). As the novel H1N1 flu spreads, these antiviral drugs may become in short supply. Therefore, the drugs may be given first to those people who have been hospitalized or are at high risk of severe illness from flu. The drugs work best if given within two days of becoming ill, but may be given later if illness is severe or for those at a high risk for complications.

Aspirin or aspirin-containing products (for example, bismuth subsalicylate—Pepto Bismol) should not be administered to any confirmed or suspected ill case of novel influenza A (H1N1) virus infection aged 18 years old and younger due to the risk of Reye syndrome. For relief of fever, other anti-pyretic medications are recommended such as acetaminophen or non steroidal anti-inflammatory drugs.

- Check ingredient labels on over-the-counter cold and flu medications to see if they contain aspirin.

- Children five years of age and older and teenagers with the flu can take medicines without aspirin, such as acetaminophen (Tylenol®) and ibuprofen (Advil®, Motrin®, Nuprin®), to relieve symptoms.

- Children younger than four years of age should not be given over-the-counter cold medications without first speaking with a health care provider.

Emergency Warning Signs

If you become ill and experience any of the following warning signs, seek emergency medical care.

In children, emergency warning signs that need urgent medical attention include the following:

- Fast breathing or trouble breathing

- Bluish or gray skin color

- Not drinking enough fluids

- Severe or persistent vomiting

- Not waking up or not interacting

- Being so irritable that the child does not want to be held

- Flu-like symptoms improve but then return with fever and worse cough

In adults, emergency warning signs that need urgent medical attention include the following:

- Difficulty breathing or shortness of breath
- Pain or pressure in the chest or abdomen
- Sudden dizziness
- Confusion
- Severe or persistent vomiting
- Flu-like symptoms improve but then return with fever and worse cough

Protect Yourself, Your Family, and Community

- Stay informed. Health officials will provide additional information as it becomes available.
- Cover your nose and mouth with a tissue when you cough or sneeze. Throw the tissue in the trash after you use it.
- Wash your hands often with soap and water, especially after you cough or sneeze. Alcohol-based hand cleaners are also effective.
- Avoid touching your eyes, nose and mouth. Germs spread this way.
- Try to avoid close contact with sick people.
- If you are sick with a flu-like illness, stay home for seven days after your symptoms begin or until you have been symptom-free for 24 hours, whichever is longer, except to seek medical care or for other necessities. Keep away from other household members as much as possible. This is to keep you from infecting others and spreading the virus further.
- If you are sick and sharing a common space with other household members in your home, wear a face mask, if available and tolerable, to help prevent spreading the virus to others.
- Follow public health advice regarding school closures, avoiding crowds, and other social distancing measures.
- If you don't have one yet, consider developing a family emergency plan as a precaution. This should include storing a supply of extra food, medicines, and other essential supplies.

Novel H1N1 Flu: Global Situation

On June 11, 2009, the World Health Organization (WHO) raised the worldwide pandemic alert level to Phase 6 in response to the ongoing global spread of the novel influenza A (H1N1) virus. A Phase 6 alert level means that a global pandemic is underway and that there are now ongoing community level outbreaks in multiple parts of world. The Phase 6 pandemic alert level is a reflection of the spread of the virus, not the severity of illness caused by the virus.

Recommendations for Travel to Areas Reporting Novel H1N1 Flu

CDC recommends that travelers at high risk for complications from any form of flu discuss their travel plans with their doctor. Together, they should look carefully at the H1N1 flu situation in their destination and the available health care options in the area. They should discuss their specific health situations and possible increased risk of traveling to the area affected by novel H1N1 flu.

Travelers at high risk for complications include the following:

- Children less than five years of age

- Persons aged 65 years or older

- Children and adolescents (less than 18 years) who are receiving long-term aspirin therapy and who might be at risk for experiencing Reye syndrome after influenza virus infection

- Pregnant women

- Adults and children who have chronic pulmonary, cardiovascular, hepatic, hematological, neurologic, neuromuscular, or metabolic disorders

- Adults and children who have immunosuppression (including immunosuppression caused by medications or by human immunodeficiency virus [HIV])

Do not travel if you are sick: If you have flu-like symptoms, you should stay home and avoid travel for seven days after you get sick or for at least 24 hours after you stop having symptoms, whichever is longer. This is to keep others from getting the virus.

- Symptoms of novel H1N1 flu virus are similar to the symptoms of seasonal flu and include fever, cough, sore throat, runny or stuffy nose, body aches, headache, chills, and fatigue.

- Some people also have diarrhea and vomiting.

Follow local guidelines: Pay attention to announcements from the local government and monitor the local health and security situation; follow any movement restrictions and prevention recommendations; and be aware that some countries are checking the health of arriving and/or exiting passengers and screening them for illness due to novel H1N1 flu to prevent others from getting sick.

Practice healthy habits to help stop the spread of novel H1N1 flu: Wash your hands, cover your mouth and nose when you cough or sneeze, and avoid close contact with sick people.

What to do if you feel sick: It is expected that most people will recover without needing medical care. If you have severe illness or you are at high risk for flu complications, seek medical care.

After your trip: Closely monitor your health for seven days. If you become ill with fever and other symptoms of novel H1N1 flu such as a cough, sore throat, and possibly vomiting and diarrhea, seek help from your health care provider.

CDC Advisors Make Recommendations for Use of Vaccine against Novel H1N1

The Centers for Disease Control and Prevention's Advisory Committee on Immunization Practices (ACIP) met July 29, 2009 to make recommendations for use of vaccine against novel influenza A (H1N1).

The committee met to develop recommendations on who should receive vaccine against novel influenza A (H1N1) when it becomes available, and to determine which groups of the population should be prioritized if the vaccine is initially available in extremely limited quantities.

The committee recommended the vaccination efforts focus on five key populations. Vaccination efforts are designed to help reduce the impact and spread of novel H1N1. The key populations include those who are at higher risk of disease or complications, those who are likely to come in contact with novel H1N1, and those who could infect young infants. When vaccine is first available, the committee recommended that programs and providers try to vaccinate:

- pregnant women,

- people who live with or care for children younger than six months of age,

- health care and emergency services personnel,

- persons between the ages of six months through 24 years of age, and

- people from ages 25 through 64 years who are at higher risk for novel H1N1 because of chronic health disorders or compromised immune systems.

These groups total approximately 159 million people in the United States.

The committee does not expect that there will be a shortage of novel H1N1 vaccine, but availability and demand can be unpredictable. There is some possibility that initially the vaccine will be available in limited quantities. In this setting, the committee recommended that the following groups receive the vaccine before others:

- pregnant women,

- people who live with or care for children younger than six months of age,

- health care and emergency services personnel with direct patient contact,

- children six months through four years of age, and

- children five through 18 years of age who have chronic medical conditions.

The committee recognized the need to assess supply and demand issues at the local level. The committee further recommended that once the demand for vaccine for these prioritized groups has been met at the local level, programs and providers should begin vaccinating everyone from ages 25 through 64 years. Current studies indicate the risk for infection among persons age 65 or older is less than the risk for younger age groups. Therefore, as vaccine supply and demand for vaccine among younger age groups is being met, programs and providers should offer vaccination to people over the age of 65.

The committee also stressed that people over the age of 65 receive the seasonal vaccine as soon as it is available. Even if novel H1N1 vaccine is initially only available in limited quantities, supply and availability will continue, so the committee stressed that programs and providers continue to vaccinate unimmunized patients and not keep vaccine in reserve for later administration of the second dose.

The novel H1N1 vaccine is not intended to replace the seasonal flu vaccine. It is intended to be used alongside seasonal flu vaccine to protect people. Seasonal flu and novel H1N1 vaccines may be administered on the same day.

Chapter 30

Lice

Chapter Contents

Section 30.1

Body Lice

Text in this section is from "Body Lice Fact Sheet,"
and "Body Lice Treatment," Centers for Disease Control
and Prevention (CDC), May 16, 2008.

Body lice are parasitic insects that live on clothing and bedding used by infested persons. Body lice frequently lay their eggs on or near the seams of clothing. Body lice must feed on blood and usually only move to the skin to feed. Body lice exist worldwide and infest people of all races. Body lice infestations can spread rapidly under crowded living conditions where hygiene is poor (homeless, refugees, victims of war or natural disasters). In the United States, body lice infestations are found only in homeless transient populations who do not have access to bathing and regular changes of clean clothes. Infestation is unlikely to persist on anyone who bathes regularly and who has at least weekly access to freshly laundered clothing and bedding.

Body lice have three forms: the egg (also called a nit), the nymph, and the adult.

Nit: Nits are lice eggs. They are generally easy to see in the seams of an infested person's clothing, particularly around the waistline and under armpits. Body lice nits occasionally also may be attached to body hair. They are oval and usually yellow to white in color. Body lice nits may take 1–2 weeks to hatch.

Nymph: A nymph is an immature louse that hatches from the nit (egg). A nymph looks like an adult body louse, but is smaller. Nymphs mature into adults about 9–12 days after hatching. To live, the nymph must feed on blood.

Adult: The adult body louse is about the size of a sesame seed, has six legs, and is tan to grayish-white. Females lay eggs. To live, lice must feed on blood. If a louse falls off of a person, it dies within about 5–7 days at room temperature.

Where are body lice found?

Body lice generally are found on clothing and bedding used by infested people. Sometimes body lice are be seen on the body when they feed. Body lice eggs usually are seen in the seams of clothing or on bedding. Occasionally eggs are attached to body hair. Lice found on the head and scalp are not body lice; they are head lice.

What are the signs and symptoms of body lice?

Intense itching (pruritus) and rash caused by an allergic reaction to the louse bites are common symptoms of body lice infestation. When body lice infestation has been present for a long time, heavily bitten areas of the skin can become thickened and discolored, particularly around the midsection of the body (waist, groin, upper thighs); this condition is called vagabond's disease. As with other lice infestations, intense itching can lead to scratching which can cause sores on the body; these sores sometimes can become infected with bacteria or fungi.

Can body lice transmit disease?

Yes. Body lice can spread epidemic typhus, trench fever, and louse-borne relapsing fever. Although louse-borne (epidemic) typhus is no longer widespread, outbreaks of this disease still occur during times of war, civil unrest, natural or man-made disasters, and in prisons where people live together in unsanitary conditions. Louse-borne typhus still exists in places where climate, chronic poverty, and social customs or war and social upheaval prevent regular changes and laundering of clothing.

How are body lice spread?

Body lice are spread through direct physical contact with a person who has body lice or through contact with articles such as clothing, beds, bed linens, or towels that have been in contact with an infested person. In the United States, actual infestation with body lice tends to occur only in persons who do not have access to regular (at least weekly) bathing and changes of clean clothes, such as homeless, transient persons.

Diagnosis: Body lice infestation is diagnosed by finding eggs and crawling lice in the seams of clothing. Sometimes a body louse can be seen on the skin crawling or feeding. Although body lice and nits can be large enough to be seen with the naked eye, sometimes a magnifying lens may be necessary to find lice or nits. Diagnosis should be made by a health care provider if you are unsure about an infestation.

Treatment: A body lice infestation is treated by improving the personal hygiene of the infested person, including assuring a regular (at least weekly) change of clean clothes. Clothing, bedding, and towels used by the infested person should be laundered using hot water (at least 130° Fahrenheit) and machine dried using the hot cycle.

Sometimes the infested person also is treated with a pediculicide [peh-DICK-you-luh-side]), a medicine that can kill lice; however, a pediculicide generally is not necessary if hygiene is maintained and items are laundered appropriately at least once a week. If used, a pediculicide should be applied exactly as directed on the bottle or by your physician.

Section 30.2

Head Lice

This section includes text from "Lice: Head Lice Fact Sheet" and "Lice: Head Lice Treatment," Centers for Disease Control and Prevention (CDC), May 16, 2008.

The head louse, or *Pediculus humanus capitis*, is a parasitic insect that can be found on the head, eyebrows, and eyelashes of people. Head lice feed on human blood several times a day and live close to the human scalp. Head lice are not known to spread disease.

Head lice are found worldwide. In the United States, infestation with head lice is most common among preschool children attending child care, elementary school children, and the household members of infested children. Although reliable data on how many people in the United States get head lice each year are not available, an estimated six million to 12 million infestations occur each year in the United States among children 3–11 years of age. In the United States, infestation with head lice is much less common among African-Americans than among persons of other races, possibly because the claws of the of the head louse found most frequently in the United States are better adapted for grasping the shape and width of the hair shaft of other races.

Head lice move by crawling; they cannot hop or fly. Head lice are spread by direct contact with the hair of an infested person. Anyone who comes in head-to-head contact with someone who already has head lice is at greatest risk. Spread by contact with clothing (such as hats, scarves, coats) or other personal items (such as combs, brushes, or towels) used by an infested person is uncommon. Personal hygiene or cleanliness in the home or school has nothing to do with getting head lice.

Head lice have three forms: the egg (also called a nit), the nymph, and the adult.

Egg (also called a nit): Nits are lice eggs laid by the adult female head louse at the base of the hair shaft nearest the scalp. Nits are firmly attached to the hair shaft and are oval-shaped and very small (about the size of a knot in thread) and hard to see. Nits often appear yellow or white although live nits sometimes appear to be the same color as the hair of the infested person. Nits are often confused with dandruff, scabs, or hair spray droplets. Head lice nits usually take about 8–9 days to hatch. Eggs that are likely to hatch are usually located no more than ¼ inch (or one centimeter) from the base of the hair shaft.

Nymph: A nymph is an immature louse that hatches from the nit. A nymph looks like an adult head louse, but is smaller. To live, a nymph must feed on blood. Nymphs mature into adults about 9–12 days after hatching from the nit.

Adult: The fully grown and developed adult louse is about the size of a sesame seed, has six legs, and is tan to grayish-white in color. Adult head lice may look darker in persons with dark hair than in persons with light hair. To survive, adult head lice must feed on blood. An adult head louse can live about 30 days on a person's head but will die within one or two days if it falls off a person. Adult female head lice are usually larger than males and can lay about six eggs each day.

Where are head lice most commonly found?

Head lice and head lice nits are found almost exclusively on the scalp, particularly around and behind the ears and near the neckline at the back of the head. Head lice or head lice nits sometimes are found on the eyelashes or eyebrows but this is uncommon. Head lice hold tightly to hair with hook-like claws at the end of each of their six legs; head lice nits are cemented firmly to the hair shaft and can be difficult to remove.

What are the signs and symptoms of head lice infestation?

- Tickling feeling of something moving in the hair.
- Itching, caused by an allergic reaction to the bites of the head louse.
- Irritability and difficulty sleeping; head lice are most active in the dark.
- Sores on the head caused by scratching. These sores can sometimes become infected with bacteria found on the person's skin.

How did my child get head lice?

Head-to-head contact with an already infested person is the most common way to get head lice. Head-to-head contact is common during play at school, at home, and elsewhere (sports activities, playground, slumber parties, and camp).

Uncommonly, head lice may be spread by sharing clothing or belongings onto which lice or nits may have crawled or fallen. The risk of getting an infestation by a louse or nit that has fallen onto a carpet or furniture is very small. Dogs, cats, and other pets do not play a role in the spread of human lice.

Diagnosis: The diagnosis of a head lice infestation is best made by finding a live nymph or adult louse on the scalp or hair of a person. Because nymphs and adult lice are very small, move quickly, and avoid light, they can be difficult to find. Use of a magnifying lens and a fine-toothed comb may be helpful to find live lice. If crawling lice are not seen, finding nits firmly attached within a ¼ inch of base of the hair shafts strongly suggests, but does not confirm, that a person is infested and should be treated. Nits that are attached more than ¼ inch from the base of the hair shaft are almost always dead or already hatched. Nits are often confused with other things found in the hair such as dandruff, hair spray droplets, and dirt particles. If no live nymphs or adult lice are seen, and the only nits found are more than ¼-inch from the scalp, the infestation is probably old and no longer active and does not need to be treated. If you are not sure if a person has head lice, the diagnosis should be made by their health care provider, local health department, or other person trained to identify live head lice.

Treatment: Treatment for head lice is recommended for persons diagnosed with an active infestation. All household members and other close contacts should be checked, and those persons with evidence of an active infestation should be treated. Some experts believe prophylactic treatment is prudent for persons who share the same bed with actively infested individuals. All infested persons (household members and close contacts) and anyone who shares a bed with the infested person should be treated at the same time.

Retreatment of head lice usually is recommended because no approved pediculicide (peh-DICK-you-luh-side) is completely ovicidal. To be most effective, retreatment should occur after all eggs have hatched but before new eggs are produced. The retreatment schedule can vary depending on the pediculicide used.

When treating head lice, supplemental measures can be combined with recommended medicine (pharmacologic treatment); however, such additional (non-pharmacologic) measures generally are not required to eliminate a head lice infestation. For example, hats, scarves, pillow cases, bedding, clothing, and towels worn or used by the infested person in the two-day period just before treatment is started can be machine washed and dried using the hot water and hot air cycles because lice and eggs are killed by exposure for five minutes to temperatures greater than 53.5° Celsius (128.3° Fahrenheit). Items that cannot be laundered may be dry-cleaned or sealed in a plastic bag for two weeks. Items such as hats, grooming aids, and towels that come in contact with the hair of an infested person should not be shared. Vacuuming furniture and floors can remove an infested person's hairs that might have viable nits attached.

Treating the infested person(s) requires using an over-the-counter (OTC) or prescription medication. Do not use a creme rinse, combination shampoo/conditioner, or conditioner before using lice medicine, and do not re-wash the hair for 1–2 days after the lice medicine is removed. Have the infested person put on clean clothing after treatment. After each treatment, checking the hair and combing with a nit comb to remove nits and lice every 2–3 days may decrease the chance of self-reinfestation. Continue to check for 2–3 weeks to be sure all lice and nits are gone.

If you aren't sure which medicine to use or how to use a particular medicine, always ask your physician, pharmacist, or other health care provider. When using a medicine, always carefully follow the instructions contained in the package or written on the label, unless the physician and pharmacist direct otherwise.

Other Tips for Treating Head Lice

1. Do not use extra amounts of any lice medication unless instructed to do so by your physician and pharmacist. The drugs used to treat lice are insecticides and can be dangerous if they are misused or overused.

2. Do not treat an infested person more than 2–3 times with the same medication if it does not seem to be working. This may be caused by using the medicine incorrectly or by resistance to the medicine. Always seek the advice of your health care provider if this should happen.

3. Do not use different head lice drugs at the same time unless instructed to do so by your physician and pharmacist.

Section 30.3

Pubic Lice

This section includes text from "Lice: Pubic 'Crab' Lice Fact Sheet," and "Lice: Pubic 'Crab' Lice Treatment," Centers for Disease Control and Prevention (CDC), May 16, 2008.

Also called crab lice or crabs, pubic lice are parasitic insects found primarily in the pubic or genital area of humans. Pubic lice infestation is found worldwide and occurs in all races, ethnic groups, and levels of society. Pubic lice have three forms: the egg (also called a nit), the nymph, and the adult.

Nit: Nits are lice eggs. They can be hard to see and are found firmly attached to the hair shaft. They are oval and usually yellow to white. Pubic lice nits take about 6–10 days to hatch.

Nymph: The nymph is an immature louse that hatches from the nit (egg). A nymph looks like an adult pubic louse but it is smaller.

Pubic lice nymphs take about 2–3 weeks after hatching to mature into adults capable of reproducing. To live, a nymph must feed on blood.

Adult: The adult pubic louse resembles a miniature crab when viewed through a strong magnifying glass. Pubic lice have six legs; their two front legs are very large and look like the pincher claws of a crab. This is how they got the nickname crabs. Pubic lice are tan to grayish-white in color. Females lay nits and are usually larger than males. To live, lice must feed on blood. If the louse falls off a person, it dies within 1–2 days.

Where are pubic lice found?

Pubic lice usually are found in the genital area on pubic hair; but they may occasionally be found on other coarse body hair, such as hair on the legs, armpits, mustache, beard, eyebrows, or eyelashes. Pubic lice on the eyebrows or eyelashes of children may be a sign of sexual exposure or abuse. Lice found on the head are generally head lice, not pubic lice. Animals do not get or spread pubic lice.

What are the signs and symptoms of pubic lice?

Signs and symptoms of pubic lice include, itching in the genital area and visible nits (lice eggs) or crawling lice.

How did I get pubic lice?

Pubic lice usually are spread through sexual contact and are most common in adults. Pubic lice found on children may be a sign of sexual exposure or abuse. Occasionally, pubic lice may be spread by close personal contact or contact with articles such as clothing, bed linens, or towels that have been used by an infested person. A common misunderstanding is that pubic lice are spread easily by sitting on a toilet seat. This would be extremely rare because lice cannot live long away from a warm human body and they do not have feet designed to hold onto or walk on smooth surfaces such as toilet seats.

Diagnosis: A pubic lice infestation is diagnosed by finding a crab louse or egg (nit) on hair in the pubic region or, less commonly, elsewhere on the body (eyebrows, eyelashes, beard, mustache, armpit, perianal area, groin, trunk, scalp). Pubic lice may be difficult to find because there may be only a few. Pubic lice often attach themselves to more than one hair and generally do not crawl as quickly as head and body lice. If crawling lice are not seen, finding nits in the pubic area strongly suggests that a person is infested and should be treated. If you are unsure about infestation, or if treatment is not successful, see a health care provider for a diagnosis. Persons infested with pubic lice should be investigated for the presence of other sexually transmitted diseases. Although pubic lice and nits can be large enough to be seen with the naked eye, a magnifying lens may be necessary to find lice or eggs.

Treatment: A lice-killing lotion containing 1% permethrin or a mousse containing pyrethrins and piperonyl butoxide can be used to treat pubic (crab) lice. These products are available over-the-counter without a prescription at a local drug store or pharmacy. These medications are safe and effective when used exactly according to the instructions in the package or on the label.

When treating pubic lice infestations, carefully follow the instructions in the package or on the label. Following treatment, most nits will still be attached to hair shafts. Nits may be removed with fingernails or by using a fine-toothed comb. Put on clean underwear and clothing after treatment. To kill any lice or nits remaining on clothing, towels, or bedding, machine-wash and machine-dry those items that the infested person used during the 2–3 days before treatment. Use hot water (at least 130° Fahrenheit) and the hot dryer cycle.

All sex partners from within the previous month should be informed that they are at risk for infestation and should be treated. Persons should avoid sexual contact with their sex partner(s) until both they and their partners have been successfully treated and reevaluated to rule out persistent infestation. Persons with pubic lice should be evaluated for other sexually transmitted diseases (STD).

Chapter 31

Measles

Measles is an infectious viral disease that occurs most often in the late winter and spring. It begins with a fever that lasts for a couple of days, followed by a cough, runny nose, and conjunctivitis (pink eye). A rash starts on the face and upper neck, spreads down the back and trunk, then extends to the arms and hands, as well as the legs and feet. After about five days, the rash fades the same order in which it appeared.

Measles is highly contagious. Infected people are usually contagious from about four days before their rash starts to four days afterwards. The measles virus resides in the mucus in the nose and throat of infected people. When they sneeze or cough, droplets spray into the air and the droplets remain active and contagious on infected surfaces for up to two hours.

Measles itself is unpleasant, but the complications are dangerous. Six to 20 percent of the people who get the disease will get an ear infection, diarrhea, or even pneumonia. One out of 1000 people with measles will develop inflammation of the brain, and about one out of 1000 will die.

Why is vaccination necessary?

In the decade before the measles vaccination program began, an estimated 3–4 million persons in the United States were infected each year, of whom 400–500 died, 48,000 were hospitalized, and another 1,000 developed chronic disability from measles encephalitis. Widespread use of measles vaccine has led to a greater than 99%

Text in this chapter is from "Measles: Q and A about Disease and Vaccine," Centers for Disease Control and Prevention (CDC), August 20, 2008.

reduction in measles cases in the United States compared with the pre-vaccine era.

However, measles is still common in other countries. The virus is highly contagious and can spread rapidly in areas where vaccination is not widespread. It is estimated that in 2006 there were 242,000 measles deaths worldwide—that equals about 663 deaths every day or 27 deaths every hour. If vaccinations were stopped, measles cases would return to pre-vaccine levels and hundreds of people would die from measles-related illnesses.

We still see measles among visitors to the United States and among U.S. travelers returning from other countries. The measles viruses these travelers bring into our country sometimes cause outbreaks; however, because most people in the United States have been vaccinated, these outbreaks are usually small.

In the last decade, measles vaccination in the United States has decreased the number of cases to the lowest point ever reported. Widespread use of the measles vaccine has led to a greater than 99% reduction in measles compared with the decade before the measles vaccination program began.

What kind of vaccine is given to prevent measles?

The measles, mumps, rubella (MMR) vaccine prevents measles and two other viral diseases—mumps and rubella. These three vaccines are safe given together. MMR is an attenuated (weakened) live virus vaccine. This means that after injection, the viruses grows and causes a harmless infection in the vaccinated person with very few, if any, symptoms. The person's immune system fights the infection caused by these weakened viruses and immunity develops which lasts throughout that person's life.

How effective is MMR vaccine?

More than 95% of the people who receive a single dose of MMR will develop immunity to all three viruses. A second vaccine dose gives immunity to almost all of those who did not respond to the first dose.

Recommendations

Why is MMR vaccine given after the first birthday?

Most infants born in the United States will receive passive protection against measles, mumps, and rubella in the form of antibodies from their mothers. These antibodies can destroy the vaccine virus if they are present when the vaccine is given and, thus, can cause the vaccine to be ineffective. By 12 months of age, almost all infants have lost this passive protection.

What is the best age to give the second dose of MMR vaccine?

The second dose of MMR can be given at any time, as long as the child is at least 12 months old and it has been at least 28 days since the first dose. However, the second dose is usually administered before the child begins kindergarten or first grade (4–5 years of age) or before entry to middle school (11–12 years of age). The age at which the second dose is required is generally mandated by state school entry requirements.

As an adult, do I need the MMR vaccine?

You do not need the MMR vaccine if you:

- had blood tests that show you are immune to measles, mumps, and rubella;
- are someone born before 1957;
- already had two doses of MMR or one dose of MMR plus a second dose of measles vaccine; or
- already had one dose of MMR and are not at high risk of measles exposure.

You should get the measles vaccine if you are not among the listed categories, and:

- are a college student, trade school student, or other student beyond high school;
- work in a hospital or other medical facility;
- travel internationally, or are a passenger on a cruise ship; or
- are a woman of childbearing age.

Do people who received MMR in the 1960s need to have their dose repeated?

Not necessarily. People who have documentation of receiving live measles vaccine in the 1960s do not need to be revaccinated. People who were vaccinated prior to 1968 with either inactivated (killed) measles vaccine or measles vaccine of unknown type should be revaccinated with at least one dose of live attenuated measles vaccine. This recommendation is intended to protect those who may have received killed measles vaccine, which was available in 1963–1967 and was not effective.

Precautions and Possible Reactions

I am two months pregnant. Is it safe for me to have my 15-month-old child vaccinated with the MMR vaccine?

Yes. Measles, mumps, and rubella vaccine viruses are not transmitted from the vaccinated person, so MMR does not pose a risk to a pregnant household member.

I am breast feeding my two-month-old baby. Is it safe for me to receive the MMR vaccine?

Yes. Breast feeding does not interfere with the response to MMR vaccine, and your baby will not be affected by the vaccine through your breast milk.

My 15-month-old child was exposed to chickenpox yesterday. Is it safe for him to receive the MMR vaccine today?

Yes. Disease exposure, including chickenpox, should not delay anyone from receiving the benefits of the MMR or any other vaccine.

What is the most common reaction following MMR vaccine?

Most people have no reaction. However, 5–10 percent of the people receiving the MMR vaccine experience a low-grade fever and a mild rash.

Chapter 32

Meningitis

What is meningitis?

Meningitis is an inflammation of the membranes that cover the brain and spinal cord. People sometimes refer to it as spinal meningitis. Meningitis is usually caused by a viral or bacterial infection. Knowing whether meningitis is caused by a virus or bacterium is important because the severity of illness and the treatment differ depending on the cause. Viral meningitis is generally less severe and clears up without specific treatment. But bacterial meningitis can be quite severe and may result in brain damage, hearing loss, or learning disabilities. For bacterial meningitis, it is also important to know which type of bacteria is causing the meningitis because antibiotics can prevent some types from spreading and infecting other people. Before the 1990s, *Haemophilus influenzae* type b (Hib) was the leading cause of bacterial meningitis. Hib vaccine is now given to all children as part of their routine immunizations. This vaccine has reduced the number of cases of Hib infection and the number of related meningitis cases. Today, *Streptococcus pneumoniae* and *Neisseria meningitidis* are the leading causes of bacterial meningitis.

This chapter includes text from "Viral (Aseptic) Meningitis FAQs," Centers for Disease Control and Prevention (CDC), updated June 24, 2009; and "Meningitis on Campus," © 2008 American College Health Association (www.acha.org). Reprinted with permission.

What are the signs and symptoms of meningitis?

High fever, headache, and stiff neck are common symptoms of meningitis in anyone over the age of two years. These symptoms can develop over several hours, or they may take 1–2 days. Other symptoms may include nausea, vomiting, discomfort looking into bright lights, confusion, and sleepiness. In newborns and small infants, the classic symptoms of fever, headache, and neck stiffness may be absent or difficult to detect. Infants with meningitis may appear slow or inactive, have vomiting, be irritable, or be feeding poorly. As the disease progresses, patients of any age may have seizures.

How is meningitis diagnosed?

Early diagnosis and treatment are very important. If symptoms occur, the patient should see a doctor immediately. The diagnosis is usually made by growing bacteria or identifying a virus from a sample of spinal fluid. The spinal fluid is obtained by performing a spinal tap, in which a needle is inserted into an area in the lower back where fluid in the spinal canal can be collected. Identification of the type of bacteria responsible is important for selection of correct antibiotics.

Can bacterial meningitis be treated?

Bacterial meningitis can be treated with a number of effective antibiotics. It is important, however, that treatment be started early in the course of the disease. Appropriate antibiotic treatment of most common types of bacterial meningitis should reduce the risk of dying from meningitis to below 15%, although the risk is higher among the elderly.

Is bacterial meningitis contagious?

Yes, some forms of bacterial meningitis are contagious. The bacteria can mainly be spread from person to person through the exchange of respiratory and throat secretions. This can occur through coughing, kissing, and sneezing. Fortunately, none of the bacteria that cause meningitis are as contagious as things like the common cold or the flu. Also, the bacteria are not spread by casual contact or by simply breathing the air where a person with meningitis has been.

However, sometimes the bacteria that cause meningitis have spread to other people who have had close or prolonged contact with a patient with meningitis caused by *Neisseria meningitidis* (also called meningococcal meningitis) or Hib. People in the same household or daycare center, or anyone with direct contact with a patient's oral secretions (such as a boyfriend or girlfriend) would be considered at increased risk of getting the infection. People who qualify as close contacts of a person with meningitis caused by *N. meningitidis* should receive antibiotics to prevent them from getting the disease. This is known as prophylaxis. Prophylaxis for household contacts of someone with Hib disease is only recommended if there is one household contact younger than 48 months who has not been fully immunized against Hib or an immunocompromised child (a child with a weakened immune system) of any age is in the household. The entire household, regardless of age, should receive prophylaxis in these cases.

Are there vaccines against bacterial meningitis?

Yes, there are vaccines against Hib, against some serogroups of *N. meningitidis* and many types of *Streptococcus pneumoniae*. The vaccines are safe and highly effective. There are also vaccines to prevent meningitis due to *S. pneumoniae* (also called pneumococcal meningitis), which can also prevent other forms of infection due to *S. pneumoniae*.

What is viral meningitis?

Viral infections are the most common cause of meningitis; bacterial infections are the second most common cause. Other, rarer causes of meningitis include fungi, parasites, and non-infectious causes, including those that are related to drugs. Meningitis caused by viral infections is sometimes called aseptic meningitis.

Is viral meningitis a serious disease?

Viral (aseptic) meningitis is serious but rarely fatal in people with normal immune systems. Usually, the symptoms last from 7–10 days and the patient recovers completely. Bacterial meningitis, on the other hand, can be very serious and result in disability or death if not treated promptly. Often, the symptoms of viral meningitis and bacterial meningitis are the same. For this reason, if you think you or your child has meningitis, see your doctor as soon as possible.

What causes viral meningitis?

Different viral infections can lead to viral meningitis. But most cases in the United States, particularly during the summer and fall months, are caused by enterovirus (which include enterovirus, coxsackievirus, and echoviruses). Most people who are infected with enterovirus either have no symptoms or only get a cold, rash, or mouth sores with low-grade fever. And, only a small number of people with enterovirus infections go on to develop meningitis.

Other viral infections that can lead to meningitis include mumps, herpesvirus (such as Epstein-Barr virus, herpes simplex viruses, and varicella-zoster virus—the cause of chickenpox and shingles), measles, and influenza.

Arboviruses, which mosquitoes and other insects spread, can also cause infections that can lead to viral meningitis. And lymphocytic choriomeningitis virus, which is spread by rodents, is a rare cause of viral meningitis.

How is viral meningitis treated?

There is no specific treatment for viral meningitis. Most patients completely recover on their own within two weeks. Antibiotics do not help viral infections, so they are not useful in the treatment of viral meningitis. Doctors often will recommend bed rest, plenty of fluids, and medicine to relieve fever and headache. A hospital stay may be necessary in more severe cases or for people with weak immune systems.

How is the virus spread?

Different viruses that cause viral meningitis are spread in different ways. Enteroviruses, the most common cause of viral meningitis, are most often spread through direct contact with an infected person's stool. The virus is spread through this route mainly among small children who are not yet toilet trained. It can also be spread this way to adults changing the diapers of an infected infant.

Enteroviruses and other viruses (such as mumps and varicella-zoster virus) can also be spread through direct or indirect contact with respiratory secretions (saliva, sputum, or nasal mucus) of an infected person. This usually happens through kissing or shaking hands with an infected person or by touching something they have handled and then rubbing your own nose or mouth. The viruses can also stay on surfaces for days and can be transferred from objects. Viruses also can spread directly when infected people cough or sneeze and send droplets containing the virus into the air we breathe.

The time from when a person is infected until they develop symptoms (incubation period) is usually between 3–7 days for an enterovirus. An infected person is usually contagious from the time they develop symptoms until the symptoms go away. Young children and people with low immune systems may spread the infection even after symptoms have resolved.

Can I get viral meningitis if I'm around someone who has it?

If you are around someone with viral meningitis, you may be at risk of becoming infected with the virus that made them sick. But you have only a small chance of developing meningitis as a complication of the illness.

How can I reduce my chances of becoming infected with viruses that can lead to viral meningitis?

Viral meningitis most commonly results from infection with an enterovirus. But there are other causes, such as measles, mumps, and chickenpox. Viral meningitis can also be caused by viruses that are spread by mosquitoes and other insects that bite people.

The specific measures for preventing or reducing your risk for viral meningitis depend on the cause. Following good hygiene practices can reduce the spread of viruses. Preventing the spread of virus can be difficult, especially since sometimes people are infected with a virus (like an enterovirus) but do not appear sick. In such cases, infected people can still spread the virus to others. Thus, it is important to always practice good hygiene to help reduce your chances of becoming infected with a virus or of passing one on to someone else.

Meningitis on Campus

Overview of Meningococcal Disease

Meningococcal disease is a potentially life-threatening bacterial infection that can lead to meningococcal meningitis, an inflammation of the membranes surrounding the brain and spinal cord, or meningococcal septicemia, an infection of the blood.

Meningococcal disease, caused by bacteria called *Neisseria meningitidis*, is the leading cause of bacterial meningitis in older children and young adults in the United States. It strikes 1,400 to 3,000 Americans each year and is responsible for approximately 150 to 300 deaths.

Adolescents and young adults account for nearly 30 percent of all cases of meningitis in the United States. In addition, approximately 100 to 125 cases of meningococcal disease occur on college campuses each year, and five to 15 students will die as a result. Evidence shows approximately 70 to 80 percent of cases in the college age group are caused by serogroup C, Y, or W-135, which are potentially vaccine-preventable.

Vaccination Recommendations for College Students

Because disease rates begin to climb earlier in adolescence and peak between the ages of 15 and 20 years, the vaccine is also recommended for all adolescents 11 through 18 years of age.

The American College Health Association (ACHA) recommends all first-year students living in residence halls receive the meningococcal vaccine. The ACHA recommendations further state that other college students under 25 years of age may choose to receive meningococcal vaccination to reduce their risk for the disease.

These recommendations, coupled with ample supply of a vaccine that may provide longer duration of protection, will help increase rates of immunization against meningococcal disease and will give college health professionals the guidance needed to help protect college students against meningococcal disease.

Meningococcal Disease Caused by Five Strains/Serogroups

Five predominant strains or serogroups of *N. meningitidis* account for most cases of meningococcal disease. These are A, B, C, Y, and W-135. The currently available vaccine protects against four of the five strains (A, C, Y, and W-135), and evidence shows approximately 70 to 80 percent of cases in the college age group are caused by serogroup C, Y or W-135, which are potentially vaccine-preventable. No vaccine is available for widespread vaccination against serogroup B.

Transmission and Symptoms of the Disease

Meningococcal disease is contagious and progresses very rapidly. The bacteria are spread person-to-person through the air by respiratory droplets (for example, coughing, sneezing). The bacteria also can be transmitted through direct contact with an infected person, such as kissing.

Meningococcal bacteria attach to the mucosal lining of the nose and throat, where they can multiply. When the bacteria penetrate the mucosal lining and enter the bloodstream, they move quickly throughout the body and can cause damage to various organs.

Many people in a population can be a carrier of meningococcal bacteria (up to 11 percent) in the nose and back of the throat, and usually nothing happens to a person other than acquiring natural antibodies.

Symptoms of meningococcal disease often resemble those of the flu or other minor febrile illness, making it sometimes difficult to diagnose, and may include high fever, severe headache, stiff neck, rash, nausea, vomiting, fatigue, and confusion. Students who notice these symptoms—in themselves, friends, or others—especially if the symptoms are unusually sudden or severe, should contact their college health center or local hospital.

If not treated early, meningitis can lead to death or permanent disabilities. One in five of those who survive will suffer from long-term side effects, such as brain damage, hearing loss, seizures, or limb amputation.

Persons at Risk for the Disease, Including College Students

Meningococcal disease can affect people at any age. Infants are at the highest risk for getting the disease. Disease rates fall through later childhood but begin to rise again in early adolescence, peaking between the ages of 15 and 20 years.

Due to lifestyle factors, such as crowded living situations, bar patronage, active or passive smoking, irregular sleep patterns, and sharing of personal items, college students living in residence halls are more likely to acquire meningococcal disease than the general college population.

Prior to 1971, military recruits experienced high rates of meningococcal disease, particularly serotype C disease. The United States military now routinely vaccinates new recruits. Since the initiation of routine vaccination of recruits, there has been an 87 percent reduction in sporadic cases and a virtual elimination of outbreaks of invasive meningococcal disease in the military.

In addition to increased risk because of crowded living situations, proximity to a person diagnosed with disease (being a household contact) also increases one's risk of disease. Other factors also increase risk, such as a compromised immune system (which might be caused by human immunodeficiency virus/acquired immunodeficiency syndrome [HIV/AIDS] or taking certain chemotherapy or immuno-suppressants) or having no spleen. Even something as simple as a respiratory tract infection may increase the risk of getting the disease. Certain genetic risk factors also may increase susceptibility to infection.

Vaccination to Prevent Meningococcal Disease

Meningococcal vaccination is recommended for all first-year students living in residence halls to protect against four of the five most common strains (or types) of *N. meningitidis* (A, C, Y, and W-135). In persons 15 to 24 years of age, 70 to 80 percent of cases are caused by potentially vaccine-preventable strains. All other college students younger than 25 who wish to reduce their risk of infection may choose to be vaccinated.

Because disease rates begin to climb earlier in adolescence and peak between the ages of 15 and 20 years, the vaccine is recommended for all adolescents 11 through 18 years of age.

Chapter 33

Methicillin-Resistant
Staphylococcus Aureus
(MRSA)

History

The *Staphylococcus aureus* (*S. aureus*) bacterium, commonly known as staph, was discovered in the 1880s. During this era, *S. aureus* infection commonly caused painful skin and soft tissue conditions such as boils, scalded-skin syndrome, and impetigo. More serious forms of *S. aureus* infection can progress to bacterial pneumonia and bacteria in the bloodstream—both of which can be fatal. *S. aureus* acquired from improperly prepared or stored food can also cause a form of food poisoning

In the 1940s, medical treatment for *S. aureus* infections became routine and successful with the discovery and introduction of antibiotic medication, such as penicillin. From that point on, however, use of antibiotics—including misuse and overuse—has aided natural bacterial evolution by helping the microbes become resistant to drugs designed to help fight these infections.

In the late 1940s and throughout the 1950s, *S. aureus* developed resistance to penicillin. Methicillin, a form of penicillin, was introduced to counter the increasing problem of penicillin-resistant *S. aureus*. Methicillin was one of most common types of antibiotics used

Excerpted from "Methicillin-Resistant *Staphylococcus aureus* (MRSA): History, Diagnosis, and Prevention," National Institute of Allergy and Infectious Diseases (NIAID), March 5, 2008; and "Methicillin-Resistant *Staphylococcus aureus* (MRSA): Transmission and Treatment," NIAID, July 7, 2009.

to treat *S. aureus* infections; but, in 1961, British scientists identified the first strains of *S. aureus* bacteria that resisted methicillin. This was the so-called birth of methicillin-resistant *Staphylococcus aureus* (MRSA).

The first reported human case of MRSA in the United States came in 1968. Subsequently, new strains of bacteria have developed that can now resist previously effective drugs, such as methicillin and most related antibiotics. MRSA is actually resistant to an entire class of penicillin-like antibiotics called beta-lactams. This class of antibiotics includes penicillin, amoxicillin, oxacillin, methicillin, and others.

S. aureus is evolving even more and has begun to show resistance to additional antibiotics. In 2002, physicians in the United States documented the first *S. aureus* strains resistant to the antibiotic, vancomycin, which had been one of a handful of antibiotics of last resort for use against *S. aureus*. Though it is feared that this could quickly become a major issue in antibiotic resistance, thus far, vancomycin-resistant strains are still rare at this time.

MRSA Transmission

Today, *S. aureus* has evolved to the point where experts refer to MRSA in terms ranging from a considerable public health burden to a crisis. The bacteria have been classified into two categories based on where infection is first acquired.

Hospital-Acquired (HA)-MRSA

HA-MRSA has been recognized for decades and primarily affects people in health care settings, such as those who have had surgery or medical devices surgically implanted. This source of MRSA is typically problematic for the elderly, for people with weakened immune systems, and for patients undergoing kidney dialysis or using venous catheters or prosthetics.

A study published in 2005 found that nearly one percent of all hospital inpatient stays, or 292,045 per year, were associated with *S. aureus* infection. The study reviewed nearly 14 million patient discharge diagnoses from 2000 and 2001. Patients with diagnoses of *S. aureus* infection, when compared with those without the infection, had about three times the length of stay, three times the total cost, and five times the risk of in-hospital death. Notably, the *S. aureus* infections in this hospital study resulted in 14,000 deaths.

Community-Associated (CA)-MRSA

CA-MRSA has only been known since the 1990s. CA-MRSA is of great concern to public health professionals because of who it can affect. Unlike the hospital sources, which usually can be traced to a specific exposure, the origin of CA-MRSA infection can be elusive. CA-MRSA skin infections are known to spread in crowded settings; in situations where there is close skin-to-skin contact; when personal items such as towels, razors, and sporting equipment is shared; when personal hygiene is compromised; and when health care is limited.

Outbreaks of CA-MRSA have involved bacterial strains with specific microbiologic and genetic differences from traditional HA-MRSA strains, and these differences suggest that community strains might spread more easily from person to person than HA-MRSA. While CA-MRSA is resistant to penicillin and methicillin, they can still be treated with other common-use antibiotics.

CA-MRSA most often enters the body through a cut or scrape and appears in the form of a skin or soft tissue infection, such as a boil or abscess. The involved site is red, swollen, and painful and is often mistaken for a spider bite. Though rare, CA-MRSA can develop into more serious invasive infections, such as bloodstream infections or pneumonia, leading to a variety of other symptoms including shortness of breath, fever, chills, and death. CA-MRSA can be particularly dangerous in children because their immune systems are not fully developed. You should pay attention to minor skin problems—pimples, insect bites, cuts, and scrapes—especially in children. If the wound appears to be infected, see a health care provider.

Researchers continue to study information about these cases in an attempt to determine why certain groups of people become ill when exposed to these strains. Researchers also continue to try to understand why high-incidence areas may appear. For example, for unknown reasons, severe outbreaks have occurred in Alaska, Georgia, and Louisiana.

MRSA Diagnosis

To diagnose *S. aureus*, a sample is obtained from the infection site and sent to a microbiology laboratory for testing. If *S. aureus* is found, the organism should be further tested to determine which antibiotic would be effective for treatment.

Doctors often diagnose MRSA by checking a tissue sample or nasal secretions for signs of drug-resistant bacteria. Current diagnostic procedures involve sending a sample to a lab where it is placed in a dish of nutrients that encourage bacterial growth (a culture). It takes about 48 hours for the bacteria to grow. However, newer tests that can detect staph deoxyribonucleic acid (DNA) in a matter of hours are now becoming more widely available. This will help health care providers decide on the proper treatment regimen for a patient more quickly, after an official diagnosis has been made.

In the hospital, you might be tested for MRSA if you show signs of infection, or if you are transferred to a hospital from another health care setting where MRSA is known to be present. You also might be tested if you have had a previous history of MRSA.

MRSA Treatment

Health care providers can treat many *S. aureus* skin infections by draining the abscess or boil and may not need to use antibiotics. Draining of skin boils or abscesses should only be done by a health care provider. For mild to moderate skin infections, incision and drainage by a health care provider is the first-line treatment. Before prescribing antibiotics, your provider will consider the potential for antibiotic resistance. Thus, if MRSA is suspected, your provider will avoid treating you with beta-lactam antibiotics, a class of antibiotic observed not to be effective in killing the staph bacteria. For severe infection, doctors will typically use vancomycin intravenously.

MRSA Prevention

The best defense against spreading MRSA is to practice good hygiene, as follows:

- Keep your hands clean by washing thoroughly with soap and water. Scrub them briskly for at least 15 seconds, then dry them with a disposable towel and use another towel to turn off the faucet. When you don't have access to soap and water, carry a small bottle of hand sanitizer containing at least 62 percent alcohol.

- Always shower promptly after exercising.

- Keep cuts and scrapes clean and covered with a bandage until healed. Keep wounds that are draining or have pus covered with clean, dry bandages. Follow your health care provider's instructions on proper care of the wound. Pus from infected wounds can contain *S. aureus* and MRSA, so keeping the infection covered will help prevent the spread to others. Bandages or tape can be discarded with regular trash.

- Avoid contact with other people's wounds or bandages.

- Avoid sharing personal items, such as towels, washcloths, razors, clothes, or uniforms.

- Wash sheets, towels, and clothes that become soiled with water and laundry detergent; use bleach and hot water if possible. Drying clothes in a hot dryer, rather than air-drying helps to kill bacteria in clothes.

Tell any health care providers who treat you if you have or had an *S. aureus* or MRSA skin infection. If you have a skin infection that requires treatment, ask your health care provider if you should be tested for MRSA. Many health care providers prescribe drugs that are not effective against antibiotic-resistant staph, which delays treatment and creates more resistant germs.

Health care providers are fighting back against MRSA infection by tracking bacterial outbreaks and by investing in products, such as antibiotic-coated catheters and gloves that release disinfectants.

Chapter 34

Mumps

What is mumps?

It is an infection caused by the mumps virus.

Who can get mumps?

Anyone who is not immune from either previous mumps infection or from vaccination can get mumps. Before the routine vaccination program was introduced in the United States, mumps was a common illness in infants, children, and young adults. Because most people have now been vaccinated, mumps is now a rare disease in the United States. Of those people who do get mumps, up to half have very mild, or no symptoms, and therefore do not know they were infected with mumps.

What are the symptoms of mumps?

The most common symptoms are fever, headache, muscle aches, tiredness, and loss of appetite followed by onset of parotitis (swollen and tender salivary glands under the ears—on one or both sides).

This chapter includes text from "Mumps: Q and A about the Disease," Centers for Disease Control and Prevention (CDC), April 17, 2006; and "CDC Health Information for International Travel 2010 (Yellow Book): Chapter 2: Mumps," CDC, 2009.

Are there complications of mumps?

The most common complication is the inflammation of the testicles (orchitis) in males who have reached puberty, but rarely does this lead to fertility problems.

Other rare complications include the following:

- Inflammation of the brain and/or tissue covering the brain and spinal cord (encephalitis/meningitis)

- Inflammation of the ovaries (oophoritis) and/or breasts (mastitis) in females who have reached puberty

- Spontaneous abortion particularly in early pregnancy (miscarriage)

- Deafness, usually permanent

How soon do symptoms appear?

Symptoms typically appear 16–18 days after infection, but this period can range from 12–25 after infection.

How is mumps spread?

Mumps is spread by mucus or droplets from the nose or throat of an infected person, usually when a person coughs or sneezes. Surfaces of items (such as toys) can also spread the virus if someone who is sick touches them without washing their hands, and someone else then touches the same surface and then rubs their eyes, mouth, or nose (this is called fomite transmission).

How long is an infected person able to spread the disease?

Mumps virus has been found in respiratory secretions seven days before until eight days after onset of parotitis. The highest isolation rates (~90%) occur closest to parotitis onset and decline rapidly thereafter. Most mumps transmission likely occurs before parotitis onset and within the subsequent five days. Transmission may also occur from persons who are not isolated including during the prodromal phase and from subclinical infections. Therefore, the Centers for Disease Control and Prevention (CDC) now recommends a five-day period after parotitis onset for isolation of mumps case-patients in community and health care settings and for use of standard and droplet precautions. (Updated July 13, 2009)

How long should a person with mumps be isolated?

CDC recommends isolation of mumps patients for five days after onset of parotitis. (Updated July 13, 2009)

What is the treatment for mumps?

There is no specific treatment. Supportive care should be given as needed. If someone becomes very ill, they should seek medical attention. If someone seeks medical attention, they should call their doctor in advance so that they don't have to sit in the waiting room for a long time and possibly infect other patients.

How do I protect myself (my kids/my family)?

Mumps vaccine (usually measles, mumps, rubella [MMR] vaccine), is the best way to prevent mumps. Other things people can do to prevent mumps and other infections is to wash hands well and often with soap, and to teach children to wash their hands too. Eating utensils should not be shared, and surfaces that are frequently touched (toys, doorknobs, tables, counters, and so forth) should also be regularly cleaned with soap and water, or with cleaning wipes.

Yellow Book Information about Mumps

Occurrence

- With the exception of the multistate outbreak in 2006, mumps is an uncommon disease in the United States because of a successful vaccination program.

- Mumps virus remains endemic in many countries throughout the world because mumps vaccine is used in only 57% of the World Health Organization member countries.

Risk for Travelers

The risk of exposure to mumps among travelers can be high in most countries of the world, especially for travelers less than 12 months of age who do not have evidence of mumps immunity. Although some countries have had variable successes with a national vaccination program—including Finland, which has declared elimination—the risk of contacting imported mumps in these countries is still a concern.

Diagnosis

• Mumps may occur in epidemics; mumps virus is the only cause of epidemic parotitis.

• Diagnosis is usually clinical, based on the presence of parotitis and associated signs, symptoms, or complications.

• Clinical case definition: An illness with acute onset of unilateral or bilateral tender, self-limited swelling of the parotid glands, other salivary gland(s), or both, lasting at least two days, and without other apparent cause.

Preventive Measures for Travelers

• Although vaccination against mumps is not a requirement for entry into any country (including the United States), travelers leaving the United States or living abroad should ensure they are immune to mumps.

• Mumps vaccine contains live, attenuated mumps virus. It is available as a monovalent formulation and in combination formulations, such as MMR. Combined MMR vaccine is recommended whenever one or more of the individual components is indicated to provide optimal protection against measles and rubella. Mumps vaccine is highly, but not 100%, effective in preventing mumps. One dose of mumps vaccine is approximately 80%–85% effective in preventing clinical mumps with parotitis, and two doses are approximately 90% effective.

• Mumps vaccine has not been demonstrated to be effective in preventing infection after exposure; however, it can be administered postexposure to provide protection against subsequent exposures. Immune globulin is not effective in preventing mumps infection following an exposure and is not recommended.

Chapter 35

Non-Polio Enterovirus

What are enteroviruses?

Enteroviruses are small viruses that are made of ribonucleic acid (RNA) and protein. This group includes the polioviruses, coxsackieviruses, echoviruses, and other enteroviruses. In addition to the three different polioviruses, there are 62 non-polio enteroviruses that can cause disease in humans: 23 Coxsackie A viruses, 6 Coxsackie B viruses, 28 echoviruses, and five other enteroviruses.

How common are infections with these viruses?

Non-polio enteroviruses are very common. They are second only to the common cold viruses, the rhinoviruses, as the most common viral infectious agents in humans. The enteroviruses cause an estimated 10–15 million or more symptomatic infections a year in the United States. All three types of polioviruses have been eliminated from the Western Hemisphere, as well as Western Pacific and European regions, by the widespread use of vaccines.

Who is at risk of infection and illness from these viruses?

Everyone is at risk of infection. Infants, children, and adolescents are more likely to be susceptible to infection and illness from these

"Non-Polio Enterovirus Infections," Centers for Disease Control and Prevention (CDC), September 5, 2006.

viruses, because they are less likely to have antibodies and be immune from previous exposures to them, but adults can also become infected and ill if they do not have immunity to a specific enterovirus.

How does someone become infected with one of these viruses?

Enteroviruses can be found in the respiratory secretions (saliva, sputum, or nasal mucus) and stool of an infected person. Other persons may become infected by direct contact with secretions from an infected person or by contact with contaminated surfaces or objects, such as a drinking glass or telephone. Parents, teachers, and childcare center workers may also become infected by contamination of the hands with stool from an infected infant or toddler during diaper changes.

What time of year is someone at risk for infection/illness?

In the United States, infections caused by the enteroviruses are most likely to occur during the summer and fall.

What illnesses do these viruses cause?

Most people who are infected with an enterovirus have no disease at all. Infected persons who become ill usually develop mild upper respiratory symptoms (a summer cold), a flu-like illness with fever and muscle aches, or an illness with rash. Less commonly, some persons have aseptic or viral meningitis. Rarely, a person may develop an illness that affects the heart (myocarditis) or the brain (encephalitis) or causes paralysis. Enterovirus infections are suspected to play a role in the development of juvenile-onset diabetes mellitus (sugar diabetes). Newborns infected with an enterovirus may rarely develop severe illness and die from infection.

Are there any long-term complications from these illnesses?

Usually, there are no long-term complications from the mild illnesses or from aseptic meningitis. Some patients who have paralysis or encephalitis, however, do not fully recover. Persons who develop heart failure (dilated cardiomyopathy) from myocarditis require long-term care for their conditions.

What are the risks of enterovirus infections in pregnancy?

Because enteroviruses are very common, pregnant women are frequently exposed to them, especially during summer and fall months.

As for any other adults, the risk of infection is higher for pregnant women who do not have antibodies from earlier exposures to enteroviruses currently circulating in the community, and are exposed to young children—the primary spreaders of these viruses.

Most enterovirus infections during pregnancy cause mild or no illness in the mother. Although the available information is limited, currently there is no clear evidence that maternal enteroviral infection causes adverse outcomes of pregnancy such as abortion, stillbirth, or congenital defects. However, mothers infected shortly before delivery, may pass the virus to the newborn. Babies born to mothers who have symptoms of enteroviral illness around the time of delivery are more likely to be infected. Newborns infected with an enterovirus usually have mild illness, but rarely they may develop an overwhelming infection of many organs, including liver and heart, and die from the infection. The risk of this severe illness is higher for the newborns infected during the first two weeks of life.

Strict adherence to generally recommended good hygienic practices by pregnant women may help to decrease the risk of infection during pregnancy and around the time of delivery.

Are these infections more severe in some years than in others?

There are no predictable patterns of circulation of these viruses or of diseases such as aseptic meningitis. There are occasional national or regional outbreaks of aseptic meningitis, such as the echovirus 30 outbreaks in the United States between 1989 and 1992 and in 2003, and echovirus 13 and echovirus 18 outbreaks in 2001. However, there is significant yearly variation, and no long-term trends have been identified.

Can these infections be prevented?

No vaccine is currently available for the non-polio enteroviruses. Because most persons who are infected with enteroviruses do not become sick, it can be difficult to prevent the spread of the virus. General cleanliness and frequent handwashing are probably effective in reducing the spread of these viruses. Also, cleaning contaminated surfaces and soiled articles first with soap and water, and then disinfecting them with a dilute solution of chlorine-containing bleach (made by mixing approximately ¼ cup of bleach with one gallon of water) can be a very effective way to inactivate the virus, especially in institutional settings such as child care centers.

Do the Centers for Disease Control and Prevention (CDC) and state health departments keep track of these viruses?

State health department laboratories report to CDC the enteroviruses they identify by testing specimens from patients. Aseptic meningitis is no longer a nationally notifiable disease in the United States. Other forms of meningitis and poliomyelitis are notifiable, which means that any doctor or laboratory that diagnoses a case must report it to the public health department.

Chapter 36

Norovirus

What are noroviruses?

Noroviruses are a group of viruses that cause the stomach flu, or gastroenteritis (GAS-tro-en-ter-I-tis), in people. The term norovirus was recently approved as the official name for this group of viruses. Several other names have been used for noroviruses, including:

- Norwalk-like viruses (NLVs),
- caliciviruses (because they belong to the virus family *Caliciviridae*), and
- small round structured viruses.

Viruses are very different from bacteria and parasites, some of which can cause illnesses similar to norovirus infection. Like all viral infections, noroviruses are not affected by treatment with antibiotics, and cannot grow outside of a person's body.

What are the symptoms of illness caused by noroviruses?

The symptoms of norovirus illness usually include nausea, vomiting, diarrhea, and some stomach cramping. Sometimes people additionally have a low-grade fever, chills, headache, muscle aches, and a general sense of tiredness. The illness often begins suddenly, and the

Text in this chapter is from "Norovirus: Q and A," Centers for Disease Control and Prevention (CDC), August 3, 2006.

infected person may feel very sick. In most people the illness is self-limiting with symptoms lasting for about one or two days. In general, children experience more vomiting than adults.

What is the name of the illness caused by noroviruses?

Illness caused by norovirus infection has several names, including the following:

- Stomach flu: This "stomach flu" is not related to the flu (or influenza), which is a respiratory illness caused by influenza virus

- Viral gastroenteritis: The most common name for illness caused by norovirus (Gastroenteritis refers to an inflammation of the stomach and intestines.)

- Acute gastroenteritis

- Non-bacterial gastroenteritis

- Food poisoning (although there are other causes of food poisoning)

- Calicivirus infection

How serious is norovirus disease?

People may feel very sick and vomit many times a day, but most people get better within one or two days, and they have no long-term health effects related to their illness. However, sometimes people are unable to drink enough liquids to replace the liquids they lost because of vomiting and diarrhea. These persons can become dehydrated (lose too much water from their body) and may need special medical attention. During norovirus infection, this problem with dehydration is usually only seen among the very young, the elderly, and people with other illness.

How do people become infected with noroviruses?

Noroviruses are found in the stool or vomit of infected people. People can become infected with the virus in several ways, including:

- eating food or drinking liquids that are contaminated with norovirus;

- touching surfaces or objects contaminated with norovirus, and then placing their hand in their mouth; or

- having direct contact with another person who is infected and showing symptoms (for example, when caring for someone with illness, or sharing foods or eating utensils with someone who is ill).

Persons working in daycare centers or nursing homes should pay special attention to children or residents who have norovirus illness. This virus is very contagious and can spread rapidly throughout such environments.

When do symptoms appear?

Symptoms of norovirus illness usually begin about 24 to 48 hours after ingestion of the virus, but they can appear as early as 12 hours after exposure.

Are noroviruses contagious?

Noroviruses are very contagious and can spread easily from person to person. Both stool and vomit are infectious. Particular care should be taken with young children in diapers who may have diarrhea.

How long are people contagious?

People infected with norovirus are contagious from the moment they begin feeling ill to at least three days after recovery. Some people may be contagious for as long as two weeks after recovery. Therefore, it is particularly important for people to use good handwashing and other hygienic practices after they have recently recovered from norovirus illness.

Who gets norovirus infection?

Anyone can become infected with these viruses. There are many different strains of norovirus, which makes it difficult for a person's body to develop long-lasting immunity. Therefore, norovirus illness can recur throughout a person's lifetime. In addition, because of differences in genetic factors, some people are more likely to become infected and develop more severe illness than others.

Is there a treatment for norovirus infection?

There is no vaccine to prevent norovirus infection. And there is no drug to treat people who are infected with the virus. Antibiotic drugs will not help if you have norovirus infection. This is because they fight against bacteria not viruses.

Norovirus illness is usually brief in people who are otherwise healthy. But, the infection can cause severe vomiting and diarrhea. This can lead to dehydration (loss of too much water from the body). During norovirus infection, young children, the elderly, and people with other illnesses are most at risk for dehydration. Symptoms of dehydration in adults and children include a decrease in urination, a dry mouth and throat, and feeling dizzy when standing up. A dehydrated child may also cry with few or no tears and be unusually sleepy or fussy.

Dehydration can lead to other serious problems. And severe dehydration may require hospitalization for treatment with intravenous (IV) fluids. Thus it is important to prevent dehydration during norovirus illness. The best way to protect against dehydration is to drink plenty of liquids. The most helpful fluids for this purpose are oral rehydration fluids (ORF). Other drinks that do not contain caffeine or alcohol can also help with mild dehydration. However, these drinks may not replace important nutrients and minerals lost due to vomiting and diarrhea.

Severe dehydration can be serious. If you think you or someone you are caring for is severely dehydrated, contact your health care provider.

Can norovirus infections be prevented?

You can decrease your chance of coming in contact with noroviruses by following these preventive steps:

- Frequently wash your hands, especially after toilet visits and changing diapers and before eating or preparing food.

- Carefully wash fruits and vegetables, and steam oysters before eating them.

- Thoroughly clean and disinfect contaminated surfaces immediately after an episode of illness by using a bleach-based household cleaner.

- Immediately remove and wash clothing or linens that may be contaminated with virus after an episode of illness (use hot water and soap).

- Flush or discard any vomitus and/or stool in the toilet and make sure that the surrounding area is kept clean.

Persons who are infected with norovirus should not prepare food while they have symptoms and for three days after they recover from their illness. Food that may have been contaminated by an ill person should be disposed of properly.

Chapter 37

Pinworms

Alternative Names

Alternative Names

Enterobiasis; oxyuriasis; threadworm; seatworm; *Enterobius vermicularis*; *E vermicularis*; helminthic infection

Definition

Pinworms are small worms that infect the intestines.

Causes

Pinworms are the most common worm infection in the United States. They are most common in school-age children.

Pinworm eggs are spread directly from person to person. They can also be spread by touching bedding, food, or other items contaminated with the eggs.

Typically, children are infected by unknowingly touching pinworm eggs and putting their fingers in their mouths. The eggs are swallowed, and eventually hatch in the small intestine. The worms mature in the colon.

Female worms then move to the child's anal area, especially at night, and deposit more eggs. This may cause intense itching. The area may even become infected. When the child scratches the itching anal area, the eggs can get under the child's fingernails. These eggs can

---

"Pinworms," © 2009 A.D.A.M., Inc. Reprinted with permission.

be transferred to other children, family members, and items in the house.

Symptoms

- Difficulty sleeping due to the itching that occurs during the night
- Intense itching around the anus
- Irritability due to itching and interrupted sleep
- Irritated or infected skin around the anus, from constant scratching
- Irritation or discomfort of the vagina in young girls (if an adult worm enters the vagina rather than the anus)
- Loss of appetite and weight (uncommon, but can occur in severe infections)

Exams and Tests

Pinworms can be spotted in the anal area, especially at night when the worms lay their eggs there.

Your doctor may have you do a tape test. A piece of cellophane tape is pressed against the skin around the anus, and removed. This should be done in the morning before bathing or using the toilet, because bathing and wiping may remove eggs. The doctor will stick the tape to a slide and look for eggs using a microscope.

Treatment

The main treatment is a single dose of either mebendazole or albendazole (anti-parasitic medication). These are available over-the-counter and by prescription.

More than one household member is likely to be infected, so the entire household is often treated. The single-dose treatment is often repeated after two weeks. This treats eggs that hatched since the first treatment.

To control the eggs:

- Clean toilet seats daily
- Keep fingernails short and clean
- Wash all bed linens twice a week
- Wash hands before meals and after using the toilet

Avoid scratching the infected area around the anus. This can contaminate your fingers and everything else that you touch afterwards.

Keep your hands and fingers away from your nose and mouth unless they are freshly washed. Carry out these measures while family members are being treated for pinworms.

Outlook (Prognosis)

Pinworm infection is fully treatable.

Possible Complications

- Pelvic inflammatory disease
- Repeated infection with the parasite (re-infestation)
- Vaginitis

When to Contact a Medical Professional

Call for an appointment with your health care provider if:

- you or your child has symptoms of pinworm infection; or
- you have seen pinworms on your child.

Prevention

Wash hands after using the bathroom and before preparing food. Wash bedding and underclothing frequently, especially those of any affected family members.

Chapter 38

Pneumonia

Overview

Pneumonia is an infection in one or both of the lungs. Many small germs, such as bacteria, viruses, and fungi, can cause pneumonia. The infection causes your lungs' air sacs, called alveoli, to become inflamed. The air sacs may fill up with fluid or pus, causing symptoms such as a cough (with phlegm), fever, chills, and trouble breathing.

Pneumonia and its symptoms can vary from mild to severe. Many factors affect how serious pneumonia is, such as the type of germ causing the infection and your age and overall health.

Pneumonia tends to be more serious for:

- infants and young children.;

- older adults (people 65 years or older);

- people who have other health problems like heart failure, diabetes, or chronic obstructive pulmonary disease (COPD);

- people who have weak immune systems as a result of diseases or other factors, such as human immunodeficiency virus/acquired immunodeficiency syndrome (HIV/AIDS), chemotherapy, or an organ or bone marrow transplant.

Pneumonia is common in the United States. Treatment for pneumonia depends on its cause, how severe symptoms are, and age and overall

Excerpted from "Pneumonia," National Heart, Lung, and Blood Institute (NHLBI), August 2008.

health. Many people can be treated at home, often with oral antibiotics. Children usually start to feel better in one to two days. For adults, it usually takes two to three days. Anyone whose symptoms get worse should be checked by a doctor. People who have more severe symptoms or underlying health problems may need treatment in a hospital. It may take three weeks or more before they can go back to their normal routines. Fatigue (tiredness) from pneumonia can last for a month or more.

Types of Pneumonia

Pneumonia is named for the way in which a person gets the infection or for the germ that causes it.

Community-Acquired Pneumonia

Community-acquired pneumonia (CAP) occurs outside of hospitals and other health care settings. Most people get CAP by breathing in germs (especially while sleeping) that live in the mouth, nose, or throat. CAP is the most common type of pneumonia. Most cases occur during the winter. About four million people get this form of pneumonia each year. About one out of every five people who has CAP needs to be treated in a hospital.

Hospital-Acquired Pneumonia

Some people catch pneumonia during a hospital stay for another illness. This is called hospital-acquired pneumonia (HAP). You're at higher risk for getting HAP if you're on a mechanical ventilator (a machine that helps you breathe). HAP tends to be more serious than CAP. This is because you're already sick. Also, hospitals tend to have more germs that are resistant to antibiotics—a treatment for pneumonia.

Health Care-Associated Pneumonia

Patients also may get pneumonia in other health care settings, such as nursing homes, dialysis centers, and outpatient clinics. This is called health care-associated pneumonia.

Other Common Types of Pneumonia

Aspiration Pneumonia

This type of pneumonia occurs when you accidentally inhale food, drink, vomit, or saliva from your mouth into your lungs. This usually happens when something disturbs your normal gag reflex, such as a brain injury, swallowing problem, or excessive use of alcohol or drugs.

Aspiration pneumonia can cause pus to form in a cavity in the lung. This is called a lung abscess.

Atypical Pneumonia

Several types of bacteria—*Legionella pneumophila, mycoplasma pneumonia,* and *Chlamydia pneumoniae*—cause this type of CAP. Atypical pneumonia is passed from person to person.

Other Names for Pneumonia

- Pneumonitis
- Bronchopneumonia
- Nosocomial pneumonia—another name for hospital-acquired pneumonia
- Walking pneumonia—a pneumonia that's mild enough that you're not bedridden
- Double pneumonia—a pneumonia that affects both lobes of the lungs

What Causes Pneumonia?

Many different germs can cause pneumonia. These include different kinds of bacteria, viruses, and, less often, fungi. Most of the time, the body filters germs out of the air that we breathe to protect the lungs from infection. Sometimes, though, germs manage to enter the lungs and cause infections. This is more likely to occur when:

- your immune system is weak,
- a germ is very strong, and
- your body fails to filter germs out of the air that you breathe.

Your mouth and airways are exposed to germs as you inhale air through your nose and mouth. Your immune system, the shape of your nose and throat, your ability to cough, and fine, hair-like structures called cilia help stop the germs from reaching your lungs. For example, coughing is one way the body keeps germs from reaching the lungs. Some people may not be able to cough because, for example, they've had a stroke or are sedated (given medicine to make them sleepy). This means germs may remain in the airways rather than being coughed out. When germs do reach your lungs, your immune system goes into action. It sends many kinds of cells to attack the germs. These cells cause the alveoli (air sacs) to become red and inflamed and to fill up with fluid and pus. This causes the symptoms of pneumonia.

Germs That Can Cause Pneumonia

Bacteria

Bacteria are the most common cause of pneumonia in adults. Some people, especially the elderly and those who are disabled, may get bacterial pneumonia after having the flu or even a common cold. Dozens of different types of bacteria can cause pneumonia. Bacterial pneumonia can occur on its own or develop after you've had a cold or the flu. This type of pneumonia often affects one lobe, or area, of a lung. When this happens, the condition is called lobar pneumonia. The most common cause of pneumonia in the United States is the bacterium *Streptococcus pneumoniae*, or *pneumococcus*.

Another type of bacterial pneumonia is called atypical pneumonia. Atypical pneumonia includes the following:

- *Legionella pneumophila:* This is sometimes called Legionnaires disease. This type of pneumonia has caused serious outbreaks. Outbreaks have been linked to exposure to cooling towers, whirlpool spas, and decorative fountains.

- *Mycoplasma pneumonia*: This is a common type of pneumonia that usually affects people younger than 40. People who live or work in crowded places like schools, homeless shelters, and prisons are most likely to get it. It's usually mild and responds well to treatment with antibiotics. But, it can be very serious in some people. It may be associated with a skin rash and hemolysis (the breakdown of red blood cells).

- *Chlamydia pneumoniae*: This kind of pneumonia can occur all year and is often mild. The infection is most common in people 65 to 79 years of age.

Viruses

Respiratory viruses cause up to one-third of the pneumonia cases in the United States each year. These viruses are the most common cause of pneumonia in children younger than five years. Most cases of viral pneumonia are mild. They get better in about 1–3 weeks without treatment. Some cases are more serious and may require treatment in a hospital. If you have viral pneumonia, you run the risk of getting bacterial pneumonia also.

The flu virus is the most common cause of viral pneumonia in adults. Other viruses that cause pneumonia include respiratory syncytial virus, rhinovirus, herpes simplex virus, severe acute respiratory syndrome (SARS), and more.

Fungi

Three types of fungi in the soil in some parts of the United States can cause pneumonia. These fungi are coccidioidomycosis in Southern California and the desert Southwest, histoplasmosis in the Ohio and Mississippi River Valleys, and cryptococcus. Most people exposed to these fungi don't get sick, but some do and require treatment.

Serious fungal infections are most common in people who have weak immune systems as a result of long-term use of medicines to suppress their immune systems or having HIV/AIDS. *Pneumocystis jirovecii*, formerly *Pneumocystis carinii*, is sometimes considered a fungal pneumonia. However, it's not treated with the usual antifungal medicines. It usually affects people who:

- have HIV/AIDS or cancer,
- have had an organ and/or bone marrow transplant, or
- take medicines that affect their immune systems.

Other kinds of fungal infections also can lead to pneumonia.

Signs and Symptoms of Pneumonia

The symptoms of pneumonia vary from mild to severe. Many factors affect how serious pneumonia is, including the type of germ causing the infection and your age and overall health. See your doctor promptly if you:

- have a high fever;
- have shaking chills;
- have a cough with phlegm, which doesn't improve or worsens;
- develop shortness of breath with normal daily activities;
- have chest pain when you breathe or cough; or
- feel suddenly worse after a cold or the flu.

People with pneumonia may have other symptoms, including nausea (feeling sick to your stomach), vomiting, and diarrhea. Symptoms may vary in certain populations.

Complications of Pneumonia

Often, people who have pneumonia can be treated successfully and not have complications. But some patients, especially those in high-risk groups, may have complications such as:

- Bacteremia: This serious complication occurs when the infection moves into your bloodstream. From there, it can quickly spread to other organs, including your brain.

- Lung abscess: An abscess occurs when pus forms in a cavity in the lung. An abscess usually is treated with antibiotics. In some cases, surgery or needle drainage is needed to remove it.

- Pleural effusion: Pneumonia may cause fluid to build up in the pleural space, which is the space between your lungs and chest wall. Pneumonia can cause the fluid to become infected—a condition called empyema. If this happens, you may need to have the fluid drained through a chest tube or removed through surgery.

Diagnosing Pneumonia

Pneumonia can be hard to diagnose because it may seem like a cold or the flu. People may not realize it's more serious until it lasts longer than these other conditions. Your doctor will diagnose pneumonia based on your medical history and the results from a physical exam and tests which may include:

- chest x ray,
- blood tests,
- sputum test,
- chest computed tomography (CT) scan,
- pleural fluid culture,
- pulse oximetry, and
- bronchoscopy.

Pneumonia Treatment

Treatment for pneumonia depends on the type of pneumonia you have and how severe it is. Most people who have community-acquired pneumonia—the most common type of pneumonia—are treated at home. The goals of treatment are to cure the infection and prevent complications.

It's important to follow your treatment plan, take all medicines as prescribed, and get ongoing medical care. Talk to your doctor about when you should schedule follow-up care. Your doctor may want you to have a chest-x-ray to make sure the pneumonia is gone.

Although you may start feeling better after a few days or weeks, fatigue (tiredness) can persist for up to a month or more. People who are treated in the hospital may need at least three weeks before they can go back to their normal routines.

Bacterial pneumonia is treated with antibiotics. You should take antibiotics as your doctor prescribes. You may start to feel better before you finish the medicine, but you should continue taking it as prescribed. If you stop too soon, the pneumonia may come back.

Viral pneumonia isn't treated with antibiotics. This type of medicine doesn't work when a virus causes the pneumonia. If you have viral pneumonia, your doctor may prescribe an antiviral medicine to treat it.

You may need to be treated in a hospital if your symptoms are severe or you are at risk for complications because of health problems.

Preventing Pneumonia

Pneumonia can be very serious and even life threatening. When possible, take steps to prevent the infection, especially if you are in a high-risk group.

Vaccines

Vaccines are available to prevent pneumococcal pneumonia and the flu. Vaccines cannot prevent all cases of infection. However, compared to people who do not get vaccinated, those who do and still get pneumonia tend to have milder cases of the infection, shorter lasting infections, and fewer serious complications.

Pneumococcal Pneumonia Vaccine

A vaccine is available to prevent pneumococcal pneumonia. In most people, one shot is good for at least five years of protection.

Influenza Vaccine

The vaccine that helps prevent the flu is good for one year. It is usually given in October or November, before peak flu season. Because many people get pneumonia after having the flu, this vaccine also helps prevent pneumonia.

Hib Vaccine

Haemophilus influenzae type b (Hib) is a type of bacteria that can cause pneumonia and meningitis (an infection of the covering of the brain and spinal cord). The Hib vaccine is given to children to help prevent these infections. The vaccine is recommended for all children in the United States who are younger than five years. It's often given to infants starting at two months of age.

Other Ways to Help Prevent Pneumonia

- Wash your hands with soap and water or alcohol-based rubs to kill germs.

- Do not smoke. Smoking damages your lungs' ability to filter out and defend against germs.

- Keep your immune system strong. Get plenty of rest and physical activity and follow a healthy diet.

If you have pneumonia, limit contact with family and friends. Cover your nose and mouth while coughing or sneezing, and dispose of tissues right away. These measures help keep the infection from spreading. If you have pneumonia, you can take steps to recover from the infection and prevent complications by doing the following:

- Get plenty of rest.

- Follow the treatment plan your doctor gives you.

- Take all medicines as your doctor prescribes. If you're using antibiotics, continue to take the medicine until it's all gone. You may start to feel better before you finish the medicine, but you should continue to take it. If you stop too soon, the pneumonia may come back.

- Talk to your doctor about when to schedule follow-up care. Your doctor may order a chest x ray to make sure the infection is gone.

It may take time to recover from pneumonia. Some people feel better and are able to return to their normal routines within a week. For other people, it can take a month or more. Most people continue to feel tired for about a month. Talk to your doctor about when you can go back to your normal activities.

Chapter 39

Polio

General Questions

What is polio?

Polio is an infectious disease caused by a virus that lives in the throat and intestinal tract. It is most often spread through person-to-person contact with the stool of an infected person and may also be spread through oral/nasal secretions. Polio used to be very common in the U.S. and caused severe illness in thousands of people each year before polio vaccine was introduced in 1955. Most people infected with the polio virus have no symptoms, however for the less than 1% who develop paralysis it may result in permanent disability and even death.

What are the symptoms of polio?

Up to about 95 percent of people infected with polio have no symptoms. However, infected persons without symptoms can still spread the virus and cause others to develop polio. About four to eight percent of infected persons have minor symptoms such as fever, sore throat, upset stomach, or flu-like symptoms, and have no paralysis or other serious symptoms. About one to two percent of infected persons develop aseptic meningitis with stiffness of the back or legs, and in some persons increased or abnormal sensations. Symptoms typically last from two to ten days, followed by complete recovery. Less than one percent

---

"Vaccines: VPD-VAC/Polio/Disease FAQs," Centers for Disease Control and Prevention (CDC), April 6, 2007.

of polio cases result in paralysis of the limbs (usually the legs). Of those cases resulting in paralysis, 5–10% die when the respiratory muscles are paralyzed. The risk of paralysis increases with age.

How common was polio in the United States?

Polio was one of the most dreaded childhood diseases of the 20th century in the United States. There were usually about 13,000 to 20,000 cases of paralytic polio reported each year in the U.S. before the introduction of Salk inactivated polio vaccine (IPV) in 1955. Polio peaked in 1952 when there were more than 21,000 reported cases. The number of cases of polio decreased dramatically following introduction of the vaccine and the development of a national vaccination program. In 1965, only 61 cases of paralytic polio were reported compared to 2,525 cases reported cases just five years earlier in 1960.

Is polio still a disease seen in the United States?

The last cases of naturally occurring paralytic polio in the United States were in 1979, when an outbreak occurred among the Amish in several Midwestern states. From 1980 through 1999, there were 152 confirmed cases of paralytic polio cases reported. Of the 152 cases, eight cases were acquired outside the United States and imported. The last imported case caused by wild poliovirus into the United States was reported in 1993. The remaining 144 cases were vaccine-associated paralytic polio (VAPP) caused by live oral polio vaccine (OPV).

What kind of polio vaccines are used in the United States?

Inactivated polio vaccine (IPV), which is given as a shot, is now used in the United States. Oral polio vaccine (OPV) has not been used in the United States since 2000 but is still used in many parts of the world.

Vaccine-Derived Poliovirus Related Questions

What is a vaccine-derived poliovirus?

A vaccine-derived poliovirus (VDPV) is a strain of polio virus, initially contained in the live OPV, that has changed over time and behaves more like a wild or naturally-occurring virus. This means it can be more easily spread to others who are unvaccinated against polio and who come in contact with the stool or oral secretions (saliva) of an infected person. These viruses may cause illness, including paralytic poliomyelitis.

Is there a difference in a disease caused by a VDPV and one cause by wild poliovirus or OPV?

No, there is no clinical difference between paralytic polio caused by wild poliovirus, OPV or a VDPV.

I've heard that a child has been found with VDPV. Is this true?

In 2005, a VDPV was found in the stool of an unvaccinated child in the state of Minnesota. The child most likely caught the virus through contact in the community with someone who received live oral vaccine in another country. For questions specifically related to this case visit www.health.state.mn.us/news/pressrel/polio100105.html.

Where do vaccine-derived polioviruses come from?

Because OPV has not been used in the United States since 2000, it is likely that any vaccine-derived poliovirus (VDPV) seen in the United States would have come from a person who received OPV in another country. OPV is used in many countries of the world, including Central and South America, Africa, and Asia.

Should I be concerned if there is a case of VDPV in the United States?

Polio vaccination can protect people against naturally occurring polioviruses and vaccine-derived polioviruses. It is unlikely that a VDPV would become widespread because most people in the United States have been vaccinated against polio. Most VDPV disappear over time without causing any clinical disease. Very rarely, usually in communities where routine polio immunization has been low, VDPV have spread beyond close contacts. Over the past decade, more than ten billion doses of OPV have been given worldwide, with only six outbreaks of circulating VDPV confirmed, resulting in only approximately 50 cases of paralytic polio. Persons who are not up to date with polio immunizations should talk with their health care provider.

Vaccine Related Questions

Who should get polio vaccine and when?

Polio vaccine or IPV is a shot, given in the leg or arm, depending on age. Polio vaccine may be given at the same time as other vaccines.

Most people should get polio vaccine when they are children. Children get four doses of IPV, at these ages:

- A dose at two months
- A dose at four months
- A dose at 6–18 months
- A booster dose at 4–6 years

Most adults do not need polio vaccine because they were vaccinated as children. But, in general, three groups of adults are at higher risk for coming into contact with polio virus and should consider polio vaccination including:

- people traveling to areas of the world where polio is common,
- laboratory workers who might handle polio virus, and
- health care workers treating patients who could have polio.

Adults in these three groups as well as those in communities where VDPV has been isolated who have never been vaccinated against polio should get three doses of IPV:

- The first dose at any time
- The second dose one to two months later
- The third dose six to twelve months after the second

As accelerated vaccination schedule can be used for unvaccinated children and adults with four week intervals between the three doses of the primary series.

Adults at high risk of coming in contact with polio virus who have received the three dose primary series should receive a booster dose of IPV. Based on available information, adults do not need more than a single lifetime booster dose with IPV.

How many children are vaccinated against polio in the United States?

According to the 2004 National Immunization Survey conducted by the Centers for Disease Control and Prevention (CDC), about 92 percent of children aged 19 to 35 months living in the United States were vaccinated against polio. About 95.5 percent of U.S. children are vaccinated against polio before school entry.

Chapter 40

Respiratory Syncytial Virus (RSV) Infection

Respiratory Syncytial Virus (RSV) Season Varies by Region and Year

Respiratory syncytial virus (RSV) is the most common cause of severe lower respiratory tract disease among infants and young children. In high-risk children and older adults, the disease can lead to more serious illnesses, such as pneumonia (inflammation of the lungs) or bronchiolitis (inflammation of the small airways in the lungs). No vaccine or effective treatment for RSV is currently available. However, palivizumab, a medication that contains virus-fighting antibodies to RSV, can help prevent severe RSV disease in high-risk children. Since these antibodies are given to protect children during RSV outbreaks in their communities, the monitoring of outbreak patterns has helped physicians determine when the drug should be given. Yearly community outbreaks of RSV usually last 3–4 months during the fall, winter, and/or spring months.

Laboratory data from the United States National Respiratory and Enteric Virus Surveillance System (NREVSS) showed that the 2006–2007 RSV season[1] varied by geographic region.[2] The season started and ended the earliest in Florida and the latest in the West. The 2006–2007 RSV seasons for Florida and for the South (excluding Florida), Northeast, Midwest, and West are summarized:

Excerpted from "CDC Data and Statistics Respiratory Syncytial Virus (RSV) Season Varies by Region and Year," Centers for Disease Control and Prevention (CDC), October 23, 2008; and "RSV: FAQ," CDC, October 17, 2008.

253

- Florida: early July to late January

- South (excluding Florida): late October to late February

- Northeast: mid-November to early February

- Midwest: mid-November to mid-March

- West: mid-December to late March

Within a region, timing of the RSV season can change from year to year. It is not known why community RSV outbreaks occur when they do, but temperature, humidity, and other environmental factors are likely to contribute to the timing of outbreaks.

Frequently Asked Questions about RSV

What is RSV?

RSV is the most common cause of bronchiolitis (inflammation of the small airways in the lung) and pneumonia in children under one year of age in the United States. Each year, 75,000 to 125,000 children in this age group are hospitalized due to RSV infection. Almost all children are infected with the virus by their second birthday, but only a small percent develop severe disease.

What are the symptoms of RSV?

Symptoms of RSV infection are similar to other respiratory infections. A person with an RSV infection might cough, sneeze, and have a runny nose, fever, and decrease in appetite. Wheezing may also occur. In very young infants, irritability, decreased activity, and breathing difficulties may be the only symptoms of infection. Most otherwise healthy infants infected with RSV do not need to be hospitalized. In most cases, even among those who need to be hospitalized, hospitalization usually last a few days, and recovery from illness usually occurs in about 1–2 weeks.

Who is at risk for severe illness?

Premature infants, children less than two years of age with congenital heart or chronic lung disease, and children with compromised (weakened) immune systems due to a medical condition or medical treatment are at highest risk for severe disease. Adults with compromised immune systems and those 65 and older are also at increased risk of severe disease.

When is the risk for infection the greatest?

RSV infections generally occur in the United States from November to April. However, the timing of the season may differ among locations and from year to year.

How can I provide care to someone with RSV?

There is no specific treatment for RSV infection. However, there are simple ways to help relieve some of the typical symptoms. Your doctor can give advice on how to make people with RSV infection more comfortable and assess whether hospitalization is needed.

How is RSV spread?

RSV can be spread when an infected person coughs or sneezes into the air. Coughing and sneezing send virus-containing droplets into the air, where they can infect a person if they inhale these droplets or these droplets come in contact with their mouth, nose, or eye.

Infection can also result from direct and indirect contact with nasal or oral secretions from infected persons. Direct contact with the virus can occur, for example, by kissing the face of a child with RSV. Indirect contact can occur if the virus gets on an environmental surface, such as a doorknob, that is then touched by other people. Direct and indirect transmissions of virus usually occur when people touch an infectious secretion and then rub their eyes or nose.

How can RSV infection be prevented?

Researchers are working to develop RSV vaccines, but none is available yet. However, there are steps that can be taken to help prevent the spread of RSV. Specifically, people who have cold-like symptoms should:

- cover their coughs and sneezes,
- wash their hands frequently and correctly (with soap and water for 15–20 seconds),
- avoid sharing their cups and eating utensils with others, and
- refrain from kissing others.

In addition, cleaning contaminated surfaces (such as doorknobs) may help stop the spread of RSV.

Special attention should be paid to protecting children who are at high risk for developing severe disease if infected with RSV. Such children include premature infants, children under two years with chronic lung or heart conditions, and children with weakened immune systems. Ideally, people with cold-like symptoms should not interact with children at high risk for severe disease. But, if this is not possible, they should carefully follow the prevention steps mentioned, and they should wash their hands before interacting with children at high risk. When possible, limiting the time that high-risk children spend in childcare centers or other potentially contagious settings may also help prevent infection and spread of the virus during the RSV season.

A drug called palivizumab is available to prevent severe RSV illness in certain infants and children who are at high risk. The drug can help prevent development of serious RSV disease, but it cannot help cure or treat children already suffering from serious RSV disease, and it cannot prevent infection with RSV. If your child is at high risk for severe RSV disease, talk to your health care provider to see if palivizumab can be used as a preventive measure.

References

1. NREVSS estimates that RSV seasons start when the median percentage of specimens testing positive for antigen is greater than or equal to ten for two consecutive weeks and ends when the median percentage of specimens testing positive is less than or equal to ten for two consecutive weeks.

2. Regions: *Northeast Region*: Connecticut, Massachusetts, New Hampshire, New Jersey, New York, and Rhode Island; *Midwest Region*: Illinois, Indiana, Minnesota, Missouri, Nebraska, North Dakota, Ohio, South Dakota, and Wisconsin; *South Region*: Alabama, Arkansas, Delaware, District of Columbia, Georgia, Kentucky, Louisiana, Maryland, Mississippi, North Carolina, Oklahoma, South Carolina, Tennessee, Texas, and Virginia; *West Region*: Alaska, Arizona, California, Colorado, Hawaii, Montana, Washington, and Wyoming; and the state of Florida.

Data Source: Respiratory syncytial virus activity–United States, July 2006–November 2007. *MMWR*. 7 Dec. 2007. 56(48);1263-1265.

Chapter 41

Rubella

Infectious Agent

Rubella virus is a member of Togaviridae family and the only member of the genus Rubivirus.

Mode of Transmission

- Rubella virus is transmitted through person-to-person contact or droplets shed from the respiratory secretions of infected persons.

- If a woman with rubella is infected during pregnancy, the virus can cross the placenta and infect the fetus.

Occurrence

- Rubella occurs worldwide.

- In the United States, endemic rubella has been eliminated. However, since 2005, an average of ten cases is reported each year. Of these cases, approximately 33% are imported or linked to importations.

"CDC Health Information for International Travel 2010 (Yellow Book): Chapter 2: The Pre-Travel Consultation: Routine Vaccine-Preventable Diseases–Rubella," Centers for Disease Control and Prevention (CDC), 2009.

Risk for Travelers

- All susceptible persons are at risk for infection from exposure to rubella during travel outside the United States.

- Because asymptomatic rubella infections are common, travelers may be unaware that they have been in contact with an infected person.

Clinical Presentation

- The average incubation period is 14 days, with a range of 12–23 days.

- Rubella usually presents as a nonspecific, maculopapular, generalized rash lasting three days or fewer (hence the term three-day measles) with generalized lymphadenopathy, particularly of the posterior auricular, suboccipital and posterior cervical lymph nodes.

- Asymptomatic rubella virus infections are common, and up to 50% of infections occur without rash.

- In adults and adolescents, the rash may be preceded by a 1- to 5-day prodrome of low-grade fever, malaise, anorexia, mild conjunctivitis, coryza, sore throat, and lymphadenopathy.

- The most important and serious consequence of rubella is infection during early pregnancy. These consequences may include miscarriages, fetal deaths/stillbirths, and an infant born with constellation of severe birth defects known as congenital rubella syndrome (CRS). The most common congenital defects are cataracts, heart defects, and hearing impairment.

Diagnosis

- Many illnesses can mimic rubella, and up to 50% of rubella infections are asymptomatic. Therefore, the only reliable evidence of acute rubella virus infection is laboratory diagnosis.

- Serologic testing for rubella-specific immunoglobulin (Ig) M antibody is the most commonly used for diagnosis of rubella.

- Diagnosis can also be made by demonstration of seroconversion of rubella-specific IgG antibody titers and by detection of virus either through virus culture or PCR.

Treatment

There is no specific antiviral therapy for rubella; basic treatment consists of supportive care.

Preventive Measures for Travelers

Vaccine

- Before international travel, persons should be immune to rubella.
- Acceptable presumptive evidence of immunity to rubella for international travelers includes the following:
  - Documentation of receipt of one or more doses of rubella-containing vaccine on or after the first birthday
  - Laboratory evidence of rubella immunity (a positive serologic test for rubella-specific IgG antibody)

References

1. CDC. Rubella. In: Atkinson W, Hamborsky J, McIntyre L, Wolfe S, editors. *Epidemiology and prevention of vaccine-preventable diseases. 10th ed.* Washington (DC): Public Health Foundation, 2008. p. 159–74.

2. Reef SE, Redd SB, Abernathy E, et al. The epidemiological profile of rubella and congenital rubella syndrome in the United States, 1998–2004: the evidence for absence of endemic transmission. *Clin Infect Dis.* 2006;43(Suppl 3):S126–32.

3. Plotkin SA, Reef SE. Rubella vaccine. In: Plotkin SA, Orenstein WA, Offit PA, editors. *Vaccines. 5th ed.* Philadelphia: Saunders Elsevier; 2008. p. 735–71.

4. Reef SE, Cochi SL. The evidence for the elimination of rubella and congenital rubella syndrome in the United States: a public health achievement. *Clin Infect Dis.* 2006;43(Suppl 3):S123–5.

5. Meissner HC, Reef SE, Cochi S. Elimination of rubella from the United States: a milestone on the road to global elimination. *Pediatrics.* 2006;117(3):933–5.

6. Robertson SE, Featherstone DA, Gacic-Dobo M, et al. Rubella and congenital rubella syndrome: global update. *Rev Panam Salud Publica.* 2003;14(5):306–15.

7. Plotinsky RN, Talbot EA, Kellenberg JE, et al. Congenital rubella syndrome in a child born to Liberian refugees: clinical and public health perspectives. *Clin Pediatr (Phila)*. 2007;46(4):349–55.

8. Watson JC, Hadler SC, Dykewicz CA, et al. Measles, mumps, and rubella-vaccine use and strategies for elimination of measles, rubella, congenital rubella syndrome and control of mumps: recommendations of the Advisory Committee on Immunization Practices (ACIP). *MMWR Recomm Rep*. 1998;47(RR-8):1–57.

9. Kroger AT, Atkinson WL, Marcuse EK, et al.; CDC. General recommendations on immunization: recommendations of the Advisory Committee on Immunization Practices (ACIP). *MMWR Recomm Rep*. 2006;55(RR-15):1–48.

Chapter 42

Scabies

What is scabies?

Scabies is an infestation of the skin by the human itch mite (*Sarcoptes scabiei* var. *hominis*). The microscopic scabies mite burrows into the upper layer of the skin where it lives and lays its eggs. The most common symptoms of scabies are intense itching and a pimple-like skin rash. The scabies mite usually is spread by direct, prolonged, skin-to-skin contact with a person who has scabies.

Scabies is found worldwide and affects people of all races and social classes. Scabies can spread rapidly under crowded conditions where close body and skin contact is frequent. Institutions such as nursing homes, extended-care facilities, and prisons are often sites of scabies outbreaks. Childcare facilities also are a common site of scabies infestations.

What is crusted (Norwegian) scabies?

Crusted scabies is a severe form of scabies that can occur in some persons who are immunocompromised (have a weak immune system), elderly, disabled, or debilitated. It is also called Norwegian scabies. Persons with crusted scabies have thick crusts of skin that contain large numbers of scabies mites and eggs. Persons with crusted scabies are very contagious to other persons and can spread the infestation

---

"Scabies Fact Sheet," Centers for Disease Control and Prevention (CDC), November 10, 2008.

easily both by direct skin-to-skin contact and by contamination of items such as their clothing, bedding, and furniture. Persons with crusted scabies may not show the usually signs and symptoms of scabies such as the characteristic rash or itching (pruritus). Persons with crusted scabies should receive quick and aggressive medical treatment for their infestation to prevent outbreaks of scabies.

How soon after infestation do symptoms of scabies begin?

If a person has never had scabies before, symptoms may take as long as 4–6 weeks to begin. It is important to remember that an infested person can spread scabies during this time, even if he or she does not have symptoms yet. In a person who has had scabies before, symptoms usually appear much sooner (1–4 days) after exposure.

What are the signs and symptoms of scabies infestation?

The most common signs and symptoms of scabies are intense itching (pruritus), especially at night, and a pimple-like (papular) itchy rash. The itching and rash each may affect much of the body or be limited to common sites such as the wrist, elbow, armpit, webbing between the fingers, nipple, penis, waist, belt-line, and buttocks. The rash also can include tiny blisters (vesicles) and scales. Scratching the rash can cause skin sores; sometimes these sores become infected by bacteria.

Tiny burrows sometimes are seen on the skin; these are caused by the female scabies mite tunneling just beneath the surface of the skin. These burrows appear as tiny raised and crooked (serpiginous) grayish-white or skin-colored lines on the skin surface. Because mites are often few in number (only 10–15 mites per person), these burrows may be difficult to find. They are found most often in the webbing between the fingers, in the skin folds on the wrist, elbow, or knee, and on the penis, breast, or shoulder blades. The head, face, neck, palms, and soles often are involved in infants and very young children, but usually not adults and older children. Persons with crusted (Norwegian) scabies may not show the usual signs and symptoms of scabies such as the characteristic rash or itching (pruritus).

How did I get scabies?

Scabies usually is spread by direct, prolonged, skin-to-skin contact with a person who has scabies. Contact generally must be prolonged; a quick handshake or hug usually will not spread scabies. Scabies is spread easily to sexual partners and household members. Scabies in adults frequently is sexually acquired. Scabies sometimes is spread indirectly by sharing articles such as clothing, towels, or bedding used by an infested person; however, such indirect spread can occur much more easily when the infested person has crusted (Norwegian) scabies.

How is scabies infestation diagnosed?

Diagnosis of a scabies infestation usually is made based on the customary appearance and distribution of the rash and the presence of burrows. Whenever possible, the diagnosis of scabies should be confirmed by identifying the mite, mite eggs, or mite fecal matter (scybala). This can be done by carefully removing a mite from the end of its burrow using the tip of a needle or by obtaining skin scraping to examine under a microscope for mites, eggs, or mite fecal matter. It is important to remember that a person can still be infested even if mites, eggs, or fecal matter cannot be found; typically fewer than 10–15 mites can be present on the entire body of an infested person who is otherwise healthy. However, persons with crusted (Norwegian) scabies can be infested with thousands of mites and should be considered highly contagious.

How long can scabies mites live?

On a person, scabies mites can live for as long as 1–2 months. Off a person, scabies mites usually do not survive more than 48–72 hours. Scabies mites will die if exposed to a temperature of 50° Celsius (122° Fahrenheit) for ten minutes.

Can scabies be treated?

Yes. Products used to treat scabies are called scabicides because they kill scabies mites; some also kill eggs. Scabicides to treat human scabies are available only with a doctor's prescription; no over-the-counter (non-prescription) products have been tested and approved for humans.

Always follow carefully the instructions provided by the doctor and pharmacist, as well as those contained in the box or printed on the label. When treating adults and older children, scabicide cream or lotion is applied to all areas of the body from the neck down to the feet and toes; when treating infants and young children, the cream or lotion also is applied to the head and neck. The medication should be left on the body for the recommended time before it is washed off. Clean clothes should be worn after treatment.

In addition to the infested person, treatment also is recommended for household members and sexual contacts, particularly those who have had prolonged skin-to-skin contact with the infested person. All persons should be treated at the same time in order to prevent re-infestation. Retreatment may be necessary if itching continues more than 2–4 weeks after treatment or if new burrows or rash continue to appear.

Never use a scabicide intended for veterinary or agricultural use to treat humans.

Who should be treated for scabies?

Anyone who is diagnosed with scabies, as well as his or her sexual partners and other contacts who have had prolonged skin-to-skin contact with the infested person, should be treated. Treatment is recommended for members of the same household as the person with scabies, particularly those persons who have had prolonged skin-to-skin contact with the infested person. All persons should be treated at the same time to prevent re-infestation.

Retreatment may be necessary if itching continues more than 2–4 weeks after treatment or if new burrows or rash continue to appear.

How soon after treatment will I feel better?

Itching may continue for 2–4 weeks after treatment, even if all the mites and eggs are killed. Additional medication may be prescribed to relieve severe itching. If itching continues more than 2–4 weeks, or if new burrows or rash continue to appear, retreatment with scabicide may be necessary; seek the advice of a physician.

Chapter 43

Shigellosis

What is shigellosis?

Shigellosis is an infectious disease caused by a group of bacteria called *Shigella*. Most people infected with *Shigella* develop diarrhea, fever, and stomach cramps starting a day or two after they are exposed to the bacteria. The diarrhea is often bloody. Shigellosis usually resolves in 5–7 days. Persons with shigellosis in the United States rarely require hospitalization. A severe infection with high fever may be associated with seizures in children less than two years old. Some persons who are infected may have no symptoms at all, but may still pass the *Shigella* bacteria to others.

What sort of germ is **Shigella?**

The *Shigella* germ is actually a family of bacteria that can cause diarrhea in humans. They are microscopic living creatures that pass from person to person. *Shigella* were discovered over 100 years ago by a Japanese scientist named Shiga, for whom they are named. There are several different kinds of *Shigella* bacteria: *Shigella sonnei*, also known as "Group D" *Shigella*, accounts for over two-thirds of shigellosis in the United States. *Shigella flexneri*, or "group B" *Shigella*, accounts for almost all the rest. Other types of *Shigella* are rare in this country, though they continue to be important causes of disease in the

"Shigellosis," Centers for Disease Control and Prevention (CDC), March 27, 2008.

developing world. One type found in the developing world, *Shigella dysenteriae* type 1, can cause deadly epidemics.

How can **Shigella** *infections be diagnosed?*

Many different kinds of germs can cause diarrhea, so establishing the cause will help guide treatment. Determining that *Shigella* is the cause of the illness depends on laboratory tests that identify *Shigella* in the stools of an infected person. The laboratory can also do special tests to determine which antibiotics, if any, would be best to treat the infection.

How can **Shigella** *infections be treated?*

Persons with mild infections usually recover quickly without antibiotic treatment. However, appropriate antibiotic treatment kills *Shigella* bacteria, and may shorten the illness by a few days. The antibiotics commonly used for treatment are ampicillin, trimethoprim/sulfamethoxazole (also known as Bactrim® or Septra®), ceftriaxone (Rocephin®), or, among adults, ciprofloxacin. Some *Shigella* bacteria have become resistant to antibiotics. This means some antibiotics might not be effective for treatment. Using antibiotics to treat shigellosis can sometimes make the germs more resistant. Therefore, when many persons in a community are affected by shigellosis, antibiotics are sometimes used to treat only the most severe cases. Antidiarrheal agents such as loperamide (Imodium®) or diphenoxylate with atropine (Lomotil®) can make the illness worse and should be avoided.

Are there long-term consequences of a **Shigella** *infection?*

Persons with diarrhea usually recover completely, although it may be several months before their bowel habits are entirely normal. About 2% of persons who are infected with one type of *Shigella, Shigella flexneri*, later develop pains in their joints, irritation of the eyes, and painful urination. This is called post-infectious arthritis. It can last for months or years, and can lead to chronic arthritis. Post-infectious arthritis is caused by a reaction to *Shigella* infection that happens only in people who are genetically predisposed to it.

Once someone has had shigellosis, they are not likely to get infected with that specific type again for at least several years. However, they can still get infected with other types of *Shigella*.

How do people catch Shigella*?*

The *Shigella* bacteria pass from one infected person to the next. *Shigella* are present in the diarrheal stools of infected persons while they are sick and for up to a week or two afterwards. Most *Shigella* infections are the result of the bacterium passing from stools or soiled fingers of one person to the mouth of another person. This happens when basic hygiene and handwashing habits are inadequate and can happen during certain types of sexual activity. It is particularly likely to occur among toddlers who are not fully toilet trained. Family members and playmates of such children are at high risk of becoming infected.

Shigella infections may be acquired from eating contaminated food. Contaminated food usually looks and smells normal. Food may become contaminated by infected food handlers who forget to wash their hands with soap after using the bathroom. Vegetables can become contaminated if they are harvested from a field with sewage in it. Flies can breed in infected feces and then contaminate food. Water may become contaminated with *Shigella* bacteria if sewage runs into it, or if someone with shigellosis swims in or plays with it (especially in splash tables, untreated wading pools, or shallow play fountains used by daycare centers). *Shigella* infections can then be acquired by drinking, swimming in, or playing with the contaminated water. Outbreaks of shigellosis have also occurred among men who have sex with men.

What can a person do to prevent this illness?

Currently, there is no vaccine to prevent shigellosis. However, the spread of *Shigella* from an infected person to other persons can be stopped by frequent and careful handwashing with soap. Frequent and careful handwashing is important among all age groups. Handwashing among children should be frequent and supervised by an adult in daycare centers and homes with children who have not been fully toilet trained.

If a child in diapers has shigellosis, everyone who changes the child's diapers should be sure the diapers are disposed of properly in a closed-lid garbage can, and should wash his or her hands and the child's hands carefully with soap and warm water immediately after changing the diapers. After use, the diaper changing area should be wiped down with a disinfectant such as diluted household bleach, Lysol® or bactericidal wipes. When possible, young children with a

Shigella infection who are still in diapers should not be in contact with uninfected children.

Basic food safety precautions and disinfection of drinking water prevents shigellosis from food and water. However, people with shigellosis should not prepare food or drinks for others until they have been shown to no longer be carrying the *Shigella* bacterium, or if they have had no diarrhea for at least two days. At swimming beaches, having enough bathrooms and handwashing stations with soap near the swimming area helps keep the water from becoming contaminated. Daycare centers should not provide water play areas.

Simple precautions taken while traveling to the developing world can prevent shigellosis. Drink only treated or boiled water, and eat only cooked hot foods or fruits you peel yourself. The same precautions prevent other types of traveler's diarrhea.

How common is shigellosis?

Every year, about 14,000 cases of shigellosis are reported in the United States. Because many milder cases are not diagnosed or reported, the actual number of infections may be twenty times greater. Shigellosis is particularly common and causes recurrent problems in settings where hygiene is poor and can sometimes sweep through entire communities. It is more common in summer than winter. Children, especially toddlers aged 2–4 years, are the most likely to get shigellosis. Many cases are related to the spread of illness in childcare settings, and many are the result of the spread of the illness in families with small children. In the developing world, shigellosis is far more common and is present in most communities most of the time.

What else can be done to prevent shigellosis?

It is important for the public health department to know about cases of shigellosis. It is important for clinical laboratories to send isolates of *Shigella* to the city, county or state public health laboratory so the specific type can be determined. If many cases occur at the same time, it may mean that a restaurant, food or water supply has a problem that needs correction by the public health department. If a number of cases occur in a daycare center, the public health department may need to coordinate efforts to improve handwashing among the staff, children, and their families. When a community-wide outbreak occurs, a community-wide approach to promote handwashing and basic hygiene among children can stop the outbreak. Improvements in worker hygiene during vegetable and fruit picking and packing may prevent shigellosis caused by contaminated produce.

Some prevention measures in place in most communities help to prevent shigellosis. Making municipal water supplies safe and treating sewage are highly effective prevention measures that have been in place for many years.

What is the government doing about shigellosis?

The Centers for Disease Control and Prevention (CDC) monitors the frequency of *Shigella* infections in the country, and assists local and state health departments in investigating outbreaks, determining means of transmission, and devising control measures. CDC also conducts research to better understand how to identify and treat shigellosis. The Food and Drug Administration (FDA) inspects imported foods, and promotes better food preparation techniques in restaurants and food processing plants. The Environmental Protection Agency (EPA) regulates and monitors the safety of our drinking water supplies. The government has also maintained active research into the development of a *Shigella* vaccine.

How can I learn more about this and other public health problems?

You can discuss any medical concerns you may have with your heath care provider. Your local city or county health department can provide more information about this and other public health problems.

Preventing Shigellosis Transmission

Some tips for preventing the spread of shigellosis:

- Wash hands with soap carefully and frequently, especially after going to the bathroom, after changing diapers, and before preparing foods or beverages
- Dispose of soiled diapers properly
- Disinfect diaper changing areas after using them
- Keep children with diarrhea out of childcare settings
- Supervise handwashing of toddlers and small children after they use the toilet

- Do not prepare food for others while ill with diarrhea
- Avoid swallowing water from ponds, lakes, or untreated pools

Chapter 44

Smallpox

What You Should Know about a Smallpox Outbreak

The thought of a smallpox outbreak is scary, but public health officials are preparing to respond quickly and effectively to such an event. The public can prepare too, by being informed. This information provides members of the public with basic information about the possible use of smallpox as a biological weapon and what to do if that happens. If a smallpox emergency occurs, more detailed information and instructions will be available on the Centers for Disease Control and Prevention (CDC) website and through other channels such as radio and television.

Why Smallpox Is a Concern

Because smallpox was wiped out many years ago, a case of smallpox today would be the result of an intentional act. A single confirmed case of smallpox would be considered an emergency.

Thanks to the success of vaccination, the last natural outbreak of smallpox in the U.S. occurred in 1949. By 1972, routine smallpox vaccinations for children in the U.S. were no longer needed. In 1980, smallpox was said to be wiped out worldwide, and no cases of naturally occurring smallpox have happened since.

"What You Should Know about a Smallpox Outbreak," Centers for Disease Control and Prevention (CDC), March 2009.

Today, the smallpox virus is kept in two approved labs in the U.S. and Russia. However, credible concern exists that the virus was made into a weapon by some countries and that terrorists may have obtained it. Smallpox is a serious, even deadly, disease. CDC calls it a category A agent. Category A agents are believed to present the greatest potential threat for harming public health.

Possible Ways of Getting Smallpox

Possible ways to become infected with smallpox include the following:

- Prolonged face-to-face contact with someone who has smallpox (usually someone who already has a smallpox rash). This was how most people became infected with smallpox in the past. However, a person can be exposed to someone who has smallpox and not become infected.

- Direct contact with infected bodily fluids or an object such as bedding or clothing that has the virus on it.

- Exposure to an aerosol release of smallpox (the virus is put in the air). On rare occasions in the past, smallpox was spread by virus carried in the air in enclosed places such as buildings, buses, and trains. The smallpox virus is not strong and is killed by sunlight and heat. In lab experiments, 90% of aerosolized smallpox virus dies within 24 hours; in the presence of sunlight, this percentage would be even greater.

Smallpox is not known to be spread by insects or animals.

Signs and Symptoms

- For the first 7–17 days after exposure, the infected person feels fine and is not contagious (cannot spread the disease).

- After 7–17 days, the first symptoms of smallpox appear. These include fever, tiredness, head and body aches, and sometimes vomiting. The fever is usually high, in the range of 101 to 104 degrees Fahrenheit. At this time, people are usually too sick to carry on their normal activities. This stage may last for 2–4 days.

- Next, a rash appears first as small red spots on the tongue and in the mouth. A rash then appears on the skin, starting on the face and spreading to the arms and legs and then to the hands and feet. Usually the rash spreads to all parts of the body within 24 hours.

- The rash becomes raised bumps and the bumps become pustules, which are raised, usually round and firm to the touch as if there's a small round object under the skin.
- The pustules begin to form a crust and then scab. By the end of the second week after the rash appears, most of the sores have scabbed over.
- The scabs begin to fall off, leaving scars. Most scabs will have fallen off three weeks after the rash first appears.

A person with smallpox is sometimes contagious when they get a fever, but the person becomes most contagious when they get a rash. The infected person is contagious until their last scab falls off. In the past, most people recovered from smallpox, but three out of every ten smallpox patients died.

Treatment and Prevention

There is no proven treatment for smallpox. Scientists are currently researching new treatments. Patients with smallpox may be helped by intravenous fluids, medicine to control fever or pain, and antibiotics for any secondary bacterial infections that may occur.

One of the best ways to prevent smallpox is through vaccination. If given to a person before exposure to smallpox, the vaccine can completely protect them. Vaccination within three days after exposure will prevent or greatly lessen the severity of smallpox in most people. Vaccination 4–7 days after exposure likely offers some protection from disease or may decrease the severity of disease. Vaccination will not protect smallpox patients who already have a rash.

Currently, the smallpox vaccine is not widely available to the general public. However, there is enough smallpox vaccine to vaccinate every person in the United States in the event of a smallpox emergency.

How Public Health Officials Will Respond to a Smallpox Outbreak

CDC has a detailed plan to protect Americans against the use of smallpox as a biological weapon. This plan includes the creation and use of special teams of health care and public health workers. If a smallpox case is found, these teams will take steps immediately to control the spread of the disease. Smallpox was wiped out through specific public health actions, including vaccination, and these actions will be used again.

- If a smallpox outbreak happens, public health officials will use television, radio, newspapers, the internet, and other channels to inform members of the public about what to do to protect themselves and their families.

- Officials will tell people where to go for care if they think they have smallpox.

- Smallpox patients will be isolated (kept away from other people who could get sick from them) and will receive the best medical care possible. Isolation prevents the virus from spreading to others.

- Anyone who has had contact with a smallpox patient will be offered smallpox vaccination as soon as possible. Then, the people who have had contact with those individuals will also be vaccinated. Following vaccination, these people will need to watch for any signs of smallpox. People who have been exposed to smallpox may be asked to take their temperatures regularly and report the results to their health department.

- The smallpox vaccine may also be offered to those who have not been exposed, but would like to be vaccinated. At local clinics, the risks and benefits of the vaccine will be explained and professionals will be available to answer questions.

- No one will be forced to be vaccinated, even if they have been exposed to smallpox.

- To prevent smallpox from spreading, anyone who has been in contact with a person with smallpox but who decides not to get the vaccine may need to be isolated for at least 18 days. During this time, they will be checked for symptoms of smallpox.

- People placed in isolation will not be able to go to work. Steps will be taken to care for their everyday needs (food and other needs).

Because smallpox does not spread as easily as measles or flu, measures like vaccination and isolation allowed public health officials to wipe out the disease.

How You Can Protect Yourself and Your Family during an Outbreak

- Stay informed. Listen to the news to learn how the outbreak is affecting your community. Public health officials will share important information including areas where smallpox cases have been found and who to call and where to go if you think you have been exposed to smallpox.

- Follow the instructions of public health authorities.

- Stay away from, and keep your children away from, anyone who might have smallpox. This is especially important if you or your children have not been vaccinated.

- If you think you have been exposed to smallpox, stay away from others and call your health department or health care provider immediately; they will tell you where to go.

Chapter 45

Staph Infections: Group A

Chapter Contents

Section 45.1

Staphylococcal Infections

"Staph Infections," March 2008, reprinted with permission from www
.kidshealth.org. Copyright © 2008 The Nemours Foundation. This information was provided by KidsHealth, one of the largest resources online
for medically reviewed health information written for parents, kids, and
teens. For more articles like this one, visit www.KidsHealth.org, or
www.TeensHealth.org.

What Are Staph Infections?

Staph infections are caused by the bacteria *Staphylococcus aureus*,
which many healthy people carry on their skin and in their noses without getting sick. But when skin is punctured or broken, staph bacteria can enter the wound and cause infections, which can lead to other
health problems.

You can help prevent staph infections in your family by encouraging regular hand washing and daily bathing, and by keeping areas that
have been cut clean or covered.

How Staph Infections Spread

Staph bacteria can spread through the air, on contaminated surfaces,
and from person to person. Kids can carry staph bacteria from one area
of their body to another—or pass it to other people—via dirty hands or
fingernails. So good hand washing is vital to preventing staph infections.

It's also important to encourage kids to keep their skin clean with a
daily bath or shower. If your child has a skin condition such as eczema
that makes frequent bathing difficult, ask your doctor for advice.

Keep areas of skin that have been injured—such as cuts, scrapes,
and rashes caused by allergic reactions or poison ivy—clean and covered, and follow any directions given by your doctor.

Complications of Staph Infections

Staph bacteria can cause toxic shock syndrome, cellulitis, and these
infections:

Folliculitis and Boils

Folliculitis is an infection of hair follicles, tiny pockets under the skin where hair shafts (strands) grow. In folliculitis, tiny white-headed pimples appear at the base of hair shafts, sometimes with a small red area around each pimple. This infection often occurs in areas where there's been friction or irritation, such as with shaving.

Folliculitis often clears up on its own with good skin hygiene. Sometimes, it can progress to become a boil. With a boil, the staph infection spreads deeper and wider, often affecting the skin's subcutaneous tissue (deeper tissue under the skin) and the oil-producing glands, which are called sebaceous glands. In the first stage, which parents and kids often miss, the area of skin either begins to itch or becomes mildly painful. Next, the skin turns red and begins to swell over the infected area. Finally, the skin above the infection becomes very tender and a whitish "head" may appear. The head may break, and the boil may begin to drain pus, blood, or an amber-colored liquid. Boils can occur anywhere on the skin, especially under the arms or on the groin or buttocks in kids.

To help relieve pain from a boil, try warm-water soaks, a heating pad, or a hot-water bottle applied to the skin for about 20 minutes, three or four times a day. Make sure that the washcloths used for the soaks are washed after each use. Boils are occasionally treated with oral antibiotics and in some cases need to be surgically drained.

Impetigo

Impetigo can affect skin anywhere on the body but commonly occurs around the nose and mouth. It usually affects preschoolers and school-age kids, especially in the summer months.

Impetigo caused by staph bacteria is characterized by large blisters containing fluid that is first clear, then cloudy. The blisters may burst, ooze fluid, and develop a honey-colored crust. Impetigo may itch and can be spread by scratching. Doctors usually prescribe a topical ointment to treat it and may, depending on the severity, add oral antibiotics.

Methicillin-Resistant Staphylococcus Aureus (MRSA)

You may have heard about methicillin-resistant *Staphylococcus aureus* (MRSA), a type of staph bacteria with a resistance to the antibiotics usually used to treat staph infections. Although MRSA infections can be harder to treat, in most cases they heal with proper care.

Most MRSA infections involve the skin, but sometimes MRSA can cause more serious problems, such as bone infections or pneumonia. MRSA pneumonia is rare, but is more of a risk for kids already sick with the flu.

Scalded Skin Syndrome

Scalded skin syndrome (SSS) most often affects newborns and kids under age five. The illness usually starts with a localized staph skin infection, but the staph bacteria manufacture a toxin that affects skin all over the body. The child has a fever, rash, and sometimes blisters. As blisters burst and the rash passes, the top layer of skin is dislodged and the skin surface becomes red and raw, like a burn.

SSS is a serious illness that needs to be treated and monitored in a hospital. It affects the body in the same way as serious burns. After treatment, most kids make a full recovery.

Treating Staph Infections

Most localized staph skin infections can be treated by washing the skin with an antibacterial cleanser, warm soaks, applying an antibiotic ointment prescribed by a doctor, and covering the skin with a clean dressing. To keep the infection from spreading, use a towel only once when you soak or clean an area of infected skin, then wash it.

Your doctor may prescribe an oral antibiotic for your child's staph skin infection. If so, give the antibiotic on schedule for as many days as the doctor directs. More serious staph infections may require hospitalization.

Call the doctor whenever your child has an area of red, irritated, or painful skin, especially if you see whitish pus-filled areas or your child has a fever or feels sick. Also, call the doctor if skin infections seem to be passing from one family member to another or if two or more family members have skin infections simultaneously.

Section 45.2

Staphylococcus Aureus *and Pregnancy*

"Staphylococcus aureus and Pregnancy," © 2007 Organization of Teratology Information Services (OTIS). Reprinted with permission. Member programs of OTIS are located throughout the U.S. and Canada. To find the Teratogen Information Service in your area, call OTIS toll-free at 866-626-OTIS (866-626-6847), or visit www.otispregnancy.org.

This section discusses the risks that exposure to S*taphylococcus aureus* can have during pregnancy. With each pregnancy, all women have a 3% to 5% chance of having a baby with a birth defect. This information should not take the place of medical care and advice from your health care provider.

What is a staph infection?

Staphylococcus aureus (staph) is a type of bacteria (germ) found on the skin or in the nose. Most of the time, people will not have problems with these bacteria. However, if staph gets inside the body through a cut or sore, it may cause painful boils or abscesses on the skin or infection in the lungs (pneumonia), bloodstream, or in a wound that is healing after surgery.

People with a higher risk of getting a staph infection include sick people in hospitals, people recovering from surgeries or other medical procedures, people living in over-crowded conditions (shelters or prisons), children in daycare, intravenous (IV) drug abusers, people with weakened immune systems, athletes, and military personnel.

Eating food that has been contaminated with staph bacteria can also cause food poisoning. Symptoms typically involve severe vomiting and diarrhea with stomach pain that will start within a few hours after exposure. This type of infection with staph bacteria usually is not serious and generally does not last for more than a day.

What medications are used to treat staph skin infections?

Draining of abscesses by your health care provider may be the only treatment needed for staph skin infections. If medication is needed, antibiotics are used. Some of the antibiotics used to treat staph infections include methicillin, penicillin, oxacillin, and amoxicillin. In rare cases, the staph bacteria do not respond to these kinds of antibiotics. This is known as methicillin resistance to *Staphylococcus aureus* or MRSA. Other medications are available for treatment in this situation.

What will a staph or MRSA skin infection look like?

Staph bacterial infections, including MRSA, can look like a pimple or a boil and can be red, swollen, and have pus or other liquids coming out of the sore.

What should I do if I think I have a staph or MRSA infection?

See your doctor. Tests will determine if the infection is staph or MRSA. If you are given an antibiotic, it is very important to follow the instructions and use all of the medication for the time indicated, even if the infection is getting better. Do not share your medicine with other people and do not save your medicine to use at another time. If the infection does not get better in a few days, or it gets worse, tell your health care provider right away.

How can I prevent staph or MRSA skin infections?

Practice good hygiene:

- Wash your hands often with soap and water, especially after using public bathrooms, handling money, or having close contact with the public.

- Clean any cuts or scrapes and cover with a bandage until a scab forms.

- Don't touch other people's cuts or their bandages.

I am pregnant and have a staph or MRSA skin infection. Will it hurt the baby?

A staph or MRSA infection has not been shown to increase the chance of having a baby with a birth defect. There have also been no reports of this infection causing miscarriage. Any infection can make it easier for you to catch other infections, so treating the staph infection will help you have a healthier pregnancy.

I am pregnant and I have a staph infection. Is there a safe treatment?

Yes. Many types of antibiotics can be used during all trimesters of pregnancy. If needed, an antibiotic in the class of penicillin may be prescribed. Studies looking at use of a penicillin or penicillin derivative during pregnancy show that these antibiotics do not appear to cause birth defects or any other problems during pregnancy. Some people are allergic to penicillins and should not take penicillin or antibiotics derived from penicillin such as methicillin. You might be allergic if you start taking the antibiotic and get a rash, hives, or diarrhea. If these or other side effects happen after taking an antibiotic, contact your doctor as soon as possible.

I am pregnant and have a MRSA infection. Is there a safe treatment?

Yes. There are many antibiotics that can be used during pregnancy to treat MRSA skin infections. Your doctor will determine which antibiotic will work for your infection.

I am pregnant. What if the father of the baby, other family member, or friend has a confirmed staph or MRSA skin infection? Should I avoid contact with him or her?

Yes. Contact with a person who has staph or MRSA should be limited.

- Don't share towels, soap, razors, or other personal items.
- If you need to wash the person's laundry, rubber gloves should be used to handle his or her clothes and bedding.
- Don't touch the person's sores, cuts, or bandages.
- Wash your hands with soap and water after direct contact with anyone who has any skin infection.

In general, exposures a father has are not likely to increase the risk to a pregnancy because, unlike the mother, the father does not share a blood connection with the developing baby.

I am breastfeeding. Can I take antibiotics for a staph or MRSA infection?

Yes. Most breastfed babies do not have problems when their mothers take antibiotics. However, some babies can have an allergy to the drug. If your baby has hives or a rash or if there is a change in the baby's stools, call the baby's pediatrician right away. You may need to take a different antibiotic to treat the skin infection if your baby is allergic.

Can my breastfed baby get a staph or MRSA infection from me?

It is possible that a staph infection may spread from mother to baby, or from baby to mother, during breastfeeding. As mentioned, individuals can carry *Staphylococcus aureus* in their nasal passage. Because of this, if your newborn has staph in his nasal passage, you may be at increased risk to develop mastitis (breast infection), particularly if you have some nipple damage. Additionally, there are some reports of infants getting a staph or MRSA infection through expressed (pumped) breast milk that was contaminated. Therefore, it is important to thoroughly wash and sterilize pumping equipment and storage containers, as well as your hands when pumping breast milk.

Your baby could also get the infection if you have an infected wound and the baby comes into contact with your wound or any pus that may have come from the wound, even if you are not breastfeeding. It is important that you keep your wound covered with bandages so that the baby does not touch the wound or any discharge from it. The baby could also become infected if she comes in contact with clothing, bedding or other materials that were in contact with the infected area.

References

Amir LH, et al. 2006. A case-control study of mastitis: nasal carriage of *Staphylococcus aureus*. *BMC Family Practice* 7:57.

Behari P, et al. 2004. Transmission of methicillin-resistant *Staphylococcus aureus* to preterm infants through breast milk. *Infect Control Hosp Epidemiol* 25(9):778–780.

Briggs G. 2005. *Drugs in Pregnancy and Lactation, a reference guide to fetal and neonatal risk.* 7ᵗʰ Ed. Baltimore, MD: Williams and Williams.

Centers for Disease Control and Prevention, Division of Healthcare Quality Promotion, National Center for Infectious Diseases. *CA-MRSA Information for the Public.* http://www.cdc.gov/ncidod/dhqp/ar_mrsa _ca_public.html. [Accessed September 28, 2007].

Elston DM 2007. Community acquired methicillin-resistant *Staphylococcus aureus*. *J Am Acad Dermatol* 56(1):1–16.

Frank A, et al. 1999. Community-acquired and clindamycin susceptible methicillin-resistant *Staphylococcus aureus* in children. *Ped Inf Dis J* 18:993–1000.

Gastelum DT, et al. 2005. Transmission of community-associated methicillin-resistant *Staphylococcus aureus* from breast milk in the neonatal intensive care unit. *Pediatr Infect Dis J*. 24(12):1122–1124.

Goto H, et al. 2003. Susceptibilities of bacteria isolated from patients with lower respiratory infectious diseases to antibiotics. *Jpn J Antibiot*. 58(3):326–58.

Kawada M, et al. 2003. Transmission of *Staphylococcus aureus* between healthy, lactating mothers and their infants by breastfeeding. *J Hum Lact* 19(4):411–417.

Laibl V, et al. 2005. Clinical Presentation of Community-Acquired Methicillin-Resistant *Staphylococcus aureus* in Pregnancy. *Obstet Gynecol* 106 (3):461–5.

Maglio D, et al. 2005. Simulation of antibiotic pharmacodynamic exposure for the empiric treatment of nosocomial bloodstream infections: a report from the OPTAMA program. *Clin Ther*. 27(7):1032–42.

Price M, et al. 1998. Prevalence of methicillin-resistant *Staphylococcus aureus* in a dermatology outpatient population. *South Med J* 91:369–71.

Saravolatz L, et al. 1982. Methicillin-resistant *Staphylococcus aureus*: epidemiologic observations during a community-acquired outbreak. *Ann Intern Med*. 96:11–16.

Section 45.3

Vancomycin-Intermediate/Resistance S. Aureus *(VISA/VRSA)*

Excerpted from "VISA/VRSA: Vancomycin-Intermediate/Resistance *Staphylococcus Aureus*," Centers for Disease Control and Prevention (CDC), October 2007.

What is Staphylococcus aureus?

Staphylococcus aureus, often simply referred to simply as staph, are bacteria commonly found on the skin and in the noses of healthy people. Occasionally, staph can cause infection; staph bacteria are one of the most common causes of skin infections in the United States. Most of these infections are minor (such as pimples, boils, and other skin conditions) and most can be treated without antimicrobial agents (also known as antibiotics or antibacterial agents). However, staph bacteria can also cause serious and sometimes fatal infections (such as bloodstream infections, surgical wound infections, and pneumonia). In the past, most serious staph bacterial infections were treated with a type of antimicrobial agent related to penicillin. Over the past 50 years, treatment of these infections has become more difficult because staph bacteria have become resistant to various antimicrobial agents, including the commonly used penicillin-related antibiotics.

What are Vancomycin-Intermediate S. Aureus *(VISA) and Vancomycin-Resistant* S. Aureus *(VRSA)?*

VISA and VRSA are specific types of antimicrobial-resistant staph bacteria. While most staph bacteria are susceptible to the antimicrobial agent vancomycin some have developed resistance. VISA and VRSA cannot be successfully treated with vancomycin because these organisms are no longer susceptible to vancomycin. However, to date, all VISA and VRSA isolates have been susceptible to other Food and Drug Administration (FDA) approved drugs.

How do VISA and VRSA get their names?

Staph bacteria are classified as VISA or VRSA based on laboratory tests. Laboratories perform tests to determine if staph bacteria are resistant to antimicrobial agents that might be used for treatment of infections. For vancomycin and other antimicrobial agents, laboratories determine how much of the agent it requires to inhibit the growth of the organism in a test tube. The result of the test is usually expressed as a minimum inhibitory concentration (MIC) or the minimum amount of antimicrobial agent that inhibits bacterial growth in the test tube. Therefore, staph bacteria are classified as VISA if the MIC for vancomycin is 4–8 micrograms per milliliter (µg/ml), and classified as VRSA if the vancomycin MIC is greater than 16µg/ml.

Who gets VISA and VRSA infections?

Persons that developed VISA and VRSA infections had several underlying health conditions (such as diabetes and kidney disease), previous infections with methicillin-resistant *Staphylococcus aureus* (MRSA), tubes going into their bodies (such as intravenous [IV] catheters), recent hospitalizations, and recent exposure to vancomycin and other antimicrobial agents.

What should I do if I think I have a staph, MRSA, VISA, or VRSA infection?

See your health care provider.

Are VISA and VRSA infections treatable?

Yes. To date, all VISA and VRSA isolates have been susceptible to several Food and Drug Administration (FDA) approved drugs.

How can the spread of VISA and VRSA be prevented?

Use of appropriate infection control practices (such as wearing gloves before and after contact with infectious body substances and adherence to hand hygiene) by health care personnel can reduce the spread of VISA and VRSA.

Because VISA and VRSA are only part of the larger problem of antimicrobial resistance in health care settings, CDC has started a Campaign to Prevent Antimicrobial Resistance. The campaign centers around four strategies that clinicians can use to prevent antimicrobial resistance: prevent infections; diagnose, and treat infections effectively; use antimicrobials wisely; and prevent transmission. A series of evidence-based steps are described that can reduce the development and spread of resistant organisms such as VISA and VRSA.

What should I do if a family member or close friend has VISA or VRSA?

VISA and VRSA are types of antibiotic-resistant staph bacteria. Therefore, as with all staph bacteria, spread occurs among people having close physical contact with infected patients or contaminated material like bandages. Therefore, persons having close physical contact with infected patients while they are outside of the health care setting should: (1) keep their hands clean by washing thoroughly with soap and water, (2) avoid contact with other people's wounds or material contaminated from wounds. If you visit a friend or family member who is infected with VISA or VRSA while they are hospitalized, follow the hospital's recommended precautions.

Chapter 46

Streptococcal Infections: Group A

Chapter Contents

Section 46.1

Strep Throat

Alternative Names

Pharyngitis–streptococcal; Streptococcal pharyngitis

Definition

Strep throat is caused by Group A *Streptococcus* bacteria. It is the most common bacterial infection of the throat.

Causes

Strep throat is most common in children between the ages of five and fifteen, although it can happen in younger children and adults. Children younger than three can get strep infections, but these usually don't affect the throat.

Strep throat is most common in the late fall, winter, and early spring. The infection is spread by person-to-person contact with nasal secretions or saliva, often among family or household members.

People with strep throat get sick 2–5 days after they are exposed. The illness usually begins suddenly. The fever often is highest on the second day. Many people also have sore throat, headache, stomach ache, nausea, or chills.

Strep throat may be very mild, with only a few of these symptoms, or it may be severe. There are many strains of strep. Some strains can lead to a scarlet fever rash. This rash is thought to be an allergic reaction to toxins made by the strep germ. On rare occasions, strep throat can lead to rheumatic fever if it is not treated. Strep throat may also cause a rare kidney complication.

Symptoms

- Difficulty swallowing

- Fever that begins suddenly
- General discomfort, uneasiness or ill feeling
- Loss of appetite
- Nausea
- Rash
- Red throat, sometimes with white patches
- Sore throat
- Tender, swollen lymph nodes in the neck

Additional symptoms that may be associated with this disease:

- Abnormal taste
- Headache
- Joint stiffness
- Muscle pain
- Nasal congestion
- Nasal discharge
- Neck pain

Exams and Tests

A throat swab can be tested (cultured) to see if strep grows from it. A rapid test is quicker, but misses a few of the cases. Negative rapid tests should be followed by a culture, to find all the cases that might have been missed.

Treatment

Be aware that most sore throats are caused by viruses, not strep. Sore throats should only be treated with antibiotics if the strep test is positive. Strep cannot be accurately diagnosed by symptoms or a physical exam alone.

Even though strep throat usually gets better on its own, antibiotics are taken to prevent rare but more serious complications, such as rheumatic fever. Penicillin or amoxicillin has been traditionally recommended and is still very effective. There has been resistance reported to azithromycin and related antibiotics.

Most sore throats are soon over. In the meantime, the following remedies may help:

- Drink warm liquids. Honey or lemon tea is a time-tested remedy.
- Gargle several times a day with warm salt water (1/2 tsp of salt in one cup water).
- Drink cold liquids or suck on popsicles to soothe the sore throat.
- Suck on hard candies or throat lozenges. This is often as effective as more expensive remedies, but should not be used in young children because of the choking risk.
- Use a cool-mist vaporizer or humidifier to moisten and soothe a dry and painful throat.
- Try over-the-counter pain medications, such as acetaminophen. Do not give aspirin to children.

Outlook (Prognosis)

The probable outcome is good. Nearly all symptoms resolve in one week. Treatment prevents serious complications associated with streptococcal infections.

Possible Complications

- Ear infection
- Sinusitis
- Mastoiditis
- Peritonsillar abscess
- Rheumatic fever
- Glomerulonephritis
- Scarlet fever

When to Contact a Medical Professional

Call if you develop the symptoms of strep throat, whether or not you think you were exposed to someone with strep throat. Also, call if you are being treated for strep throat and are not feeling better within 24–48 hours.

Prevention

Most people with strep are contagious until they have been on antibiotics 24–48 hours. Thus, they should stay home from school, daycare, or work until they have been on antibiotics for at least a day.

Get a new toothbrush after you are no longer contagious, but before finishing the antibiotics. Otherwise the bacteria can live in the toothbrush and re-infect you when the antibiotics are done. Also, keep your family's toothbrushes and utensils separate, unless they have been washed.

If repeated cases of strep still occur in a family, you might check to see if someone is a strep carrier. Carriers have strep in their throats, but the bacteria do not make them sick. Sometimes, treating them can prevent others from getting strep throat.

References

This article uses information by permission from Alan Greene, MD, © Greene Ink, Inc.

Alcaide ML, Bisno AL. Pharyngitis and epiglottitis. *Infect Dis Clin North Am*. 2007;21:449–469.

Del Mar C, Glasziou PP, Spinks A. Antibiotics for sore throat. *Cochrane Database Syst Rev*. 2006 Oct 18;(4):CD000023.

Institute for Clinical Systems Improvement. *Health care guideline: Diagnosis and treatment of respiratory illness in children and adults*. February 2008. Accessed November 9, 2008.

Section 46.2

Scarlet Fever

"Scarlet Fever, General Information," Centers for
Disease Control and Prevention (CDC), April 13, 2008.

What is scarlet fever?

Scarlet fever, sometimes called scarlatina, is a disease caused by a bacteria called group A *Streptococcus* or group A strep, the same bacteria that causes strep throat. Scarlet fever is a rash that sometimes occurs in people that have strep throat. People with scarlet fever typically also have a high fever and a strawberry-like appearance of the tongue. The rash of scarlet fever is usually seen in children under the age of 18.

How do you get scarlet fever?

This illness can be caught from contact with the sick person because this germ is carried in the mouth and nasal fluids. The disease can be spread through contact with droplets shed when an infected person coughs or sneezes. If you touch your mouth, nose, or eyes after touching something that has these fluids on them, you may become ill. Also, if you drink from the same glass or eat from the same plate as the sick person, you could also become ill. The best way to keep from getting sick is to wash your hands often and avoid sharing eating utensils. It is especially important for anyone with a sore throat to wash his or her hands often and not share eating or drinking utensils.

What are the symptoms of scarlet fever?

Scarlet fever begins with a rash that shows up as tiny red bumps. It most often begins on the chest and stomach but can then spread all over the body. It looks like a sunburn and feels like a rough piece of sandpaper. Most of the time, it is redder in the creases of the elbows, arm pits, and groin areas. The rash lasts about 2–7 days. After the rash is gone, the skin on the tips of the fingers and toes begins to peel. Some other common signs of scarlet fever are:

- a flush face with a pale area around the lips,

- a red and sore throat that can have white or yellow patches,

- a fever of 101 degrees Fahrenheit (38.3 degrees Celsius) or higher,

- swollen glands in the neck, and

- a whitish coating can appear on the surface of the tongue. The tongue itself looks like a strawberry because the normal bumps on the tongue look bigger.

Other less common signs of illness include:

- feeling sick to your stomach (nausea) and throwing up (vomiting),

- having a headache, and

- having body aches.

How is scarlet fever diagnosed?

To diagnose the cause of your child's rash or sore throat, your doctor or health care provider will examine your child and swab the back of the throat with a cotton swab. The swab will be then used for a throat culture or a rapid antigen test (sometimes called a rapid strep test) to see if there is a group A strep infection.

What is the treatment for scarlet fever?

If your doctor or health care provider diagnoses you or your child with scarlet fever, the doctor will give you a drug that fights germs (antibiotic) for your child. Be sure to give your child the drug as the doctor tells you. Never share any of the drugs with anyone else. Also, be sure to ask your doctor about drugs you can buy in the store for sore throat pain.

Is there anything else I can do to make my child feel better?

Warm liquids like soup or cold foods like popsicles or milkshakes help to ease the pain of the sore throat. Offer these to your child often, especially when he or she has a fever since the body needs a lot of fluid when it is sick with a fever. A cool mist humidifier will help to keep the air in your child's room moist which will keep the throat from getting too dry or more painful. Your child needs plenty of rest.

What should I do if I think my child has scarlet fever?

If you think your child has scarlet fever, take your child to his or her doctor right away. The doctor may give your child drugs that fight germs (antibiotics). Do not let your child return to daycare or school until he or she has taken the antibiotics for at least 24 hours.

Section 46.3

Severe/Invasive Group A Streptococcal (GAS) Disease

Text in this section is from "Group A Streptococcal (GAS) Disease, General Information," Centers for Disease Control and Prevention (CDC), April 3, 2008.

Group A *Streptococcus* is a bacterium often found in the throat and on the skin. People may carry group A streptococci in the throat or on the skin and have no symptoms of illness. Most GAS infections are relatively mild illnesses such as strep throat, or impetigo. Occasionally these bacteria can cause severe and even life-threatening diseases.

Severe, sometimes life-threatening, GAS disease may occur when bacteria get into parts of the body where bacteria usually are not found, such as the blood, muscle, or the lungs. These infections are termed invasive GAS disease. Two of the most severe, but least common, forms of invasive GAS disease are necrotizing fasciitis and streptococcal toxic shock syndrome. Necrotizing fasciitis (occasionally described by the media as "the flesh-eating bacteria") is a rapidly progressive disease which destroys muscles, fat, and skin tissue. Streptococcal toxic shock syndrome (STSS) results in a rapid drop in blood pressure and causes organs (for example, kidney, liver, lungs) to fail. STSS is not the same as the "toxic shock syndrome" due to the bacteria *Staphylococcus aureus* which has been associated with tampon usage. While 10%–15% of patients with invasive group A streptococcal disease die from their infection, approximately 25% of patients with necrotizing fasciitis and more than 35% with STSS die.

These bacteria are spread through direct contact with mucus from the nose or throat of persons who are infected or through contact with infected wounds or sores on the skin. Ill persons, such as those who have strep throat or skin infections, are most likely to spread the infection. Persons who carry the bacteria but have no symptoms are much less contagious. Treating an infected person with an antibiotic for 24 hours or longer generally eliminates their ability to spread the bacteria. However, it is important to complete the entire course of antibiotics as prescribed. It is not likely that household items like plates, cups, or toys spread these bacteria.

About 9,000–11,500 cases of invasive GAS disease occur each year in the United States, resulting in 1,000–1,800 deaths annually. STSS and necrotizing fasciitis each comprise an average of about 6%–7% of these invasive cases. In contrast, there are several million cases of strep throat and impetigo each year.

Invasive GAS infections occur when the bacteria get past the defenses of the person who is infected. This may occur when a person has sores or other breaks in the skin that allow the bacteria to get into the tissue, or when the person's ability to fight off the infection is decreased because of chronic illness or an illness that affects the immune system. Also, some virulent strains of GAS are more likely to cause severe disease than others.

Few people who come in contact with GAS will develop invasive GAS disease. Most people will have a throat or skin infection, and some may have no symptoms at all. Although healthy people can get invasive GAS disease, people with chronic illnesses like cancer, diabetes, and chronic heart or lung disease, and those who use medications such as steroids have a higher risk. Persons with skin lesions (such as cuts, chicken pox, surgical wounds), the elderly, and adults with a history of alcohol abuse or injection drug use also have a higher risk for disease.

Early signs and symptoms of necrotizing fasciitis are severe pain and swelling, often rapidly increasing, fever; and redness at a wound site.

Early signs and symptoms of STSS are fever, abrupt onset of generalized or localized severe pain, often in an arm or leg, dizziness, influenza-like syndrome, confusion, and a flat red rash over large areas of the body (only occurs in 10% of cases).

How is invasive group A streptococcal disease treated?

GAS infections can be treated with many different antibiotics. For STSS and necrotizing fasciitis, high dose penicillin and clindamycin are recommended. For those with very severe illness, supportive care in an intensive care unit may also be needed. For persons with necrotizing fasciitis, early and aggressive surgery is often needed to remove damaged tissue and stop disease spread. Early treatment may reduce the risk of death from invasive group A streptococcal disease. However, even the best medical care does not prevent death in every case.

What can be done to help prevent group A streptococcal infections?

The spread of all types of GAS infection can be reduced by good hand washing, especially after coughing and sneezing and before preparing foods or eating. Persons with sore throats should be seen by a doctor who can perform tests to find out whether the illness is strep throat. If the test result shows strep throat, the person should stay home from work, school, or day care until 24 hours after taking an antibiotic. All wounds should be kept clean and watched for possible signs of infection such as redness, swelling, drainage, and pain at the wound site. A person with signs of an infected wound, especially if fever occurs, should immediately seek medical care. It is not necessary for all persons exposed to someone with an invasive group A strep infection (necrotizing fasciitis or strep toxic shock syndrome) to receive antibiotic therapy to prevent infection. However, in certain circumstances, antibiotic therapy may be appropriate. That decision should be made after consulting with your doctor.

Chapter 47

Streptococcal Infections: Group B

Chapter Contents

Section 47.1

Streptococcus Pneumoniae

This section begins with an excerpt from "VPD Surveillance Manual, 4th Ed. 2008: Pneumococcal Disease: Chapter 11," Centers for Disease Control and Prevention (CDC); followed by the sub-heading "*Streptococcus Pneumoniae* Facts" from "Pneumococcal Disease," National Institute of Allergy and Infectious Diseases (NIAID), July 14, 2009.

Pneumococcal Disease

Streptococcus pneumoniae is a leading cause worldwide of illness and death for young children, persons with underlying medical conditions, and the elderly. The pneumococcus is the most commonly identified cause of bacterial pneumonia; since the widespread use of vaccines against *Haemophilus influenzae* type b, it has become the most common cause of bacterial meningitis in the United States. The Centers for Disease Control and Prevention (CDC)'s Active Bacterial Core Surveillance (ABC) system has tracked invasive pneumococcal disease (IPD) in selected regions of the United States since 1994. ABC data suggest that rates of invasive disease are highest among persons younger than two years of age and those 65 years of age or older.

Cross-sectional studies suggest that pneumococci can be found in the upper respiratory tract of 15% of well adults; in childcare settings, up to 65% of children are colonized. Although pneumococcal carriage can lead to invasive disease (for example, meningitis or bacteremia), acute otitis media (AOM) is the most common clinical manifestation of pneumococcal infection among children and the most common outpatient diagnosis resulting in antibiotic prescriptions in that group.

Each year in the United States, pneumococcal disease accounts for a substantial number of cases of meningitis, bacteremia, pneumonia, and AOM. Approximately 12% of all patients with invasive pneumococcal disease die of their illness, but case-fatality rates are higher for the elderly and patients with certain underlying illnesses.

Streptococcus Pneumoniae *Facts*

The primary causes of death from pneumococcus are:

- pneumonia, in which fluid fills the lungs, hindering oxygen from reaching the bloodstream;

- meningitis, an infection of the fluid surrounding the spinal cord and brain; and

- sepsis, an overwhelming infection of the bloodstream by toxin-producing bacteria.

Diagnosis

Pneumonia can be diagnosed in a number of different ways. A chest x-ray is the most specific way to diagnose pneumonia. Health care providers can also diagnose many cases by using a stethoscope and/or observing a child's respiratory rate and breathing patterns.

Antibiotic Resistance, Human Immunodeficiency Virus (HIV) Worsen Threat

Pneumococcal infections are becoming more difficult to treat as bacteria become resistant to some of the most commonly used antibiotics.

Table 47.1. Incidence of pneumococcal infections in the United States

Type of bacterial infection	Number of cases per year
Meningitis*	2,000
Bloodstream infection†	8,000
Pneumonia (hospitalized)§	106,000–175,000
Acute otitis media in children under five years**	3,100,000

* S. pneumoniae isolated from cerebrospinal fluid or clinical diagnosis of meningitis with pneumococcus isolated from another sterile site.

† Bacteremia without focus.

§ Estimates before introduction of pneumococcal conjugate vaccine for children in 2000.

** The number of doctor visits per year for acute otitis media in children younger than five years is estimated to be 14,106,159. Approximately 30% of these visits probably represent otitis media with effusion and do not require antibiotics. Recent data from etiologic studies of otitis media in two different areas of the United States suggest that approximately 31% of acute otitis media episodes are caused by S. pneumoniae. [14.1 million x 70% x 31% = 3.1 million].

301

Antibiotic resistance has economic as well as clinical consequences. Overuse of antibiotics leads to increased resistance and threatens the effectiveness of existing therapy, which in turn increases the cost of treatment by requiring the use of more expensive antibiotics.

Data from a recently published study suggest that the problem of pneumococcal disease will increase in the wake of increasing HIV infection. Data from a South African study show that children with HIV/ acquired immunodeficiency syndrome (AIDS) are 20 to 40 times more likely to get pneumococcal disease than children without HIV/AIDS.

Saving Lives with Vaccines

New, lifesaving pneumococcal vaccines are safe and highly effective in preventing pneumococcal disease. Since 2000, when U.S. infants began receiving routine vaccination against pneumococcal disease, the country has nearly eliminated childhood pneumococcal disease caused by vaccine serotypes. In addition, vaccination of infants has reduced the spread of pneumococcal bacteria so that adults have less contact with pneumococci and are thus indirectly protected from pneumococcal disease.

Quick Facts about Pneumococcal Disease and Vaccination

- According to the World Health Organization (WHO), pneumococcal pneumonia and meningitis are responsible for 800,000– 1 million child deaths each year.

- More than 90 percent of pneumococcal pneumonia deaths in children occur in developing countries.

- In developing countries, pneumococcal meningitis kills or disables 40–75 percent of children who get it.

- Children with HIV/AIDS are 20 to 40 times more likely to get pneumococcal disease than children without HIV/AIDS.

- Increasing rates of drug-resistant pneumococcal infections threaten the effectiveness of antibiotic treatment.

- Conjugate pneumococcal vaccination is safe and effective for preventing severe childhood pneumococcal disease caused by serotypes included in the vaccine.

- Conjugate vaccines containing 7–11 pneumococcal serotypes are expected to prevent 50%–80% of all serious childhood pneumococcal disease worldwide.

- High-risk infants and children, including those with HIV infection, can be safely and effectively vaccinated with pneumococcal conjugate vaccines.

- Conjugate pneumococcal vaccines represent an effective tool for preventing antibiotic-resistant infections.

- Routine pneumococcal conjugate vaccination in developing countries could contribute to achieving the United Nations Millennium Development Goal to decrease childhood deaths by two-thirds by the year 2015.

Section 47.2

Group B Strep in Pregnancy and Newborns

"General Public, Frequently Asked Questions: Group B Strep Prevention," Centers for Disease Control and Prevention (CDC), April 20, 2008.

Group B streptococcus (group B strep) is a type of bacteria that causes illness in newborn babies, pregnant women, the elderly, and adults with other illnesses, such as diabetes or liver disease. Group B strep is the most common cause of life-threatening infections in newborns.

Newborns and Group B Strep

How common is group B strep disease in newborns?

Group B strep is the most common cause of sepsis (blood infection) and meningitis (infection of the fluid and lining around the brain) in newborns. Group B strep is a frequent cause of newborn pneumonia and is more common than other, more well-known, newborn problems such as rubella, congenital syphilis, and spina bifida. In the year 2001, there were about 1,700 babies in the U.S. less than one week old who got early-onset group B strep disease.

How does group B strep disease affect newborns?

About half of the cases of group B strep disease among newborns happen in the first week of life (early-onset disease), and most of these cases start a few hours after birth. Sepsis, pneumonia (infection in the lungs), and meningitis (infection of the fluid and lining around the brain) are the most common problems. Premature babies are more at risk of getting a group B strep infection, but most babies who become sick from group B strep are full-term. Group B strep disease may also develop in infants one week to several months after birth (late-onset disease). Meningitis is more common with late-onset group B strep disease. Only about half of late-onset group B strep disease among newborns comes from a mother who is a group B strep carrier; the source of infection for others with late-onset group B strep disease can be hard to figure out. Late-onset disease is slightly less common than early-onset disease.

Can group B strep disease among newborns be prevented?

Yes. Most early-onset group B strep disease in newborns can be prevented by giving pregnant women antibiotics (medicine) through the vein (intravenous [IV]) during labor. Antibiotics help to kill some of the strep bacteria that are dangerous to the baby during birth. The antibiotics help during labor only—they can't be taken before labor, because the bacteria can grow back quickly. Any pregnant woman who had a baby with group B strep disease in the past, or who now has a bladder (urinary tract) infection caused by group B strep should receive antibiotics during labor.

Pregnant women who carry group B strep (test positive during this pregnancy) should be given antibiotics at the time of labor or when their water breaks.

What are the symptoms of group B strep in a newborn?

The symptoms for early-onset group B strep can seem like other problems in newborns. Some symptoms are fever, difficulty feeding, irritability, or lethargy (limpness or hard to wake up the baby). If you think your newborn is sick, get medical help right away.

How is group B strep disease diagnosed and treated in babies?

If a mother received antibiotics for group B strep during labor, the baby will be observed to see if he or she should get extra testing or treatment. If the doctors suspect that a baby has group B strep infection, they will take a sample of the baby's sterile body fluids, such as blood or spinal fluid. Group B strep disease is diagnosed when the bacteria are grown from cultures of those fluids. Cultures take a few days to grow. Group B strep infections in both newborns and adults are usually treated with antibiotics (for example, penicillin or ampicillin) given through a vein (IV).

Pregnancy and Group B Strep Prevention

How will I know if I need antibiotics to prevent passing group B strep to my baby?

You should get a screening test late in pregnancy to see if you carry group B strep. If your test comes back positive, you should get antibiotics through the vein (IV) during labor. If you had a previous baby who got sick with group B strep disease, or if you had a urinary tract infection (bladder infection) during this pregnancy caused by group B strep, you also need to get antibiotics through the vein (IV) when your labor starts.

How do you find out if you carry group B strep during pregnancy?

The Centers for Disease Control and Prevention (CDC) have revised guidelines that recommend that a pregnant woman be tested for group B strep in her vagina and rectum when she is 35 to 37 weeks pregnant. The test is simple and does not hurt. A sterile swab (Q-tip) is used to collect a sample from the vagina and the rectum. This is sent to a laboratory for testing.

What happens if my pregnancy screening test is positive for group B strep?

To prevent group B strep bacteria from being passed to the newborn, pregnant women who carry group B strep should be given antibiotics through the vein (IV) at the time of labor or when their water breaks.

Are there any symptoms if you are a group B strep carrier?

• Most pregnant women have no symptoms when they are carriers for group B strep bacteria.

• Sometimes, group B strep can cause bladder infections during pregnancy, or infections in the womb during labor or after delivery.

Being a carrier (testing positive for group B strep, but having no symptoms) is quite common. Around 25% of women may carry the bacteria at any time. This does not mean that they have group B strep disease, but it does mean that they are at higher risk for giving their baby a group B strep infection during birth.

What if I do not know whether or not I am group B strep positive when my labor starts?

Talk to your doctor about your group B strep status. Pregnant women who do not know whether or not they are group B strep positive when labor starts should be given antibiotics if they have:

- labor starting at less than 37 weeks (preterm labor);

- prolonged membrane rupture (water breaking more than 18 hours before labor starts); or

- fever during labor.

What are the risks of taking antibiotics to prevent group B strep disease in my newborn?

Penicillin is the most common antibiotic that is given. If you are allergic to penicillin, there are other antibiotics that can be given. Penicillin is very safe and effective at preventing group B strep disease in newborns. There can be side effects from penicillin for the woman, including a mild reaction to penicillin (about a 10% chance). There is a rare chance (about 1 in 10,000) of the mother having a severe allergic reaction that requires emergency treatment.

However, a pregnant woman who is a group B strep carrier (tested positive) at full-term delivery who gets antibiotics can feel confident knowing that she has only a one in 4000 chance of delivering a baby with group B strep disease. If a pregnant woman who is a group B strep carrier does not get antibiotics at the time of delivery, her baby has a one in 200 chance of developing group B strep disease. This means that those infants whose mothers are group B strep carriers and do not get antibiotics have over 20 times the risk of developing disease than those who do receive treatment.

Can group B strep cause stillbirth, pre-term delivery, or miscarriage?

There are many different factors that lead to stillbirth, pre-term delivery, or miscarriage. Most of the time, the cause is not known. Group B strep can cause some stillbirths, and pre-term babies are at greater risk of group B strep infections. However, the relationship between group B strep and premature babies is not always clear.

Will a cesarean section (C-section) prevent group B strep in a newborn?

A C-section should not be used to prevent early-onset group B strep infection in infants. If you need to have a C-section for other reasons, and you are group B strep positive, you will not need antibiotics for group B strep only, unless you begin labor or your water breaks before the surgery begins.

What should I do if my water breaks early?

If your water breaks before term, get to the hospital right away. If your group B strep test has not been done, or if you don't know if you have been tested, you should talk with your doctor about group B strep disease prevention. If you have already tested positive for group B strep, remind the doctors and nurses during labor.

Can I breastfeed my baby if I am group B strep positive?

Yes. Women who are group B strep positive can breastfeed safely. There are many benefits for both the mother and child.

More about Group B Strep

Do people who are group B strep carriers feel sick?

Many people carry group B strep in their bodies, but they do not become sick or have any symptoms. Adults can have group B strep in the bowel, vagina, bladder, or throat. About 25% of pregnant women carry group B strep in the rectum or vagina. A person who is a carrier has the bacteria in her body but may not feel sick. However, her baby may come into contact with group B strep during birth. Group B strep bacteria may come and go in people's bodies without symptoms. A person does not have to be a carrier all of her life.

How does someone get group B strep?

- The bacteria that cause group B strep disease normally live in the intestine, vagina, or rectal areas.
- Group B strep colonization is not a sexually transmitted disease (STD).

Approximately 25% (one in four) of pregnant women carry group B strep bacteria in their vagina or rectum. For most women there are no symptoms of carrying group B strep bacteria.

Will group B strep go away with antibiotics?

Antibiotics that are given when labor starts help to greatly reduce the number of group B strep bacteria present during labor. This reduces the chances of the newborn becoming exposed and infected. However, for women who are group B strep carriers, antibiotics before labor starts are not a good way to get rid of group B strep bacteria. Since they naturally live in the gastrointestinal tract (guts), the bacteria can come back after antibiotics. A woman may test positive at certain times and not at others. That's why it's important for all pregnant women to be tested for group B strep carriage between 35 to 37 weeks of every pregnancy. Talk to your doctor or nurse about the best way to prevent group B strep disease,

What if I'm allergic to some antibiotics?

Tell your doctor or nurse about your allergies during your checkup. Try to make a plan for delivery. When you get to the hospital, remind your doctor if you are allergic to any medicines. There are a variety of different antibiotics that can be used, even if you are allergic to some.

Is there a vaccine for group B strep?

There is not a vaccine right now to prevent group B strep. The federal government is supporting research on a vaccine for the prevention of group B strep disease.

Are yeast infections caused by group B strep?

Yeast infections are not caused by group B strep bacteria. Taking antibiotics can sometimes increase the chances of having a yeast infection. When bacteria that are normally found in the vagina are killed by antibiotics, yeast may have a chance to grow more quickly than usual.

Is group B strep the same as strep throat?

No. Strep throat is caused by group A streptococcus bacteria. Group A and group B streptococcus are different kinds of bacteria. They both belong to the same family, but they are different species.

Section 47.3

Late Onset Group B Strep Disease

"General Public, Adult Late-Onset: Group B Strep Prevention," Centers for Disease Control and Prevention (CDC), April 20, 2008.

What is late-onset group B strep disease?

Late-onset group B strep disease is disease that occurs in infants one week to several months after birth. Such babies may appear healthy at birth and only first develop symptoms of group B strep disease after the first week of life.

How common is late-onset group B strep disease?

Approximately three babies out of every 10,000 births develop late-onset group B strep disease. Late-onset disease used to be less common than group B strep disease in the first week of life. Now that prevention efforts have reduced cases of early newborn disease, about half of all infant group B strep infections are in the late-onset category.

How do babies get late-onset group B strep disease?

Early studies suggest that only about half of late-onset group B strep disease among newborns comes from a mother who is a group B strep carrier. The source of infection for others with late-onset group B strep disease can be hard to figure out. The Centers for Disease Control and Prevention (CDC) is involved in some research studies to try to better understand the causes of late-onset disease.

At what age do most babies develop late-onset group B strep infections?

About 80% of all late-onset group B strep infections occur in the first two months of life. Most occur in the first month of life.

What serious problems in babies are caused by late-onset group B strep?

Late-onset group B strep disease most commonly causes bloodstream infections, pneumonia (infection of the lungs), or meningitis (infection of the fluid and lining surrounding the brain). Meningitis is more common among babies with late-onset disease than those who get sick during the first week of life.

What babies are more at risk for late-onset group B strep disease?

Late-onset group B strep disease is more common among babies who are born prematurely (less than 37 weeks). The rates of late-onset disease are also higher among male infants, and among African American babies.

Is there a way to prevent late-onset group B strep disease?

Unfortunately, the method we recommend to prevent group B strep disease in the first week of life (giving women who are carriers of the bacteria antibiotics through the vein (intravenous [IV]) during labor) does not prevent late-onset disease. Although rates of disease in the first week of life have declined, rates of late-onset disease have remained fairly stable in the 1990s. Researchers are currently working on developing a group B strep vaccine which may one day be available to the public as a way to prevent late-onset group B strep disease.

Section 47.4

Adult Group B Strep Disease

Excerpted from "General Public, Adult Disease: Group B Strep Prevention," Centers for Disease Control and Prevention (CDC), April 20, 2008.

Beyond newborns and mothers—some facts about group B strep disease in the rest of the population.

What is the rate of serious group B strep infections among non-pregnant adults?

The rates of serious group B strep infections are much higher among newborns than among any other age group. Nonetheless, serious group B strep infections occur in other age groups in both men and women. Among non-pregnant adults, rates of serious disease range from 4.1 to 7.2 cases per 100,000 people.

How serious is this infection in adults?

The average death rate for invasive infections (infections where the bacteria have entered a part of the body that is normally not exposed to bacteria) is 8–10% for adults ages 18–64, and 15–25% for adults 65 years of age and over. Mortality rates are lower among younger adults, and adults who do not have other medical conditions.

Who is more at risk for adult group B strep disease?

The rate of serious group B strep disease increases with age. The average age of cases in non-pregnant adults is about 60 years old. Most adult group B strep disease occurs in adults who have serious medical conditions. These include: diabetes mellitus; liver disease; history of stroke; history of cancer; or bed sores.

Among the elderly, rates of serious group B strep disease are more common among residents of nursing facilities, and among bedridden hospitalized patients. Group B strep disease among non-pregnant adults may often be acquired after recent trauma, or after having certain invasive hospital procedures like surgery.

311

What are the symptoms of group B strep disease in adults?

Sometimes group B strep can cause mild disease in adults, such as urinary tract infections (UTIs, also called bladder infections). These are treated the same way urinary tract infections caused by other bacteria are treated, with antibiotics, and are usually not that serious.

Serious, invasive disease (infections where the bacteria have entered a part of the body that is normally not exposed to bacteria) can present in a number of different ways. The most common problems in adults are: bloodstream infections, pneumonia, skin and soft-tissue infections, and bone and joint infections. Rarely in adults, group B strep can cause meningitis (infection of the fluid and lining surrounding the brain).

How are serious group B strep infections diagnosed?

If doctors suspect a patient has an invasive group B strep infection, they will take a sample of sterile body fluids, such as blood or spinal fluid. Group B strep disease is diagnosed when the bacteria are grown from cultures of those fluids. Cultures take a few days to grow.

How are serious group B strep infections treated?

Group B strep bacteria are usually treated with penicillin or other common antibiotics. Sometimes soft tissue and bone infections may need surgery. Your treatment will vary according to the kind of infection with group B strep you have, and you should ask your doctors about specific treatment options.

Is there any way to prevent group B strep disease in adults?

Standard infection control measures, particularly for patients who are hospitalized or in nursing homes, help reduce the risk of bacterial infections, including those caused by group B strep. Researchers are currently working on developing a group B strep vaccine which may one day be available to the public as a way to prevent serious group B strep infections among adults, particularly among the elderly.

Chapter 48

Syphilis

What is syphilis?

Syphilis is a sexually transmitted disease (STD) caused by the bacterium *Treponema pallidum*. It has often been called the great imitator because so many of the signs and symptoms are indistinguishable from those of other diseases.

How common is syphilis?

In the United States, health officials reported over 36,000 cases of syphilis in 2006, including 9,756 cases of primary and secondary syphilis. In 2006, half of all primary and secondary syphilis cases were reported from 20 counties and two cities; and most primary and secondary syphilis cases occurred in persons 20 to 39 years of age. The incidence of primary and secondary syphilis was highest in women 20 to 24 years of age and in men 35 to 39 years of age. Reported cases of congenital syphilis in newborns increased from 2005 to 2006, with 339 new cases reported in 2005 compared to 349 cases in 2006.

Between 2005 and 2006, the number of reported primary and secondary syphilis cases increased 11.8 percent. Primary and secondary rates have increased in males each year between 2000 and 2006 from 2.6 to 5.7 and among females between 2004 and 2006. In 2006, 64%

Text in this chapter is from "STD Facts: Syphilis," Centers for Disease Control and Prevention (CDC), January 4, 2008.

of the reported primary and secondary syphilis cases were among men who have sex with men (MSM).

How do people get syphilis?

Syphilis is passed from person to person through direct contact with a syphilis sore. Sores occur mainly on the external genitals, vagina, anus, or in the rectum. Sores also can occur on the lips and in the mouth. Transmission of the organism occurs during vaginal, anal, or oral sex. Pregnant women with the disease can pass it to the babies they are carrying. Syphilis cannot be spread through contact with toilet seats, doorknobs, swimming pools, hot tubs, bathtubs, shared clothing, or eating utensils.

What are the signs and symptoms in adults?

Many people infected with syphilis do not have any symptoms for years, yet remain at risk for late complications if they are not treated. Although transmission occurs from persons with sores who are in the primary or secondary stage, many of these sores are unrecognized. Thus, transmission may occur from persons who are unaware of their infection.

Primary Stage

The primary stage of syphilis is usually marked by the appearance of a single sore (called a chancre), but there may be multiple sores. The time between infection with syphilis and the start of the first symptom can range from 10–90 days (average 21 days). The chancre is usually firm, round, small, and painless. It appears at the spot where syphilis entered the body. The chancre lasts 3–6 weeks, and it heals without treatment. However, if adequate treatment is not administered, the infection progresses to the secondary stage.

Secondary Stage

Skin rash and mucous membrane lesions characterize the secondary stage. This stage typically starts with the development of a rash on one or more areas of the body. The rash usually does not cause itching. Rashes associated with secondary syphilis can appear as the chancre is healing or several weeks after the chancre has healed. The characteristic rash of secondary syphilis may appear as rough, red, or reddish brown spots both on the palms of the hands and the bottoms of the feet. However, rashes with a different appearance may occur on other parts of the body, sometimes resembling rashes caused by other diseases. Sometimes rashes associated with secondary syphilis are so faint that they are not noticed. In addition to rashes, symptoms of secondary syphilis may include fever, swollen lymph glands, sore throat, patchy hair loss, headaches, weight loss, muscle aches, and fatigue. The signs and symptoms of secondary syphilis will resolve with or without treatment, but without treatment, the infection will progress to the latent and possibly late stages of disease.

Late and Latent Stages

The latent (hidden) stage of syphilis begins when primary and secondary symptoms disappear. Without treatment, the infected person will continue to have syphilis even though there are no signs or symptoms; infection remains in the body. This latent stage can last for years. The late stages of syphilis can develop in about 15% of people who have not been treated for syphilis, and can appear 10–20 years after infection was first acquired. In the late stages of syphilis, the disease may subsequently damage the internal organs, including the brain, nerves, eyes, heart, blood vessels, liver, bones, and joints. Signs and symptoms of the late stage of syphilis include difficulty coordinating muscle movements, paralysis, numbness, gradual blindness, and dementia. This damage may be serious enough to cause death.

How does syphilis affect a pregnant woman and her baby?

The syphilis bacterium can infect the baby of a woman during her pregnancy. Depending on how long a pregnant woman has been infected, she may have a high risk of having a stillbirth (a baby born dead) or of giving birth to a baby who dies shortly after birth. An infected baby may be born without signs or symptoms of disease. However, if not treated immediately, the baby may develop serious problems within a few weeks. Untreated babies may become developmentally delayed, have seizures, or die.

How is syphilis diagnosed?

Some health care providers can diagnose syphilis by examining material from a chancre (infectious sore) using a special microscope called a dark-field microscope. If syphilis bacteria are present in the sore, they will show up when observed through the microscope.

A blood test is another way to determine whether someone has syphilis. Shortly after infection occurs, the body produces syphilis antibodies that can be detected by an accurate, safe, and inexpensive blood test. A low level of antibodies will likely stay in the blood for months or years even after the disease has been successfully treated. Because untreated syphilis in a pregnant woman can infect and possibly kill her developing baby, every pregnant woman should have a blood test for syphilis.

What is the link between syphilis and human immunodeficiency virus (HIV)?

Genital sores (chancres) caused by syphilis make it easier to transmit and acquire HIV infection sexually. There is an estimated 2- to 5-fold increased risk of acquiring HIV if exposed to that infection when syphilis is present.

Ulcerative STDs that cause sores, ulcers, or breaks in the skin or mucous membranes, such as syphilis, disrupt barriers that provide protection against infections. The genital ulcers caused by syphilis can bleed easily, and when they come into contact with oral and rectal mucosa during sex, increase the infectiousness of and susceptibility to HIV. Having other STDs is also an important predictor for becoming HIV infected because STDs are a marker for behaviors associated with HIV transmission.

What is the treatment for syphilis?

Syphilis is easy to cure in its early stages. A single intramuscular injection of penicillin, an antibiotic, will cure a person who has had syphilis for less than a year. Additional doses are needed to treat someone who has had syphilis for longer than a year. For people who are allergic to penicillin, other antibiotics are available to treat syphilis. There are no home remedies or over-the-counter drugs that will cure syphilis. Treatment will kill the syphilis bacterium and prevent further damage, but it will not repair damage already done.

Because effective treatment is available, it is important that persons be screened for syphilis on an on-going basis if their sexual behaviors put them at risk for STDs.

Persons who receive syphilis treatment must abstain from sexual contact with new partners until the syphilis sores are completely healed. Persons with syphilis must notify their sex partners so that they also can be tested and receive treatment if necessary.

Will syphilis recur?

Having syphilis once does not protect a person from getting it again. Following successful treatment, people can still be susceptible to re-infection. Only laboratory tests can confirm whether someone has syphilis. Because syphilis sores can be hidden in the vagina, rectum, or mouth, it may not be obvious that a sex partner has syphilis. Talking with a health care provider will help to determine the need to be re-tested for syphilis after being treated.

How can syphilis be prevented?

The surest way to avoid transmission of sexually transmitted diseases, including syphilis, is to abstain from sexual contact or to be in a long-term mutually monogamous relationship with a partner who has been tested and is known to be uninfected.

Avoiding alcohol and drug use may also help prevent transmission of syphilis because these activities may lead to risky sexual behavior. It is important that sex partners talk to each other about their HIV status and history of other STDs so that preventive action can be taken.

Genital ulcer diseases, like syphilis, can occur in both male and female genital areas that are covered or protected by a latex condom, as well as in areas that are not covered. Correct and consistent use of latex condoms can reduce the risk of syphilis, as well as genital herpes and chancroid, only when the infected area or site of potential exposure is protected.

Condoms lubricated with spermicides (especially Nonoxynol-9 or N-9) are no more effective than other lubricated condoms in protecting against the transmission of STDs. Use of condoms lubricated with N-9 is not recommended for STD/HIV prevention. Transmission of an STD, including syphilis cannot be prevented by washing the genitals, urinating, and/or douching after sex. Any unusual discharge, sore, or rash, particularly in the groin area, should be a signal to refrain from having sex and to see a doctor immediately.

Sources

Centers for Disease Control and Prevention. Sexually transmitted diseases treatment guidelines 2006. *MMWR* 2006;55(no. RR-1).

Centers for Disease Control and Prevention. *Sexually Transmitted Disease Surveillance, 2006*. Atlanta, GA: U.S. Department of Health and Human Service, November 2007.

K. Holmes, P. Mardh, P. Sparling et al (eds). *Sexually Transmitted Diseases, 3rd Edition*. New York: McGraw-Hill, 1999, chapters 33–37.

Chapter 49

Tinea Infections (Ringworm, Jock Itch, Athlete's Foot)

If your kids are active, locker-room showers and heaps of sweaty clothes probably are part of their everyday lives—and so is the risk of getting fungal skin infections.

Jock itch, athlete's foot, and ringworm are all types of fungal skin infections known collectively as tinea. They're caused by fungi called dermatophytes that live on skin, hair, and nails and thrive in warm, moist areas.

Symptoms of these infections can vary depending on where they appear on the body. The source of the fungus might be soil, an animal (most often a cat, dog, or rodent), or in most cases, another person. Minor trauma to the skin (such as scratches) and poor skin hygiene increase the potential for infection.

It's important to teach kids to take precautions to prevent fungal skin infections, which can be itchy and uncomfortable. If they do get one, most can be treated with over-the-counter medication, though some might require treatment by a doctor.

"Tinea (Ringworm, Jock Itch, Athlete's Foot)," October 2008, reprinted with permission from www.kidshealth.org. Copyright © 2008 The Nemours Foundation. This information was provided by KidsHealth, one of the largest resources online for medically reviewed health information written for parents, kids, and teens. For more articles like this one, visit www.KidsHealth.org, or www.TeensHealth.org.

Ringworm

Ringworm isn't a worm, but a fungal infection of the scalp or skin that got its name from the ring or series of rings that it can produce.

Symptoms of Ringworm

Ringworm of the scalp may start as a small sore that resembles a pimple before becoming patchy, flaky, or scaly. These flakes may be confused with dandruff. It can cause some hair to fall out or break into stubble. It can also cause the scalp to become swollen, tender, and red.

Sometimes, there may be a swollen, inflamed mass known as a kerion, which oozes fluid. These symptoms can be confused with impetigo or cellulitis. The distinctive features of ringworm are itching, redness on the skin, and a circular patchy lesion that spreads along its borders and clears at the center.

Ringworm of the nails may affect one or more nails on the hands or feet. The nails may become thick, white or yellowish, and brittle.

If you suspect that your child has ringworm, call your doctor.

Treating Ringworm

Ringworm is fairly easy to diagnose and treat. Most of the time, the doctor can diagnose it by looking at it or by scraping off a small sample of the flaky infected skin to test for the fungus. The doctor may recommend an antifungal ointment for ringworm of the skin or an oral medication for ringworm of the scalp and nails.

Preventing Ringworm

A child usually gets ringworm from another infected person, so it's important to encourage kids to avoid sharing combs, brushes, pillows, and hats with others.

Jock Itch

Jock itch, an infection of the groin and upper thighs, got its name because cases are commonly seen in active kids who sweat a lot while playing sports. But the fungus that causes the jock itch infection can thrive on the skin of any kids who spend time in hot and humid weather, wear tight clothing like bathing suits that cause friction, share towels and clothing, and don't completely dry off their skin. It can last for weeks or months if it goes untreated.

Symptoms of Jock Itch

Symptoms of jock itch may include:

- itching, chafing, or burning in the groin, thigh, or anal area;
- skin redness in the groin, thigh, or anal area;
- flaking, peeling, or cracking skin.

Treating Jock Itch

Jock itch can usually be treated with over-the-counter antifungal creams and sprays. When using one of these, kids should:

- Wash and then dry the area with a clean towel.
- Apply the antifungal cream, powder, or spray as directed on the label.
- Change clothing, especially the underwear, every day.
- Continue this treatment for two weeks, even if symptoms disappear, to prevent the infection from recurring.

If the ointment or spray is not effective, call your doctor, who can prescribe other treatment.

Preventing Jock Itch

Jock itch can be prevented by keeping the groin area clean and dry, particularly after showering, swimming, and sweaty activities.

Athlete's Foot

Athlete's foot typically affects the soles of the feet, the areas between the toes, and sometimes the toenails. It can also spread to the palms of the hands, the groin, or the underarms if your child touches the affected foot and then touches another body part. It got its name because it affects people whose feet tend to be damp and sweaty, which is often the case with athletes.

Symptoms of Athlete's Foot

The symptoms of athlete's foot may include itching, burning, redness, and stinging on the soles of the feet. The skin may flake, peel, blister, or crack.

Treating Athlete's Foot

A doctor can often diagnose athlete's foot simply by examining the foot or by taking a small scraping of the affected skin to detect the presence of the fungus that causes athlete's foot.

Over-the-counter antifungal creams and sprays may effectively treat mild cases of athlete's foot within a few weeks. Athlete's foot can recur or be more serious. If that's the case, ask your doctor about trying a stronger treatment.

Preventing Athlete's Foot

Because the fungus that causes athlete's foot thrives in warm, moist areas, infections can be prevented by keeping feet and the space between the toes clean and dry.

Athlete's foot is contagious and can be spread in damp areas, such as public showers or pool areas, so it's wise to take extra precautions. Encourage kids to:

- wear waterproof shoes or flip-flops in public showers, like those in locker rooms;

- alternate shoes or sneakers to prevent moisture buildup and fungus growth;

- avoid socks that trap moisture or make the feet sweat and instead choose cotton or wool socks or socks made of fabric that wicks away the moisture;

- choose sneakers that are well ventilated with small holes to keep the feet dry.

By taking the proper precautions and teaching them to your kids, you can prevent these uncomfortable skin infections from putting a crimp in your family's lifestyle.

Chapter 50

Trichomoniasis

Trichomoniasis is a common sexually transmitted disease (STD) that affects both women and men, although symptoms are more common in women.

How common is trichomoniasis?

Trichomoniasis is the most common curable STD in young, sexually active women. An estimated 7.4 million new cases occur each year in women and men.

How do people get trichomoniasis?

Trichomoniasis is caused by the single-celled protozoan parasite, *Trichomonas vaginalis*. The vagina is the most common site of infection in women, and the urethra (urine canal) is the most common site of infection in men.

The parasite is sexually transmitted through penis-to-vagina intercourse or vulva-to-vulva (the genital area outside the vagina) contact with an infected partner. Women can acquire the disease from infected men or women, but men usually contract it only from infected women.

This chapter includes text from "Trichomoniasis Fact Sheet," Centers for Disease Control and Prevention (CDC), December 17, 2007.

What are the signs and symptoms of trichomoniasis?

Most men with trichomoniasis do not have signs or symptoms; however, some men may temporarily have an irritation inside the penis, mild discharge, or slight burning after urination or ejaculation.

Some women have signs or symptoms of infection which include a frothy, yellow-green vaginal discharge with a strong odor. The infection also may cause discomfort during intercourse and urination, as well as irritation and itching of the female genital area. In rare cases, lower abdominal pain can occur. Symptoms usually appear in women within 5–28 days of exposure.

What are the complications of trichomoniasis?

The genital inflammation caused by trichomoniasis can increase a woman's susceptibility to human immunodeficiency virus (HIV) infection if she is exposed to the virus. Having trichomoniasis may increase the chance that an HIV-infected woman passes HIV to her sex partner(s).

How does trichomoniasis affect a pregnant woman and her baby?

Pregnant women with trichomoniasis may have babies who are born early or with low birth weight (low birth weight is less than 5.5 pounds).

How is trichomoniasis diagnosed?

For both men and women, a health care provider must perform a physical examination and laboratory test to diagnose trichomoniasis. The parasite is harder to detect in men than in women. In women, a pelvic examination can reveal small red ulcerations (sores) on the vaginal wall or cervix.

What is the treatment for trichomoniasis?

Trichomoniasis can usually be cured with prescription drugs, either metronidazole or tinidazole, given by mouth in a single dose. The symptoms of trichomoniasis in infected men may disappear within a few weeks without treatment. However, an infected man, even a man who has never had symptoms or whose symptoms have stopped, can continue to infect or re-infect a female partner until he has been treated. Therefore, both partners should be treated at the same time to eliminate the parasite. Persons being treated for trichomoniasis should avoid sex until they and their sex partners complete treatment and have no symptoms. Metronidazole can be used by pregnant women.

Having trichomoniasis once does not protect a person from getting it again. Following successful treatment, people can still be susceptible to re-infection.

How can trichomoniasis be prevented?

The surest way to avoid transmission of sexually transmitted diseases is to abstain from sexual contact, or to be in a long-term mutually monogamous relationship with a partner who has been tested and is known to be uninfected. Latex male condoms, when used consistently and correctly, can reduce the risk of transmission of trichomoniasis.

Any genital symptom such as discharge or burning during urination or an unusual sore or rash should be a signal to stop having sex and to consult a health care provider immediately. A person diagnosed with trichomoniasis (or any other STD) should receive treatment and should notify all recent sex partners so that they can see a health care provider and be treated. This reduces the risk that the sex partners will develop complications from trichomoniasis and reduces the risk that the person with trichomoniasis will become re-infected. Sex should be stopped until the person with trichomoniasis and all of his or her recent partners complete treatment for trichomoniasis and have no symptoms.

Sources

Centers for Disease Control and Prevention. Sexually transmitted diseases treatment guidelines 2006. *MMWR 2006*: 55 (No. RR-11).

Krieger JN and Alderete JF. Trichomonas vaginalis and trichomoniasis. In: K. Holmes, P. Markh, P. Sparling et al (eds). *Sexually Transmitted Diseases, 3rd Edition*. New York: McGraw-Hill, 1999, 587–604.

Weinstock H, Berman S, Cates W. Sexually transmitted disease among American youth: Incidence and prevalence estimates, 2000. *Perspectives on Sexual and Reproductive Health 2004*; 36: 6–10.

Chapter 51

Tuberculosis

Tuberculosis (TB) Overview

In developed countries, such as the United States, many people think tuberculosis (TB) is a disease of the past. TB, however, is still a leading killer of young adults worldwide. Some two billion people—one-third of the world's population—are thought to be infected with TB bacteria, *Mycobacterium tuberculosis* (*Mtb*).

TB is a chronic bacterial infection. It is spread through the air and usually infects the lungs, although other organs and parts of the body can be involved as well. Most people who are infected with *Mtb* harbor the bacterium without symptoms (have latent TB), but some will develop active TB disease. According to World Health Organization (WHO) estimates, each year, eight million people worldwide develop active TB and nearly two million die.

One in ten people who are infected with *Mtb* may develop active TB at some time in their lives. The risk of developing active disease is greatest in the first year after infection, but active disease often does not occur until many years later.

TB in the United States

In 2006, the Centers for Disease Control and Prevention (CDC) reported 13,799 cases of active TB. While the overall rate of new TB cases

This chapter includes "Tuberculosis (TB) Overview," National Institute of Allergy and Infectious Diseases (NIAID), June 23, 2008; and text from "Tuberculosis: Getting Healthy, Staying Healthy," NIAID, NIH Publication No. 08–5725, June 2008.

continues to decline in the United States since national reporting began in 1953, the annual decrease in TB cases has slowed from an average of 7.1 percent (1993–2000) to the current average of 3.8 percent (2001–2005), according to CDC. In addition to those with active TB, an estimated 10–15 million people in the United States have latent TB.

Minorities are affected disproportionately by TB, which occurs among foreign-born individuals nearly nine times as frequently as among people born in the United States. This is partially because they were often exposed to *Mtb* in their country of origin before moving to the United States. In 2004, a very high percentage of Asians (95 percent) and Hispanics (75 percent) who were born outside the United States were reported to have TB.

Tuberculosis: Getting Healthy, Staying Healthy

What is tuberculosis (TB)?

Tuberculosis (TB) is a disease caused by a germ. You can get this germ from another person. The TB germ can invade your lungs and make you very sick.

The germ can do two things in your body:

- It can sleep quietly without you noticing it (this is called a TB infection)

- Or it can wake up and make you sick (this is called TB disease)

In addition, there are now two more serious types of TB disease.

- The first is called multidrug-resistant TB (MDR TB). MDR TB is hard to treat because the two best medicines for TB don't get rid of the germ.

- The second is called extensively drug-resistant TB (XDR TB). XDR TB is a rare kind of MDR TB that is very hard to treat. Most of the medicines used to get rid of the TB germ don't work very well.

What is TB infection?

TB infection means that the TB germ is asleep in your body. You have TB infection because someone with TB disease has given the TB germ to you.

TB infection can turn into TB disease if the germ wakes up. You can stop this from happening by taking medicines to get rid of the TB germs in your body.

Can I give TB infection to someone else?

No. You cannot spread the germ to others when you only have a TB infection.

How can my doctor tell if I have TB infection?

Your doctor will do different tests to see whether you have TB infection in your body. One is called a TB skin test, or purified protein derivative (PPD) test. Your doctor will inject a drop of liquid in the skin on your arm. If you have the TB germ, you will get a skin bump after a few days. This skin bump will then go away. Your doctor will also take a picture of your lungs with a chest x-ray. Your doctor will know that you have a sleeping TB germ in your body if you get a skin bump after your PPD test, but there are no spots or shadows on the x-ray of your lungs.

How does my doctor treat TB infection?

Your doctor may give you medicines called antibiotics. You will have to take these medicines for many months to make sure all the TB germs are gone from your body. You have to take all your medicines until your doctor tells you that you are finished, even if the medicines make you feel sick. You should eat well and get lots of rest while you are taking your medicines. If you stop taking your medicines, the TB germs may stay in your body, wake up, and make you sick with TB disease.

When you are finished taking your medicines, the TB germ should be gone from your body. A PPD test may give you a skin bump because your body remembers that you have once been infected with the TB germ. If the medicines did not work well and not all the germs are gone from your body, you could get sick with TB disease.

What is TB disease?

TB can become a disease in your body and your lungs when the TB germs wake up and become active to make you sick. You may have a fever, cough, lose weight, and have night sweats.

Can I give TB disease to someone else?

Yes. The TB germ can go through the air from your lungs to other people. To protect others from TB:

- cover your mouth when you speak, laugh, or cough; and

- do not go to school or work until your doctor tells you that you will no longer spread the germs.

How can my doctor tell if I have TB disease?

Your doctor will look at how sick you are. You will get a PPD test and an x-ray of your chest to look at your lungs. Your doctor will know that you have TB disease if you get a skin bump after your PPD test and you have spots or shadows on the x-ray of your lungs.

How does my doctor treat TB disease?

Your doctor will give you medicines, called antibiotics, that may cure your TB. You will have to take different pills for many months to make sure all the TB germs are gone from your body. Some kinds of TB disease are hard to treat with medicines. If you have a more serious TB illness, such as MDR TB, or XDR TB, your doctor may give you different kinds of medicines that you will take for a longer period of time. It is very important that you take all your TB medicines.

You have to take your medicines until your doctor tells you that you are finished, even if the medicines make you feel sick. You may have to see a nurse who will give the medicine to you every day. You should eat well and get lots of rest while you are taking your medicines. If you do not take your medicine every day, the TB germs may not go away and you could get very sick or die from TB.

After you finish all your medicines, the TB germ should be gone. Because your body remembers that you have had the TB germ, a new PPD test may still give you a skin bump. If the medicines did not kill all the TB germs, you could get TB disease again. If you think you have TB disease again, you need to go to your doctor or clinic and say that you had TB before.

Chapter 52

Typhoid Fever

Infectious Agent

Typhoid fever is an acute, life-threatening febrile illness caused by the bacterium *Salmonella (S.) enterica* serotype Typhi. Paratyphoid fever is a similar illness caused by *S. paratyphi* A, B, or C.

Mode of Transmission

- Humans are the only source. No animal or environmental reservoirs have been identified.

- Typhoid and paratyphoid fever are most often acquired through consumption of water or food that have been contaminated by feces of an acutely infected or convalescent individual or a chronic asymptomatic carrier.

- Transmission through sexual contact, especially among men who have sex with men, has rarely been documented.

Occurrence

- An estimated 22 million cases of typhoid fever and 200,000 related deaths occur worldwide each year; an additional six

---

This chapter includes text from "CDC Health Information for International Travel 2010 (Yellow Book) Chapter 2: Typhoid Fever," Centers for Disease Control and Prevention (CDC), U.S. Department of Health and Human Services, Public Health Service, 2009.

million cases of paratyphoid fever are estimated to occur annually.

- Approximately 400 cases of typhoid fever and 150 cases of paratyphoid fever are reported to the Centers for Disease Control and Prevention (CDC) each year among persons with onset of illness in the United States, most of whom are recent travelers.

Risk for Travelers

- Risk is greatest for travelers to South Asia (6–30 times higher than all other destinations). Other areas of risk include East and Southeast Asia, Africa, the Caribbean, and Central and South America.

- Travelers to South Asia are at highest risk for infections that are nalidixic acid-resistant or multidrug-resistant (for example, resistant to ampicillin, chloramphenicol, and trimethoprim–sulfamethoxazole).

- Travelers who are visiting friends or relatives are at increased risk.

- Although the risk of acquiring typhoid or paratyphoid fever increases with the duration of stay, travelers have acquired typhoid fever even during visits of less than one week to countries where the disease is endemic.

Clinical Presentation

- The incubation period of typhoid and paratyphoid infections is 6–30 days. The onset of illness is insidious, with gradually increasing fatigue and a fever that increases daily from low-grade to as high as 102° Fahrenheit (F)–104° F (38.5° Celsius (C)–40° C) by the third to fourth day of illness. Headache, malaise, and anorexia are nearly universal. Hepatosplenomegaly (enlargement of the liver and spleen) can often be detected. A transient, macular rash of rose-colored spots can occasionally be seen on the trunk.

- Fever is commonly lowest in the morning, reaching a peak in late afternoon or evening. Untreated, the disease can last for a month. The serious complications of typhoid fever generally occur only after 2–3 weeks of illness, mainly intestinal hemorrhage or perforation, which can be life threatening.

Diagnosis

- Infection with typhoid or paratyphoid fever results in a very low-grade septicemia (blood poisoning). Blood culture is usually positive in only half the cases. Stool culture is not usually positive during the acute phase of the disease. Bone-marrow culture increases the diagnostic yield to about 80% of cases.

- The Widal test is an old serologic assay for detecting immunoglobulin (Ig) M and IgG antibodies to the O and H antigens of *Salmonella*. The test is unreliable, but is widely used in developing countries because of its low cost. Newer serologic assays are somewhat more sensitive and specific than the Widal test, but are infrequently available.

- Because there is no definitive test for typhoid or paratyphoid fever, the diagnosis often has to be made clinically. The combination of a history of being at risk for infection and a gradual onset of fever that increases in severity over several days should raise suspicion of typhoid or paratyphoid fever.

Treatment

- Specific antimicrobial therapy shortens the clinical course of typhoid fever and reduces the risk for death.

- Empiric treatment of typhoid or paratyphoid fever in most parts of the world would utilize a fluoroquinolone, most often ciprofloxacin. However, resistance to fluoroquinolones is highest in the Indian subcontinent and increasing in other areas. Injectable third-generation cephalosporins are often the empiric drug of choice when the possibility of fluoroquinolone resistance is high.

- Patients treated with an appropriate antibiotic still require 3–5 days to defervesce (fever to abate) completely, although the height of the fever decreases each day. Patients may actually feel worse during the time that the fever is starting to go away. If fever does not subside within five days, alternative antimicrobial agents or other foci of infection should be considered.

Preventive Measures for Travelers

Vaccine

- CDC recommends typhoid vaccine for travelers to areas where there is a recognized increased risk of exposure to *S. typhi.*

- The typhoid vaccines currently available do not offer protection against *S.* Paratyphi infection.

- Travelers should be reminded that typhoid immunization is not 100% effective, and typhoid fever could still occur.

- Two typhoid vaccines are currently available in the United States.

  - Oral live, attenuated vaccine (Vivotif vaccine, manufactured from the Ty21a strain of *S. typhi* by Crucell/Berna) (Updated July 27, 2009)

  - Vi capsular polysaccharide vaccine (ViCPS) (Typhim Vi, manufactured by Sanofi Pasteur) for intramuscular use

- Both vaccines protect 50%–80% of recipients.

- Primary vaccination with oral Ty21a vaccine consists of four capsules, one taken every other day. The capsules should be kept refrigerated (not frozen), and all four doses must be taken to achieve maximum efficacy. Each capsule should be taken with cool liquid no warmer than 37° C (98.6° F), approximately one hour before a meal. This regimen should be completed one week before potential exposure. The vaccine manufacturer recommends that Ty21a not be administered to infants or children less than six years of age.

- Primary vaccination with ViCPS consists of one 0.5 mL dose administered intramuscularly. One dose of this vaccine should be given at least two weeks before expected exposure. The manufacturer does not recommend the vaccine for infants and children less than two years of age.

Vaccine Safety and Adverse Reactions

Information is not available on the safety of these vaccines in pregnancy; it is prudent on theoretical grounds to avoid vaccinating pregnant women. Live, attenuated Ty21a vaccine should not be given to immunocompromised travelers, including those infected with human immunodeficiency virus (HIV). The intramuscular vaccine presents a theoretically safer alternative for this group. The only contraindication to vaccination with ViCPS vaccine is a history of severe local or systemic reactions after a previous dose. Neither of the available vaccines should be given to persons with an acute febrile illness.

Precautions and Contraindications

Theoretical concerns have been raised about the immunogenicity of live, attenuated Ty21a vaccine in persons concurrently receiving antimicrobials (including antimalarial chemoprophylaxis), Ig, or viral vaccines. The growth of the live Ty21a strain is inhibited in vitro by various antibacterial agents. Vaccination with Ty21a should be delayed for over 72 hours after the administration of any antibacterial agent. Available data do not suggest that simultaneous administration of oral polio or yellow fever vaccine decreases the immunogenicity of Ty21a. If typhoid vaccination is warranted, it should not be delayed because of administration of viral vaccines. Simultaneous administration of Ty21a and Ig does not appear to pose a problem.

Chapter 53

Vaginal and Reproductive Tract Infections

Bacterial Vaginosis

What is bacterial vaginosis?

Bacterial vaginosis (BV) is the name of a condition in women where the normal balance of bacteria in the vagina is disrupted and replaced by an overgrowth of certain bacteria. It is sometimes accompanied by discharge, odor, pain, itching, or burning.

How common is bacterial vaginosis?

Bacterial vaginosis (BV) is the most common vaginal infection in women of childbearing age. In the United States, BV is common in pregnant women.

How do people get bacterial vaginosis?

The cause of BV is not fully understood. BV is associated with an imbalance in the bacteria that are normally found in a woman's vagina. The vagina normally contains mostly "good" bacteria, and fewer "harmful" bacteria. BV develops when there is an increase in harmful bacteria.

This chapter includes text from "STD Facts: Bacterial Vaginosis," Centers for Disease Control and Prevention (CDC), February 2008; "STD Facts: Pelvic Inflammatory Disease (PID)," CDC, April 7, 2008; and "Vaginal Yeast Infections: FAQ," Women's Health Information Center, September 23, 2008.

Not much is known about how women get BV. There are many unanswered questions about the role that harmful bacteria play in causing BV. Any woman can get BV. However, some activities or behaviors can upset the normal balance of bacteria in the vagina and put women at increased risk including having a new sex partner or multiple sex partners, or douching.

It is not clear what role sexual activity plays in the development of BV. Women do not get BV from toilet seats, bedding, swimming pools, or from touching objects around them. Women who have never had sexual intercourse may also be affected.

What are the signs and symptoms of bacterial vaginosis?

Women with BV may have an abnormal vaginal discharge with an unpleasant odor. Some women report a strong fish-like odor, especially after intercourse. Discharge, if present, is usually white or gray; it can be thin. Women with BV may also have burning during urination or itching around the outside of the vagina, or both. However, most women with BV report no signs or symptoms at all.

What are the complications of bacterial vaginosis?

In most cases, BV causes no complications. But there are some serious risks from BV including the following:

- BV can increase a woman's susceptibility to human immunodeficiency virus (HIV) infection if she is exposed to the HIV virus.

- BV increases the chances that an HIV-infected woman can pass HIV to her sex partner.

- BV has been associated with an increase in the development of an infection following surgical procedures such as a hysterectomy or an abortion.

- BV while pregnant may put a woman at increased risk for some complications of pregnancy, such as preterm delivery.

- BV can increase a woman's susceptibility to other sexually transmitted diseases (STD), such as herpes simplex virus (HSV), chlamydia, and gonorrhea.

How does bacterial vaginosis affect a pregnant woman and her baby?

Pregnant women with BV more often have babies who are born premature or with low birth weight (low birth weight is less than 5.5

pounds). Also, the bacteria that cause BV can sometimes infect the uterus (womb) and fallopian tubes (tubes that carry eggs from the ovaries to the uterus). This type of infection is called pelvic inflammatory disease (PID). PID can cause infertility or damage the fallopian tubes enough to increase the future risk of ectopic pregnancy and infertility. Ectopic pregnancy is a life-threatening condition in which a fertilized egg grows outside the uterus, usually in a fallopian tube which can rupture.

How is bacterial vaginosis diagnosed?

A health care provider must examine the vagina for signs of BV and perform laboratory tests on a sample of vaginal fluid to look for bacteria associated with BV.

What is the treatment for bacterial vaginosis?

Although BV will sometimes clear up without treatment, all women with symptoms of BV should be treated to avoid complications. Male partners generally do not need to be treated. However, BV may spread between female sex partners.

Treatment is especially important for pregnant women. All pregnant women who have ever had a premature delivery or low birth weight baby should be considered for a BV examination, regardless of symptoms, and should be treated if they have BV. All pregnant women who have symptoms of BV should be checked and treated.

Some physicians recommend that all women undergoing a hysterectomy or abortion be treated for BV prior to the procedure, regardless of symptoms, to reduce their risk of developing an infection.

BV is treatable with antibiotics prescribed by a health care provider. Two different antibiotics are recommended as treatment for BV: metronidazole or clindamycin. Either can be used with non-pregnant or pregnant women, but the recommended dosages differ. Women with BV who are HIV-positive should receive the same treatment as those who are HIV-negative.

BV can recur after treatment.

How can bacterial vaginosis be prevented?

BV is not completely understood by scientists, and the best ways to prevent it are unknown. However, it is known that BV is associated with having a new sex partner or having multiple sex partners. The following basic prevention steps can help reduce the risk of upsetting the natural balance of bacteria in the vagina and developing BV:

- Be abstinent.

- Limit the number of sex partners.

- Do not douche.

- Use all of the medicine prescribed for treatment of BV, even if the signs and symptoms go away.

Pelvic Inflammatory Disease (PID)

What is PID?

Pelvic inflammatory disease (PID) is a general term that refers to infection of the uterus (womb), fallopian tubes (tubes that carry eggs from the ovaries to the uterus), and other reproductive organs. It is a common and serious complication of some sexually transmitted diseases (STDs), especially chlamydia and gonorrhea. PID can damage the fallopian tubes and tissues in and near the uterus and ovaries. PID can lead to serious consequences including infertility, ectopic pregnancy (a pregnancy in the fallopian tube or elsewhere outside of the womb), abscess formation, and chronic pelvic pain.

How common is PID?

Each year in the United States, it is estimated that more than one million women experience an episode of acute PID. More than 100,000 women become infertile each year as a result of PID, and a large proportion of the ectopic pregnancies occurring every year are due to the consequences of PID.

How do women get PID?

PID occurs when bacteria move upward from a woman's vagina or cervix (opening to the uterus) into her reproductive organs. Many different organisms can cause PID, but many cases are associated with gonorrhea and chlamydia, two very common bacterial STDs. A prior episode of PID increases the risk of another episode because the reproductive organs may be damaged during the initial bout of infection.

Sexually active women in their childbearing years are most at risk, and those under age 25 are more likely to develop PID than those older than 25. This is partly because the cervix of teenage girls and young women is not fully matured, increasing their susceptibility to the STDs that are linked to PID.

The more sex partners a woman has, the greater her risk of developing PID. Also, a woman whose partner has more than one sex partner is at greater risk of developing PID, because of the potential for more exposure to infectious agents.

Women who douche may have a higher risk of developing PID compared with women who do not douche. Research has shown that douching changes the vaginal flora (organisms that live in the vagina) in harmful ways, and can force bacteria into the upper reproductive organs from the vagina.

Women who have an intrauterine device (IUD) inserted may have a slightly increased risk of PID near the time of insertion compared with women using other contraceptives or no contraceptive at all. However, this risk is greatly reduced if a woman is tested and, if necessary, treated for STDs before an IUD is inserted.

What are the signs and symptoms of PID?

Symptoms of PID vary from none to severe. When PID is caused by chlamydial infection, a woman may experience mild symptoms or no symptoms at all, while serious damage is being done to her reproductive organs. Because of vague symptoms, PID goes unrecognized by women and their health care providers about two-thirds of the time. Women who have symptoms of PID most commonly have lower abdominal pain. Other signs and symptoms include fever, unusual vaginal discharge that may have a foul odor, painful intercourse, painful urination, irregular menstrual bleeding, and pain in the right upper abdomen (rare).

What are the complications of PID?

Prompt and appropriate treatment can help prevent complications of PID. Without treatment, PID can cause permanent damage to the female reproductive organs. Infection-causing bacteria can silently invade the fallopian tubes, causing normal tissue to turn into scar tissue. This scar tissue blocks or interrupts the normal movement of eggs into the uterus. If the fallopian tubes are totally blocked by scar tissue, sperm cannot fertilize an egg, and the woman becomes infertile. Infertility also can occur if the fallopian tubes are partially blocked or even slightly damaged. About one in ten women with PID becomes infertile, and if a woman has multiple episodes of PID, her chances of becoming infertile increase.

In addition, a partially blocked or slightly damaged fallopian tube may cause a fertilized egg to remain in the fallopian tube. If this fertilized egg begins to grow in the tube as if it were in the uterus, it is called an ectopic pregnancy. As it grows, an ectopic pregnancy can rupture the fallopian tube causing severe pain, internal bleeding, and even death.

Scarring in the fallopian tubes and other pelvic structures can also cause chronic pelvic pain (pain that lasts for months or even years). Women with repeated episodes of PID are more likely to suffer infertility, ectopic pregnancy, or chronic pelvic pain.

How is PID diagnosed?

PID is difficult to diagnose because the symptoms are often subtle and mild. Many episodes of PID go undetected because the woman or her health care provider fails to recognize the implications of mild or nonspecific symptoms. Because there are no precise tests for PID, a diagnosis is usually based on clinical findings. If symptoms such as lower abdominal pain are present, a health care provider should perform a physical examination to determine the nature and location of the pain and check for fever, abnormal vaginal or cervical discharge, and for evidence of gonorrheal or chlamydial infection. If the findings suggest PID, treatment is necessary.

The health care provider may also order tests to identify the infection-causing organism or to distinguish between PID and other problems with similar symptoms. A pelvic ultrasound is a helpful procedure for diagnosing PID. An ultrasound can view the pelvic area to see whether the fallopian tubes are enlarged or whether an abscess is present. In some cases, a laparoscopy may be necessary to confirm the diagnosis. A laparoscopy is a surgical procedure in which a thin, rigid tube with a lighted end and camera (laparoscope) is inserted through a small incision in the abdomen. This procedure enables the doctor to view the internal pelvic organs and to take specimens for laboratory studies, if needed.

What is the treatment for PID?

PID can be cured with several types of antibiotics. A health care provider will determine and prescribe the best therapy. However, antibiotic treatment does not reverse any damage that has already occurred to the reproductive organs. If a woman has pelvic pain and other symptoms of PID, it is critical that she seek care immediately. Prompt antibiotic treatment can prevent severe damage to reproductive organs. The longer a woman delays treatment for PID, the more likely she is to become infertile or to have a future ectopic pregnancy because of damage to the fallopian tubes.

Because of the difficulty in identifying organisms infecting the internal reproductive organs and because more than one organism may be responsible for an episode of PID, PID is usually treated with at least two antibiotics that are effective against a wide range of infectious agents. These antibiotics can be given by mouth or by injection. The symptoms may go away before the infection is cured. Even if symptoms go away, the woman should finish taking all of the prescribed medicine. This will help prevent the infection from returning. Women being treated for PID should be re-evaluated by their health care provider two to three days after starting treatment to be sure the antibiotics are working to cure the infection. In addition, a woman's sex partner(s) should be treated to decrease the risk of re-infection, even if the partner(s) has no symptoms. Although sex partners may have no symptoms, they may still be infected with the organisms that can cause PID.

How can PID be prevented?

Women can protect themselves from PID by taking action to prevent STDs or by getting early treatment if they do get an STD. The surest way to avoid transmission of STDs is to abstain from sexual intercourse, or to be in a long-term mutually monogamous relationship with a partner who has been tested and is known to be uninfected. Latex male condoms, when used consistently and correctly, can reduce the risk of transmission of chlamydia and gonorrhea.

The Centers for Disease Control and Prevention (CDC) recommends yearly chlamydia testing of all sexually active women age 25 or younger, older women with risk factors for chlamydial infections (those who have a new sex partner or multiple sex partners), and all pregnant women. An appropriate sexual risk assessment by a health care provider should always be conducted and may indicate more frequent screening for some women.

Treating STDs early can prevent PID. Women who are told they have an STD and are treated for it should notify all of their recent sex partners so they can see a health care provider and be evaluated for STDs. Sexual activity should not resume until all sex partners have been examined and, if necessary, treated.

Vaginal Yeast Infections

What is a vaginal yeast infection?

A vaginal yeast infection is irritation of the vagina and the area around it called the vulva (vul-vuh). Yeast is a type of fungus. Yeast infections are caused by overgrowth of the fungus *Candida albicans*. Small amounts of yeast are always in the vagina. But when too much yeast grows, you can get an infection. Yeast infections are very common. About 75 percent of women have one during their lives. And almost half of women have two or more vaginal yeast infections.

What are the signs of a vaginal yeast infection?

The most common symptom of a yeast infection is extreme itchiness in and around the vagina. Other symptoms include:

- burning, redness, and swelling of the vagina and the vulva;
- pain when passing urine;
- pain during sex;
- soreness;
- a thick, white vaginal discharge that looks like cottage cheese and does not have a bad smell; and
- a rash on the vagina.

You may only have a few of these symptoms. They may be mild or severe.

Should I call my doctor if I think I have a yeast infection?

Yes, you need to see your doctor to find out for sure if you have a yeast infection. The signs of a yeast infection are much like those of sexually transmitted infections (STIs) like chlamydia and gonorrhea. So, it's hard to be sure you have a yeast infection and not something more serious. If you've had vaginal yeast infections before, talk to your doctor about using over-the-counter medicines.

How is a vaginal yeast infection diagnosed?

Your doctor will do a pelvic exam to look for swelling and discharge. Your doctor may also use a swab to take a fluid sample from your vagina. A quick look with a microscope or a lab test will show if yeast is causing the problem.

Why did I get a yeast infection?

Many things can raise your risk of a vaginal yeast infection, such as:

- stress;

- lack of sleep;
- illness;
- poor eating habits, including eating extreme amounts of sugary foods;
- pregnancy;
- having your period;
- taking certain medicines, including birth control pills, antibiotics, and steroids;
- diseases such as poorly controlled diabetes and HIV/acquired immunodeficiency syndrome (AIDS); or
- hormonal changes during your periods.

Can I get a yeast infection from having sex?

Yes, but it is rare. Most often, women don't get yeast infections from sex. The most common cause is a weak immune system.

How are yeast infections treated?

Yeast infections can be cured with antifungal medicines available as creams, tablets, or ointments or suppositories that are inserted into the vagina. These products can be bought over the counter at the drug store or grocery store. Your doctor can also prescribe you a single dose of oral fluconazole. But do not use this drug if you are pregnant.

Infections that don't respond to these medicines are starting to be more common. Using antifungal medicines when you don't really have a yeast infection can raise your risk of getting a hard-to-treat infection in the future.

Is it safe to use over-the-counter medicines for yeast infections?

Yes, but always talk with your doctor before treating yourself for a vaginal yeast infection if you:

- are pregnant,
- have never been diagnosed with a yeast infection, or
- have repeated yeast infections.

Studies show that two-thirds of women who buy these products don't really have a yeast infection. Using these medicines the wrong way may lead to a hard-to-treat infection. Plus, treating yourself for a yeast infection when you really have something else may worsen the problem. Certain STIs that go untreated can cause cancer, infertility, pregnancy problems, and other health problems. If you decide to use these over-the-counter medicines, read and follow the directions carefully. Some creams and inserts may weaken condoms and diaphragms.

If I have a yeast infection, does my sexual partner need to be treated?

Yeast infections are not STIs, and health experts don't know for sure if they are transmitted sexually. About 12–15 percent of men get an itchy rash on the penis if they have unprotected sex with an infected woman. If this happens to your partner, he should see a doctor. Men who haven't been circumcised are at higher risk.

How can I avoid getting another yeast infection?

To help prevent vaginal yeast infections, you can:

- avoid douches;
- avoid scented hygiene products like bubble bath, sprays, pads, and tampons;
- change tampons and pads often during your period;
- avoid tight underwear or clothes made of synthetic fibers;
- wear cotton underwear and pantyhose with a cotton crotch;
- change out of wet swimsuits and exercise clothes as soon as you can; and
- avoid hot tubs and very hot baths.

If you keep getting yeast infections, be sure and talk with your doctor.

What should I do if I get repeat yeast infections?

Call your doctor. About five percent of women get four or more vaginal yeast infections in one year. This is called recurrent vulvovaginal candidiasis (RVVC). RVVC is more common in women with diabetes or weak immune systems. Doctors most often treat this problem with antifungal medicine for up to six months.

Chapter 54

Vancomycin-Resistant Enterococci (VRE)

What is vancomycin-resistant enterococci (VRE)?

Enterococci are bacteria that are normally present in the human intestines and in the female genital tract and are often found in the environment. These bacteria can sometimes cause infections. Vancomycin is an antibiotic that is often used to treat infections caused by enterococci. In some cases, enterococci have become resistant to vancomycin and are called vancomycin-resistant enterococci, or VRE. Most VRE infections occur in people in hospitals.

What types of infections does VRE cause?

VRE can live in the human intestines and female genital tract without causing disease (often called colonization). However, sometimes, it can be the cause infections of the urinary tract, the bloodstream, or of wounds.

Are certain people at risk of getting VRE?

The following persons are at an increased risk becoming infected with VRE:

- People who have been previously treated with the antibiotic vancomycin or other antibiotics for long periods of time

"VRE: Information for the Public," Centers for Disease Control and Prevention (CDC), April 7, 2008.

- People who are hospitalized, particularly when they receive antibiotic treatment for long periods of time

- People with weakened immune systems such as patients in intensive care units, or in cancer or transplant wards

- People who have undergone surgical procedures such as abdominal or chest surgery

- People with medical devices that stay in for some time such as urinary catheters or central intravenous (IV) catheters.

- People who are colonized with VRE

How common is VRE?

Information collected by the Centers for Disease Control and Prevention (CDC) during 2006 and 2007 showed that enterococci caused about one of every eight infections in hospitals and only about 30% of these are VRE. VRE can be more common in certain groups of people such as those with weakened immune systems.

What is the treatment for VRE?

People who are colonized (bacteria are present, but have no symptoms of an infection) with VRE do not usually need treatment. Most VRE infections can be treated with antibiotics other than vancomycin. Laboratory testing of the VRE can determine which antibiotics will work. For people who get VRE infections in their bladder and have urinary catheters, removal of the catheter when it is no longer needed can also help get rid of the infection.

How is VRE spread?

VRE is often passed from person to person by the hands of caregivers. VRE can get onto a caregiver's hands after they have contact with other people with VRE or after contact with contaminated surfaces. VRE can also be spread directly to people after they touch surfaces that are contaminated with VRE. VRE is not usually spread through the air by coughing or sneezing.

How can I prevent the spread of VRE?

If you or someone in your household has VRE, the following are some things you can do to prevent the spread of VRE:

- Keep your hands clean. Always wash your hands thoroughly after using the bathroom and before preparing food. Clean your hands after contact with persons who have VRE. Wash with soap and water (particularly when visibly soiled) or use alcohol-based hand rubs.

- Frequently clean areas of your home such as your bathroom that may become contaminated with VRE.

- Wear gloves if you may come in contact with body fluids that may contain VRE, such as stool or bandages from infected wounds. Always wash your hands after removing gloves.

- If you have VRE, be sure to tell health care providers caring for you that you have VRE so that they are aware of your infection. Health care facilities use special precautions to help prevent the spread of VRE to others.

What should I do if I think I have VRE?

Talk with your health care provider if you think you have VRE.

Chapter 55

Whooping Cough (Pertussis)

Whooping cough—or pertussis—is an infection of the respiratory system caused by the bacterium *Bordetella pertussis* (or *B. pertussis*). It's characterized by severe coughing spells that end in a "whooping" sound when the person breathes in. Before a vaccine was available, pertussis killed 5,000 to 10,000 people in the United States each year. Now, the pertussis vaccine has reduced the annual number of deaths to less than 30.

But in recent years, the number of cases has started to rise. By 2004, the number of whooping cough cases spiked past 25,000, the highest level it's been since the 1950s. It's mainly affected infants younger than six months old before they're adequately protected by immunizations, and kids 11 to 18 years old whose immunity has faded.

Signs and Symptoms

The first symptoms of whooping cough are similar to those of a common cold:

- runny nose
- sneezing
- mild cough
- low-grade fever

After about one to two weeks, the dry, irritating cough evolves into coughing spells. During a coughing spell, which can last for more than a minute, the child may turn red or purple. At the end of a spell, the child may make a characteristic whooping sound when breathing in or may vomit. Between spells, the child usually feels well.

Although it's likely that infants and younger children who become infected with *B. pertussis* will develop the characteristic coughing episodes with their accompanying whoop, not everyone will. However, sometimes infants don't cough or whoop as older kids do. They may look as if they're gasping for air with a reddened face and may actually stop breathing for a few seconds during particularly bad spells.

Adults and adolescents with whooping cough may have milder or atypical symptoms, such as a prolonged cough without the coughing spells or the whoop.

Contagiousness

Pertussis is highly contagious. The bacteria spread from person to person through tiny drops of fluid from an infected person's nose or mouth. These may become airborne when the person sneezes, coughs, or laughs. Others then can become infected by inhaling the drops or getting the drops on their hands and then touching their mouths or noses.

Infected people are most contagious during the earliest stages of the illness up to about two weeks after the cough begins. Antibiotics shorten the period of contagiousness to five days following the start of antibiotic treatment.

Prevention

Whooping cough can be prevented with the pertussis vaccine, which is part of the DTaP (diphtheria, tetanus, acellular pertussis) immunization. DTaP immunizations are routinely given in five doses before a child's sixth birthday. To give additional protection in case immunity fades, the American Association of Pediatrics (AAP) now recommends that kids ages 11–18 get a booster shot of the new combination vaccine (called Tdap), ideally when they're 11 or 12 years old, instead of the Td booster routinely given at this age. As is the case with all immunization schedules, there are important exceptions and special circumstances. Your doctor will have the most current information.

Experts believe that up to 80% of nonimmunized family members will develop whooping cough if they live in the same house as someone who has the infection. For this reason, anyone who comes into close contact with someone who has pertussis should receive antibiotics to prevent spread of the disease. Young kids who have not received all five doses of the vaccine may require a booster dose if exposed to an infected family member.

Incubation

The incubation period (the time between infection and the onset of symptoms) for whooping cough is usually seven to ten days, but can be as long as 21 days.

Duration

Pertussis can cause prolonged symptoms. The child usually has one to two weeks of common cold symptoms, followed by approximately two to four weeks of severe coughing, though the coughing spells can sometimes last even longer. The last stage consists of another several weeks of recovery with gradual resolution of symptoms. In some children, the recovery period may last for months.

Professional Treatment

Call the doctor if you suspect that your child has whooping cough. To make a diagnosis, the doctor will take a medical history, do a thorough physical exam, and take nose and throat mucus samples that will be examined and cultured for *B. pertussis* bacteria. Blood tests and a chest x-ray may also be done.

If your child has whooping cough, it will be treated with antibiotics, usually for two weeks. Many experts believe that the medication is most effective in shortening the infection when it's given in the first stage of the illness, before coughing spells begin. But even if antibiotics are started later, they're still important because they can stop the spread of the pertussis infection to others. Ask your doctor whether preventive antibiotics or vaccine boosters for other family members are needed.

Some kids with whooping cough need to be treated in a hospital. Infants and younger children are more likely to be hospitalized because they're at greater risk for complications such as pneumonia, which occurs in about one in five children under the age of one year who have pertussis. Up to 75% of infants younger than six months old with whooping cough will receive hospital treatment. In infants younger than six months of age, whooping cough can even be life-threatening.

While in the hospital, a child may need suctioning of thick respiratory secretions. Breathing will be monitored and oxygen given, if needed. Intravenous (IV) fluids might be required if the child shows signs of dehydration or has difficulty eating. Precautions will be taken to prevent the infection from spreading to other patients, hospital staff, and visitors.

Home Treatment

If your child is being treated for pertussis at home, follow the schedule for giving antibiotics exactly as your doctor prescribed. Giving cough medicine probably will not help, as even the strongest usually can't relieve the coughing spells of whooping cough.

During recovery, let your child rest in bed and use a cool-mist vaporizer to help loosen respiratory secretions and soothe irritated lungs and breathing passages. (Be sure to follow directions for keeping it clean and mold-free.) In addition, keep your home free of irritants that can trigger coughing spells, such as aerosol sprays, tobacco smoke, and smoke from cooking, fireplaces, and wood-burning stoves.

Kids with whooping cough may vomit or not eat or drink much because of frequent coughing. So offer smaller, more frequent meals and encourage your child to drink lots of fluids. Watch for signs of dehydration, too, including thirst, irritability, restlessness, lethargy, sunken eyes, a dry mouth and tongue, dry skin, crying without tears, and fewer trips to the bathroom to urinate (or in infants, fewer wet diapers).

When to Call the Doctor

Call the doctor if you suspect that your child has whooping cough or has been exposed to someone with whooping cough, even if your child has already received all scheduled pertussis immunizations.

Your child should be examined by a doctor if he or she has prolonged coughing spells, especially if these spells:

- make your child turn red or purple,
- are followed by vomiting,
- are accompanied by a whooping sound when your child breathes in after coughing.

If your child has been diagnosed with whooping cough and is being treated at home, seek immediate medical care if he or she has difficulty breathing or shows signs of dehydration.

Part Three

Self-Treatment for Contagious Diseases

Chapter 56

Self-Care for Colds or Flu

Chapter Contents

Section 56.1

What to Do for Colds and Flu

Text in this section is from "Get Set for Winter Illness Season,"
U.S. Food and Drug Administration (FDA), July 22, 2009.

While contagious viruses are active year-round, fall and winter are when we're all most vulnerable to them. This is due in large part to people spending more time indoors with others when the weather gets cold.

Colds and Flu

Most respiratory bugs come and go within a few days, with no lasting effects. However, some cause serious health problems. Although symptoms of colds and flu can be similar, the two are different.

Colds are usually distinguished by a stuffy or runny nose and sneezing. Other symptoms include coughing, a scratchy throat, and watery eyes. No vaccine against colds exists because they can be caused by many types of viruses. Often spread through contact with mucus, colds come on gradually.

Flu comes on suddenly, is more serious, and lasts longer than colds. The good news is that yearly vaccination can help protect you from getting the flu. Flu season in the United States generally runs from November to April.

Flu symptoms include fever, headache, chills, dry cough, body aches, fatigue, and general misery. Like colds, flu can cause a stuffy or runny nose, sneezing, and watery eyes. Young children may also experience nausea and vomiting with flu.

Prevention Tips

Get Vaccinated against Flu

Flu complications cause an average of 36,000 deaths each year, according to the Centers for Disease Control and Prevention (CDC). Flu vaccine, available as a shot or a nasal spray, remains the best way to prevent and control influenza. The best time to get a flu vaccination is from October through November, although getting it in December and January is not too late. A new flu shot is needed every year because the predominant flu viruses change every year.

Everyone—children, adolescents, adults, and elderly people— should be vaccinated. Certain people are more at risk for developing complications from flu; they should be immunized as soon as vaccine is available. These groups include:

- people 65 and older;

- residents of nursing homes or other places that house people with chronic medical conditions such as diabetes, asthma, and heart disease;

- adults and children with heart or lung disorders, including asthma;

- adults and children who have required regular medical follow-up or hospitalization during the preceding year because of chronic metabolic diseases (including diabetes), kidney dysfunction, a weakened immune system, or disorders caused by abnormalities of hemoglobin (a protein in red blood cells that carries oxygen); and

- young people ages six months to 18 years receiving long-term aspirin therapy, and who as a result might be at risk for developing Reye syndrome after being infected with influenza.

Also, flu vaccination for health care workers is urged because unvaccinated workers can be a primary cause of outbreaks in health care settings. Talk to your doctor before getting vaccinated if you have certain allergies, especially to eggs; have an illness, such as pneumonia; have a high fever; or are pregnant.

Wash Your Hands Often

Teach children to do the same. Both colds and flu can be passed through coughing, sneezing, and contaminated surfaces, including the hands. CDC recommends regular washing of your hands with warm, soapy water for about 15 seconds.

Try to Limit Exposure to Infected People

Keep infants away from crowds for the first few months of life. This is especially important for premature babies who may have underlying abnormalities such as lung or heart disease.

Practice Healthy Habits

- Eat a balanced diet.

- Get enough sleep.

- Exercise. It can help the immune system better fight off the germs that cause illness.

- Do your best to keep stress in check.

Also, people who use tobacco or who are exposed to secondhand smoke are more prone to respiratory illnesses and more severe complications than nonsmokers.

Already Sick?

Usually, colds and flu simply have to be allowed to run their course. You can try to relieve symptoms without taking medicine. Gargling with salt water may relieve a sore throat. And a cool-mist humidifier may help relieve stuffy noses.

Here are other steps to consider:

- First, call your doctor. This will ensure that the best course of treatment can be started early.

- If you are sick, try not to make others sick too. Limit your exposure to other people. Also, cover your mouth with a tissue when you cough or sneeze, and throw used tissues into the trash immediately.

- Stay hydrated and rested. Fluids can help loosen mucus and make you feel better, especially if you have a fever. Avoid alcoholic and caffeinated products. These may dehydrate you.

- Know your medicine options. If you choose to use medicine, there are over-the-counter (OTC) options that can help relieve the symptoms of colds and flu.

If you want to unclog a stuffy nose, nasal decongestants may help. Cough suppressants quiet coughs; expectorants loosen mucus so you can cough it up; antihistamines help stop a runny nose and sneezing; and pain relievers can ease fever, headaches, and minor aches. In addition, there are prescription antiviral medications approved by the U.S. Food and Drug Administration (FDA) that are indicated for treating the flu. Talk to your health care professional to find out what will work best for you.

Taking Over-the-Counter (OTC) Products

Be wary of unproven treatments: It's best to use treatments that have been approved by the FDA. Many people believe that products with certain ingredients—vitamin C or Echinacea, for example—can treat winter illnesses. Unless the FDA has approved a product for treatment of specific symptoms, you cannot assume that the product will treat those symptoms. Tell your health care professionals about any supplements or herbal remedies you use.

Read medicine labels carefully and follow directions: People with certain health conditions, such as high blood pressure, should check with a health care professional or pharmacist before taking a new cough and cold medicine. Some medicines can worsen underlying health problems.

Choose appropriate OTC medicines: Choose OTC medicines specifically for your symptoms. If all you have is a runny nose, only use a medicine that treats a runny nose. This can keep you from unnecessarily doubling up on ingredients, a practice that can prove harmful.

Check the medicine's side effects: Certain medications such as antihistamines can cause drowsiness. Medications can interact with food, alcohol, dietary supplements, and each other. The safest strategy is to make sure your health care professional and pharmacist know about every product you are taking, including nonprescription drugs and any dietary supplements such as vitamins, minerals, and herbals.

Check with a doctor before giving medicine to children: Get medical advice before treating children suffering from cold and flu symptoms. Do not give children medication that is labeled only for adults.

Don't give aspirin or aspirin-containing medicines to children and teenagers: Children and teenagers suffering from flu-like symptoms, chickenpox, and other viral illnesses shouldn't take aspirin. Reye syndrome, a rare and potentially fatal disease found mainly in children, has been associated with using aspirin to treat flu or chickenpox in kids. Reye syndrome can affect the blood, liver, and brain. Some medicine labels may refer to aspirin as salicylate or salicylic acid. Be sure to educate teenagers, who may take OTC medicines without their parents' knowledge.

When to See a Doctor

See a health care professional if you aren't getting any better or if your symptoms worsen. Mucus buildup from a viral infection can lead to a bacterial infection. With children, be alert for high fevers and for abnormal behavior such as unusual drowsiness, refusal to eat, crying a lot, holding the ears or stomach, and wheezing.

Signs of trouble for all people can include:

- a cough that disrupts sleep;
- a fever that won't go down;
- increased shortness of breath;
- face pain caused by a sinus infection; or
- worsening of symptoms, high fever, chest pain, or a difference in the mucus you're producing, all after feeling better for a short time.

Cold and flu complications may include bacterial infections (for example: bronchitis, sinusitis, ear infections, and pneumonia) that could require antibiotics.

Remember: While antibiotics are used against bacterial infections, they don't help against viral infections such as the cold or flu.

Section 56.2

Cold and Flu Guidelines: Myths and Facts

Myth: You can catch the flu from a flu shot.

Fact: The flu vaccine is made from an inactivated virus, so a person cannot get the flu from a flu shot. Some people may be sore at the spot where the vaccination was injected, and in a few cases, may develop a fever, muscle aches, and feel unwell for a day or two. In very rare cases when a person is allergic to the vaccine, there may be an immediate reaction.

Myth: One kind of flu is the "stomach flu."

Fact: About one out of three people with the flu may have an upset stomach, but this is rarely the main symptom of the flu. Other viruses and bacteria, and food poisoning are more common causes of nausea, vomiting, and diarrhea.

Myth: There is nothing you can do once you get sick with the flu except stay home in bed.

Fact: Antivirals, when started within two days after flu symptoms appear, can reduce the duration of the illness and the severity of symptoms. Symptom relief medications can also help to minimize the discomfort associated with flu symptoms.

Myth: You can catch the flu or a cold from going outdoors in cold weather.

Fact: The flu and colds are more common in the winter months because that is when the viruses spread across the country. It has nothing to do with being outside in cold weather.

Myth: Large doses of Vitamin C can keep you from catching the flu or a cold, or will quickly cure them.

Fact: These claims have not been proven. Still, it is important to one's overall health to consume the minimum daily requirement of Vitamin C (75 and 90 milligrams (mg)/day for adult women and men, respectively; smokers, require an additional 35 mg/day).

Myth: "Feed a cold and starve a fever (flu)."

Fact: This is definitely not a good idea in either case. More fluids than usual are needed when someone has the flu or a cold. It is recommended to drink plenty of water and juice, eat enough food to satisfy an appetite, and drink hot fluids to ease a cough and sore throat.

Myth: Herbal remedies are an effective treatment for colds.

Fact: Echinacea and other herbs are getting a lot of publicity as cold remedies. To date, none of these claims are solidly supported by scientific studies.

Myth: Chicken soup and hot toddies are effective treatments for the flu or colds.

Fact: A bowl of chicken soup is a popular home remedy. While hot liquids can soothe a scratchy throat or cough, chicken soup has no special power to cure the flu or a cold. As for hot toddies, another folk remedy, any beverage containing alcohol should be avoided when someone is sick.

Section 56.3

Questions and Answers about Preventing Seasonal Flu

This section includes "CDC Says 'Take 3' Steps to Fight the Flu," Centers for Disease Control and Prevention (CDC), July 20, 2009; and "Q and A: Preventing Seasonal Flu," CDC, February 15, 2007.

Three Steps to Fight the Flu

Flu is a serious contagious disease. Each year in the United States, on average, more than 200,000 people are hospitalized and 36,000 people die from seasonal flu complications. Now there is a new and very different flu virus spreading worldwide among people called novel or new H1N1 flu. This virus may cause more illness or more severe illness than usual. The Centers for Disease Control and Prevention (CDC) urges you to take the following actions to protect yourself and others from influenza (the flu):

Take Time to Get Vaccinated

- CDC recommends a yearly seasonal flu vaccine as the first and most important step in protecting against seasonal influenza.

- While there are many different flu viruses, the seasonal flu vaccine protects against the three seasonal viruses that research suggests will be most common.

- Vaccination is especially important for people at high risk of serious flu complications, including young children, pregnant women, people with chronic health conditions like asthma, diabetes or heart and lung disease, and people 65 years and older.

- Seasonal flu vaccine is also important for health care workers, and other people who live with or care for high risk people to prevent giving the flu to those at high risk.

- A seasonal vaccine will not protect you against novel H1N1.

- A new vaccine against novel H1N1 is being produced and will be available as an option for prevention of novel H1N1 infection.

- People at greatest risk for novel H1N1 infection include children, pregnant women, and people with chronic health conditions like asthma, diabetes, or heart and lung disease.

Take Everyday Preventive Actions

- Cover your nose and mouth with a tissue when you cough or sneeze. Throw the tissue in the trash after you use it.

- Wash your hands often with soap and water, especially after you cough or sneeze. Alcohol-based hand cleaners are also effective.

- Avoid touching your eyes, nose, or mouth. Germs spread this way.

- Try to avoid close contact with sick people.

- If you get the flu, CDC recommends that you stay home from work or school for seven days after symptoms begin, or until you are symptom free for 24 hours, whichever is longer.

- While sick, limit contact with others to keep from infecting them.

Take Flu Antiviral Drugs If Your Doctor Recommends Them

- If you get seasonal or novel H1N1 flu, antiviral drugs can treat the flu.

- Antiviral drugs are prescription medicines (pills, liquid, or an inhaled powder) that fight against the flu by keeping flu viruses from reproducing in your body.

- Antiviral drugs can make your illness milder and make you feel better faster. They may also prevent serious flu complications.

- Antiviral drugs are not sold over-the-counter and are different from antibiotics.

- Antiviral drugs may be especially important for people who are very sick (hospitalized) or people who are sick with the flu and who are at increased risk of serious flu complications, such as pregnant women, young children, and those with chronic health conditions.

- For treatment, antiviral drugs work best if started within the first two days of symptoms.

- Flu-like symptoms include fever (usually high), headache, extreme tiredness, dry cough, sore throat, runny or stuffy nose, muscle aches, and sometimes diarrhea and vomiting.

Preventing Seasonal Flu

What can I do to protect myself against the flu?

By far, the single best way to prevent the flu is for individuals, especially people at high risk for serious complications from the flu, to get a vaccination each fall.

What are other steps that can be taken to prevent the flu?

These are other good health habits that can help prevent the flu.

- Avoid close contact with people who are sick. When you are sick, keep your distance from others to protect them from getting sick too.

- If possible, stay home from work, school, and errands when you are sick. You will help prevent others from catching your illness.

- Cover your mouth and nose with a tissue when coughing or sneezing. It may prevent those around you from getting sick.

- Washing your hands often will help protect you from germs.

- Avoid touching your eyes, nose, or mouth. Germs are often spread when a person touches something that is contaminated with germs and then touches his or her eyes, nose, or mouth.

Also, antiviral medications may be used to prevent the flu.

Can herbal, homeopathic, or other folk remedies protect against the flu?

There is no scientific evidence that any herbal, homeopathic, or other folk remedies have any benefit against influenza.

How long can human influenza viruses remain viable on inanimate items (such as books and doorknobs)?

Studies have shown that human influenza viruses generally can survive on surfaces for between two and eight hours.

What kills influenza virus?

Influenza virus is destroyed by heat (167–212° Fahrenheit (F) [75–100° Celsius]). In addition, several chemical germicides, including chlorine, hydrogen peroxide, detergents (soap), iodophors (iodine-based antiseptics), and alcohols are effective against influenza viruses if used in proper concentration for sufficient length of time. For example, wipes or gels with alcohol in them can be used to clean hands. The gels should be rubbed until they are dry.

Section 56.4

Taking Care of Yourself When You Have Seasonal Flu

"Taking Care of Yourself When You Have Seasonal Flu,"
Centers for Disease Control and Prevention (CDC), February 23, 2009.

Flu Symptoms

The flu is a contagious respiratory illness caused by influenza viruses. It can cause mild to severe illness, and at times can lead to death.

Symptoms of flu include the following:

- Fever (usually high)
- Headache
- Extreme tiredness
- Dry cough
- Sore throat

- Runny or stuffy nose

- Muscle aches

- Stomach symptoms, such as nausea, vomiting, and diarrhea, also can occur but are more common in children than adults

While getting a flu vaccine each year is the best way to protect against flu, influenza antiviral drugs can fight against influenza, offering a second line of defense against the flu.

Antiviral Drugs

Antiviral drugs are an important second line of defense against the flu.

- If you do get the flu, antiviral drugs are an important treatment option. (They are not a substitute for vaccination.)

- Antiviral drugs are prescription medicines (pills, liquid, or an inhaler) that fight against the flu by keeping flu viruses from reproducing in your body.

- Antiviral drugs can make your illness milder and make you feel better faster. They may also prevent serious flu complications. This could be especially important for people at high risk.

- For treatment, antiviral drugs work best if started soon after getting sick (within two days of symptoms).

There are four flu antiviral drugs approved for use in the United States. The four antiviral drugs are:

1. Oseltamivir (brand name Tamiflu®) is approved to both treat and prevent influenza A and B virus infection in people one year of age and older.

2. Zanamivir (brand name Relenza®) is approved to treat influenza A and B virus infection in people seven years and older and to prevent influenza A and B virus infection in people five years and older.

3. Amantadine (Symmetrel®, generic) is approved to treat and prevent only influenza A viruses in people older than one year.

4. Rimantadine (Flumadine®, generic) is approved to prevent only influenza A virus infection among people older than one

year. It is approved to treat only influenza A virus infections in people 13 and older.

Antiviral drugs differ in terms of who can take them, how they are given, their dose (which can vary depending on a person's age or medical conditions), and side effects. For more information, consult the package insert for each drug. Your doctor can help decide whether you should take an antiviral drug this flu season and which one you should use.

If You Get Sick

Most healthy people recover from the flu without complications. If you get the flu:

- Stay home from work or school.
- Get lots of rest, drink plenty of liquids, and avoid using alcohol and tobacco.
- There are over-the-counter (OTC) medications to relieve the symptoms of the flu (but never give aspirin to children or teenagers who have flu-like symptoms, particularly fever).
- Remember that serious illness from the flu is more likely in certain groups of people including people 65 and older, pregnant women, people with certain chronic medical conditions, and young children.
- Consult your doctor early on for the best treatment, but also be aware of emergency warning signs that require urgent medical attention.

Emergency Warning Signs

Seek emergency medical care if you or someone you know is having any of following warning signs or symptoms.

In children, emergency warning signs that need urgent medical attention include the following:

- Fast breathing or trouble breathing
- Bluish skin color
- Not drinking enough fluids
- Not waking up or not interacting

- Being so irritable that the child does not want to be held
- Flu-like symptoms improve but then return with fever and worse cough
- Fever with a rash

In adults, the following emergency warning signs need urgent medical attention:

- Difficulty breathing or shortness of breath
- Pain or pressure in the chest or abdomen
- Sudden dizziness
- Confusion
- Severe or persistent vomiting

Seek emergency medical care if you or someone you know is experiencing any of the listed symptoms.

Chapter 57

Sore Throat Care

Definition

A sore throat is discomfort, pain, or scratchiness in the throat. A sore throat often makes it painful to swallow.

Considerations

Sore throats are common. Most of the time, the soreness is worse in the morning and improves as the day progresses.

Like colds, the vast majority of sore throats are caused by viral infections. This means most sore throats will not respond to antibiotics. Many people have a mild sore throat at the beginning of every cold. When the nose or sinuses become infected, drainage can run down the back of the throat and irritate it, especially at night. Or, the throat itself can be infected.

Some viruses can cause specific types of sore throat. For example, Coxsackievirus sometimes causes blisters in the throat, especially in the late summer and early fall. Mononucleosis and the flu can also cause specific viral throat infections.

Strep throat is the most common bacterial cause of sore throat. Because strep throat can occasionally lead to rheumatic fever, antibiotics are given. Strep throat often includes a fever (greater than 101° Fahrenheit [F]), white, draining patches on the throat, and swollen or tender lymph glands in the neck. Children may have a headache and stomach pain.

"Sore Throat," © 2009 A.D.A.M., Inc. Reprinted with permission.

A sore throat is less likely to be strep throat if it is a minor part of a typical cold (with runny nose, stuffy ears, cough, and similar symptoms). Strep cannot be accurately diagnosed by looking at the throat alone. It requires a laboratory test.

Sometimes breathing through the mouth will cause a sore throat in the absence of any infection. During the months of dry winter air, some people will wake up with a sore throat most mornings. This usually disappears after having something to drink.

In addition, allergies (allergic rhinitis) can cause a sore throat.

With a sore throat, sometimes the tonsils or surrounding parts of the throat are inflamed. Either way, removing the tonsils to try to prevent future sore throats is not recommended for most children.

Causes

- Breathing through the mouth (can cause drying and irritation of the throat)
- Common cold
- Endotracheal intubation (tube insertion)
- Flu
- Infectious mononucleosis
- Something stuck in the throat
- Strep throat
- Surgery such as tonsillectomy and adenoidectomy
- Viral pharyngitis

Home Care

Most sore throats are soon over. In the meantime, the following remedies may help:

- Drink warm liquids. Honey or lemon tea is a time-tested remedy.
- Gargle several times a day with warm salt water (1/2 tsp of salt in one cup water).
- Cold liquids or popsicles help some sore throats.
- Sucking on hard candies or throat lozenges can be very soothing, because it increases saliva production. This is often as effective as more expensive remedies, but should not be used in young children because of the choking risk.
- Use a cool-mist vaporizer or humidifier to moisten and soothe a dry and painful throat.

- Try over-the-counter pain medications, such as acetaminophen. Do not give aspirin to children.

When to Contact a Medical Professional

Call your health care provider if there is:

- excessive drooling in a young child;
- fever, especially 101° F or greater;
- pus in the back of the throat;
- red rash that feels rough, and increased redness in the skin folds;
- severe difficulty swallowing or breathing;
- tender or swollen lymph glands in the neck.

What to Expect at Your Office Visit

Your health care provider will perform a physical examination. He or she may want to know some details about the sore throat, such as:

- How long has the sore throat been present?
- Have other family members had recent sore throats?
- Is the pain increasing, staying the same, or decreasing?
- Are you able to swallow saliva, fluids, and food?
- Is there excessive drooling (in infants)?
- Are you hoarse?
- Is it worse at night? Are you able to sleep?
- Are you breathing through your mouth?
- Is the soreness better in the morning? Better with moist air or mist? Better with medication?
- What other symptoms are also present—noisy breathing, fever, wheezing, allergies, rash?
- Have you had a recent injury or surgery?
- Are there swollen lymph glands in your neck?
- Are there sores or pus in the back of your throat?
- Is there a sensation of gagging?
- What medications are you taking?
- What is your typical daily diet?

The following diagnostic tests may be performed:

- Complete blood count
- Monospot test (to rule out mononucleosis)
- Throat culture and rapid strep test

Treatment

Usually, treatment will be delayed until lab test results are known. Doctors will often begin treatment of a sore throat immediately if there is a family history of rheumatic fever, if the patient has scarlet fever, or if rheumatic fever is commonly occurring in the community at the time.

Antibiotics are usually not wise if the strep test or throat culture is negative, and they can have serious side effects.

When antibiotics are started, it is important to complete the entire course as directed, even after symptoms improve. Children can return to school or day care 24 hours after antibiotics are started.

For a sore throat caused by infectious mononucleosis, rest and home treatment is recommended.

For a sore throat caused by bacterial tonsillitis, antibiotic treatment may be recommended. Some tonsillitis is viral and will clear up without treatment (surgery is rarely necessary). Recurrent or persistent sore throats without bacterial infection may be due to allergies and require antiallergy treatment.

Prevention

Clean your hands frequently, especially before eating. This is a powerful way to help prevent many sore throat infections. You might avoid some sore throats by reducing contact with people with sore throats, but often these people are contagious even before they have symptoms, so this approach is less effective.

Not too long ago, tonsils were commonly removed in an attempt to prevent sore throats. This is no longer recommended in most circumstances.

A cool mist vaporizer or humidifier can prevent some sore throats caused by breathing dry air with an open mouth.

References

Alcaide ML, Bisno AL. Pharyngitis and epiglottitis. *Infect Dis Clin North Am.* 2007;21(2):449–69,vii.

Del Mar CB, Glasziou PP, Spinks A. Antibiotics for sore throat. *Cochrane Database Syst Rev.* 2008:(3):CD000023.

Chapter 58

Fever: What You Can Do

Alternative Names

Elevated temperature; Hyperthermia; Pyrexia

Definition

Fever is the temporary increase in the body's temperature, in response to some disease or illness.

A child has a fever when their temperature is at or above one of these levels:

- 100.4° Fahrenheit (F) (38° Celsius [C]) measured in the bottom (rectally)
- 99.5° F (37.5° C) measured in their mouth (orally)
- 99° F (37.2° C) measured under their arm (axillary)

An adult probably has a fever when their temperature is above 99–99.5° F (37.2–37.5° C), depending on what time of the day it is.

Considerations

Normal body temperature may change during any given day. It is usually highest in the evening. Other factors that may affect body temperature:

"Fever," © 2009 A.D.A.M., Inc. Reprinted with permission.

- In the second part of a woman's menstrual cycle, her temperature may go up by one degree or more.
- Physical activity, strong emotion, eating, heavy clothing, medications, high room temperature, and high humidity can all increase your body temperature.

Fever is an important part of the body's defense against infection. Many infants and children develop high fevers with minor viral illnesses. While a fever signals to us that a battle might be going on in the body, the fever is fighting for the person, not against.

Most bacteria and viruses that cause infections in people thrive best at 98.6° F. Many infants and children develop high fevers with minor viral illnesses. While a fever signals to us that a battle might be going on in the body, the fever is fighting for the person, not against.

Brain damage from a fever generally will not occur unless the fever is over 107.6° F (42° C). Untreated fevers caused by infection will seldom go over 105° F unless the child is overdressed or trapped in a hot place.

Febrile seizures do occur in some children. However, most febrile seizures are over quickly, do not mean your child has epilepsy, and do not cause any permanent harm. Unexplained fevers that continue for days or weeks are called fevers of undetermined origin (FUO).

Causes

Almost any infection can cause a fever. Some common infections are:

- respiratory infections such as colds or flu-like illnesses, sore throats, ear infections, sinus infections, infectious mononucleosis, and bronchitis;
- urinary tract infections;
- viral gastroenteritis and bacterial gastroenteritis; and
- more serious infections such as pneumonia, bone infections (osteomyelitis), appendicitis, tuberculosis, skin infections or cellulitis, and meningitis.

Children may have a low-grade fever for one or two days after some immunizations.

Teething may cause a slight increase in a child's temperature, but not higher than 100° F.

Autoimmune or inflammatory disorders may also cause fevers. Some examples are:

- arthritis or connective tissue illnesses such as rheumatoid arthritis, systemic lupus erythematosus;
- ulcerative colitis and Crohn disease; and
- vasculitis or periarteritis nodosa.

The first symptom of a cancer may be a fever. This is especially true of Hodgkin disease, non-Hodgkin lymphoma, and leukemia. Other possible causes of fever include:

- blood clots or thrombophlebitis; and
- medications, such as some antibiotics, antihistamines, some seizure medicines.

Home Care

A simple cold or other viral infection can sometimes cause a high fever (102–104° F, or 38.9–40° C). This does not usually mean you or your child have a serious problem. Some serious infections may cause no fever or even a very low body temperature, especially in infants.

If the fever is mild and have no other problems, you do not need treatment. Drink fluids and rest.

The illness is probably not serious if your child:

- is still interested in playing;
- is eating and drinking well;
- is alert and smiling at you;
- has a normal skin color;
- looks well when their temperature comes down.

Take steps to lower a fever if you or your child are uncomfortable, vomiting, dried out (dehydrated), or not sleeping well. Remember, the goal is to lower, not eliminate, the fever.

When trying to lower a fever:

- Do not bundle up someone who has the chills.
- Remove excess clothing or blankets. The room should be comfortable, not too hot or cool. Try one layer of lightweight clothing, and

377

one lightweight blanket for sleep. If the room is hot or stuffy, a fan may help.

- A lukewarm bath or sponge bath may help cool someone with a fever. This is especially effective after medication is given—otherwise the temperature might bounce right back up.
- Do not use cold baths, ice, or alcohol rubs. These cool the skin, but often make the situation worse by causing shivering, which raises the core body temperature.

Here are some guidelines for taking medicine to lower a fever:

- Acetaminophen (Tylenol®) and ibuprofen (Advil®, Motrin®) help reduce fever in children and adults. Sometimes doctors advise you to use both types of medicine.
- Take acetaminophen every 4–6 hours. It works by turning down the brain's thermostat.
- Take ibuprofen every 6–8 hours. Do not use ibuprofen in children younger than six months old.
- Aspirin is very effective for treating fever in adults. Do not give aspirin to children unless your child's doctor so to use it.
- Know how much you or your child weigh, and then always check the instructions on the package.
- In children under three months of age, call your doctor first before giving medicines.

Eating and drinking with a fever:

- Everyone, especially children, should drink plenty of fluids. Water, popsicles, soup, gelatin are all good choices.
- Do not give too much fruit or apple juice and avoid sports drinks in younger children.
- While eating foods with a fever is fine, foods should not be forced.

When to Contact a Medical Professional

Call a doctor right away if your child:

- is younger than three months old and has a rectal temperature of 100.4° F (38° C) or higher;
- is 3–12 months old and has a fever of 102.2° F (39° C) or higher;

- is under age two years and has a fever that lasts longer than 24–48 hours;
- is older and has a fever for longer than 48–72 hours;
- has a fever over 105° F (40.5° C), unless it comes down readily with treatment and the person is comfortable;
- has other symptoms that suggest an illness may need to be treated, such as a sore throat, earache, or cough;
- has been having fevers come and go for up to a week or more, even if they are not very high;
- has a serious medical illness, such as a heart problem, sickle cell anemia, diabetes, or cystic fibrosis;
- recently had an immunization;
- has a new rash or bruises appear;
- has pain with urination;
- has trouble with their immune system (chronic steroid therapy, after a bone marrow or organ transplant, their spleen previously has been removed, is human immunodeficiency virus (HIV)-positive, or they're being treated for cancer);
- has recently traveled to a third world country.

Call 911 if you or your child has a fever and:

- is crying and cannot be calmed down (children);
- cannot be awakened easily or at all;
- seems confused;
- cannot walk;
- has difficulty breathing, even after their nose is cleared;
- has blue lips, tongue, or nails;
- has a very bad headache;
- has a stiff neck;
- refuses to move an arm or leg (children);
- has a seizure.

Call your doctor right away if you are an adult and you:

- have a fever over 105° F (40.5° C), unless it comes down readily with treatment and you are comfortable;

- have a fever that stays at or keeps on going above 103° F;
- have a fever for longer than 48–72 hours;
- have had fevers come and go for up to a week or more, even if they are not very high;
- have a serious medical illness, such as a heart problem, sickle cell anemia, diabetes, cystic fibrosis, chronic obstructive pulmonary disease (COPD), or other chronic lung problems;
- have a new rash or bruises appear;
- have pain with urination;
- have trouble with your immune system (chronic steroid therapy, after a bone marrow or organ transplant, spleen was previously removed, HIV-positive, were being treated for cancer);
- have recently traveled to a third world country.

What to Expect at Your Office Visit

Your doctor will perform a physical examination, which may include a detailed examination of the skin, eyes, ears, nose, throat, neck, chest, and abdomen to look for the cause of the fever.

Treatment depends on the duration and cause of the fever, and on other accompanying symptoms.

The following diagnostic tests may be performed:

- Blood studies, such as a complete blood count (CBC) or blood differential
- Urinalysis
- X-ray of the chest

References

American College of Emergency Physicians Clinical Policies Subcommittee on Pediatric Fever. Clinical policy for children younger than three years presenting to the emergency department with fever. *Ann Emerg Med.* 2003;42(4):530–545.

Legget J. Approach to fever or suspected infection in the normal host. Goldman L, Ausiello D, eds. *Cecil Medicine*, 23rd ed. Philadelphia, Pa: Saunders Elsevier; 2007: chap 302.

Chapter 59

Mouth Sores: Causes and Care

Alternative Names

Aphthous stomatitis

Definition

Various types of sores can appear anywhere within the mouth, including the inner cheeks, gums, tongue, lips, or palate.

Causes

Most mouth sores are cold sores (also called fever blisters), canker sores, or other irritation caused by:

- biting your cheek, tongue, or lip;
- chewing tobacco;
- braces;
- a sharp or broken tooth or poorly fitting dentures;
- burning your mouth from hot food or drinks.

Cold sores are caused by herpes simplex virus and are very contagious. Usually, you have tenderness, tingling, or burning before the actual sore appears. Herpes sores begin as blisters and then crust over.

"Mouth Sores," © 2009 A.D.A.M., Inc. Reprinted with permission.

The herpes virus can reside in your body for years, appearing as a mouth sore only when something provokes it. Such circumstances may include another illness, especially if there is a fever, stress, hormonal changes (such as menstruation), and sun exposure.

Canker sores are not contagious and can appear as a single pale or yellow ulcer with a red outer ring, or as a cluster of such lesions. The cause of canker sores is not entirely clear, but may be related to:

- a virus,
- a temporary weakness in your immune system (for example, from cold or flu),
- hormonal changes,
- mechanical irritation,
- stress, or
- low levels of vitamin B_{12} or folate.

For unknown reasons, women seem to get canker sores more often than men. This may be related to hormonal changes.

Less commonly, mouth sores can be a sign of an underlying illness, tumor, or reaction to a medication. Such potential illnesses can be grouped into several broad categories:

- Infection (such as hand-foot-mouth syndrome)
- Autoimmune diseases (including lupus)
- Bleeding disorders
- Malignancy (cancer)
- Immunosuppression (that is, when your immune system is weakened—for example, if you have acquired immunodeficiency syndrome [AIDS] or are receiving medication after a transplant)

Drugs that might cause mouth sores include chemotherapeutic agents for cancer, aspirin, barbiturates (used for insomnia), gold (used for rheumatoid arthritis), penicillin, phenytoin (used for seizures), streptomycin, or sulfonamides.

Home Care

Mouth sores generally last 10–14 days, even if you don't do anything. They sometimes last up to six weeks. The following steps can make you feel better:

- Gargle with cool water or eat popsicles. This is particularly helpful if you have a mouth burn.
- Avoid hot beverages and foods, spicy and salty foods, and citrus.
- Take pain relievers like acetaminophen.

For canker sores:

- Rinse with salt water.
- Apply a thin paste of baking soda and water.
- Mix one part hydrogen peroxide with one part water and apply this mixture to the lesions using a cotton swab.
- For more severe cases, treatments include fluocinonide gel (Lidex) or chlorhexidine gluconate (Peridens) mouthwash.

Nonprescription preparations, like Orabase®, can protect a sore inside the lip and on the gums. Blistex® or Campho-Phenique® may provide some relief of canker sores and fever blisters, especially if applied when the sore initially appears.

Additional steps that may help cold sores or fever blisters:

- Apply ice to the lesion
- Take L-lysine tablets

Anti-viral medications for herpes lesions of the mouth may be recommended by your doctor. Some experts feel that they shorten the time that the blisters are present, while others claim that these drugs make no difference.

When to Contact a Medical Professional

Call your doctor if:

- the sore begins soon after you start a new medication;
- you have large white patches on the roof of your mouth or your tongue (this may be thrush or another type of lesion);
- your mouth sore lasts longer than two weeks;
- you are immunocompromised (for example, from human immunodeficiency virus [HIV] or cancer);
- you have other symptoms like fever, skin rash, drooling, or difficulty swallowing.

What to Expect at Your Office Visit

Your doctor will perform a physical examination, focusing on your mouth and tongue. Medical history questions may include the following:

- Are the sores on your lips, gums, tongue, lining of your cheeks, or elsewhere?

- Are the sores open ulcers?

- Are there large, white patches on the roof of the mouth or on your tongue?

- How long have you had the mouth sores? More than two weeks?

- Have you ever had sores of this type before?

- What medications do you take?

- Do you have other symptoms like fever, sore throat, or breath odor?

Treatment may depend on the underlying cause of the mouth sore.

A topical anesthetic (applied to a localized area of the skin) such as lidocaine or Xylocaine® may be used to relieve pain (but should be avoided in children).

An antifungal medication may be prescribed for oral thrush (a yeast infection).

An antiviral medication may be prescribed for herpes lesions (although, some feel that this does not shorten the length of time that the lesions are present).

Antibiotics may be prescribed for severe or persistent canker sores.

Prevention

You can reduce your chance of getting common mouth sores by:

- reducing stress and practicing relaxation techniques like yoga or meditation, and

- avoiding very hot foods or beverages.

You can avoid mechanical irritation by:

- visiting your dentist right away if you have a sharp or broken tooth or misfit dentures,

- chewing slowly,

- using a soft-bristle toothbrush.

If you seem to get canker sores often, talk to your doctor about taking folate and vitamin B_{12} to prevent outbreaks.

If you get cold sores often, taking L-lysine tablets or increasing lysine in your diet (found in fish, chicken, eggs, and potatoes) may reduce outbreaks. Do not use L-lysine if you have high cholesterol, heart disease, or high triglycerides.

To prevent the spread of herpes sores, do not kiss or have oral sex with someone with a cold sore or fever blister. Do not participate in these activities when you have an active cold sore. Do not share razors, lip balm, toothbrushes, or lipsticks.

To prevent cancerous mouth lesions:

- Do not smoke or use tobacco.

- Limit alcohol to two drinks per day.

- Wear a wide-brimmed hat to shade your lips. Wear a lip balm with sun protection factor (SPF) 15 at all times.

References

Mandell GL, Bennett JE, Dolin R. *Principles and Practice of Infectious Diseases.* 5*th* ed. London, UK: Churchill Livingstone, Inc.; 2000.

Yeung-Yue KA. Herpes simplex viruses 1 and 2. *Dermatol Clin.* 2002; 20(2): 249–266.

MacDonald J. Canker sore remedies: baking soda. *CMAJ.* 2002; 166(7): 884.

Gonsalves WC, Chi AC, Neville BW. Common oral lesions: Part I. Superficial mucosal lesions. *Am Fam Physician.* 2007;75(4):501–7.

Chapter 60

Over-the-Counter
(OTC) Medications

Chapter Contents

Section 60.1

OTC Medications and How They Work

Reprinted with permission from "OTC Medicines and How They Work," October 2003, Updated March 2008, http://familydoctor.org/online/ famdocen/home/otc-center/basics/otc.html. Copyright © 2008 American Academy of Family Physicians. All Rights Reserved.

In this section, you'll learn what you need to know to make wise choices about over-the-counter (OTC) medicines for you and your family. The following information has been adapted from the American Academy of Family Physicians (AAFP) guide for physicians, "Appropriate Use of Common OTC Analgesics and Cough and Cold Medications."

What does OTC mean?

OTC is short for over-the-counter. These are medicines you can buy without a prescription from your doctor. Chances are, you've used OTC medicines many times to relieve pain and treat symptoms of the common cold, the flu and allergies. In this section, you'll learn about four of the most common types of OTC products and how each works.

- Pain relievers
- Antihistamines
- Decongestants
- Cough medicines

Pain Relievers

The OTC products that relieve your headache, fever, or muscle aches are not all the same. That's because the pain relievers you see in the aisles of your local drug store or pharmacy are either nonsteroidal anti-inflammatory drugs (called NSAIDs, which include aspirin, ibuprofen, naproxen, and ketoprofen) or acetaminophen. Each of these drugs has a different way of working.

Aspirin and NSAIDs relieve pain by stopping the production of prostaglandins, which are natural chemicals in the body. Prostaglandins irritate nerve endings, triggering the sensation of pain. Commonly used NSAIDs include:

- Aspirin, the medicine in products such as Bayer and St. Joseph
- Ibuprofen, the medicine in products such as Advil and Motrin IB
- Naproxen, the medicine in products such as Aleve
- Ketoprofen, the medicine in products such as Orudis KT

Acetaminophen relieves pain and reduces fever. We don't completely understand the way acetaminophen relieves pain. We do know that unlike aspirin and NSAIDs (which work in the skin, muscles, and joints), acetaminophen blocks painful sensation in the brain and the spinal cord.

- Acetaminophen is in products such as Tylenol and Tempra.

Antihistamines

Antihistamines work by blocking the receptors that trigger itching, nasal irritation, sneezing, and mucus production. The three types of antihistamines are:

- diphenhydramine, the medicine in products such as Banophen, Benadryl Allergy, and Diphenhist;
- brompheniramine, the medicine in products such as Dimetapp Allergy; and
- chlorpheniramine, the medicine in products such as Aller-Chlor, Chlo-Amine, and Chlor-Trimeton Allergy.

Decongestants

Decongestants work by narrowing blood vessels in the lining of the nose. As a result, less blood is able to flow through the nasal area, and swollen tissue inside the nose shrinks. Pseudoephedrine is the only decongestant used in OTC products.

- Pseudoephedrine is in products such as Allermed, Genaphed, and Sudafed.

Cough Medicines

Cough medicines are grouped into two types: antitussives and expectorants. Antitussives, or cough suppressants, block the cough reflex.

- Dextromethorphan is a common antitussive and is in products such as Delsym, Drixoral, Pertussin CS, and Robitussin Pediatric.

Expectorants, on the other hand, are thought to thin mucus and make coughing more productive in clearing the mucus from the airway.

- Guaifenesin is the only expectorant used in OTC products and is in products such as Guiatuss, Robitussin, and Tusibron.

Timeline of Symptoms Associated with the Common Cold

There is no cure for the common cold. Medicine can only make your symptoms less bothersome until your body can fight off the virus. Medicine won't make your cold go away completely. The following are tips to help you feel better when you have a cold:

- Stay home and rest, especially while you have a fever.

Table 60.1. Over-the-Counter (OTC) Medicines for Cold Symptoms

Day	Symptoms	OTC Medicine
1	Fatigue, mild sore throat	Acetaminophen (some brand names: Panadol, Tempra, Tylenol) or nonsteroidal anti-inflammatory drug (ibuprofen [some brand names: Advil, Menadol, Motrin])
2	Runny nose	Antihistamine (diphenhydramine [some brand names: Benadryl Allergy, Banophen, Diphenhist], chlorpheniramine [some brand names: Aller-Chlor, Chlo-Amine, Chlor-Trimeton Allergy])
3	"Stopped up" nose	Decongestant (pseudoephedrine [some brand names: Allermed, Genaphed, Sudafed])
4	Dry cough	Antitussive (dextromethorphan [some brand names: Drixoral, Pertussin CS, Robitussin Pediatric])
5	Moist, productive cough	Expectorant (guaifenesin [some brand names: Guiatuss, Robitussin, Tusibron])
6	Voice "breaks" or disappears altogether	No medicine will help your voice come back sooner. Resting it is the only thing that will help.

- Don't smoke and avoid secondhand smoke.

- Drink plenty of fluids like water, fruit juices, and clear soups.

- Don't drink alcohol.

- Gargle with warm salt water a few times a day to relieve a sore throat. Throat sprays or lozenges may also help relieve the pain.

- Use salt water (saline) nose drops to help loosen mucus and moisten the tender skin in your nose.

Many cold medicines are available over-the-counter. If you decide to use an OTC medicine to treat your cold symptoms, consult Table 60.1.

How to Read an OTC Drug Label

You don't need a prescription to buy OTC medicine. But like prescription drugs, OTC medicines can also cause unwanted and sometimes dangerous side effects. Before you buy an OTC medicine, it's important to read and thoroughly understand the information on the drug label. Use the following as a guide. If you have questions about a medicine, ask your pharmacist or family doctor.

1. **Active ingredient:** The active ingredient is the chemical compound in the medicine that works to relieve your symptoms. It is always the first item on the label. There may be more than one active ingredient in a product. The label will clearly show this.

2. **Uses:** This section lists the symptoms the medicine is meant to treat. The U.S. Food and Drug Administration (FDA) must approve these uses. Uses are sometimes referred to as "indications."

3. **Warnings:** This safety information will tell you what other medicines, foods, or situations (such as driving) to avoid while taking this medicine.

4. **Directions:** Information about how much medicine you should take and how often you should take it will be listed here.

5. **Other information:** Any other important information, such as how to store the product, will be listed here.

6. **Inactive ingredients:** An inactive ingredient is a chemical compound in the medicine that isn't meant to treat a symptom.

Inactive ingredients can include preservatives, binding agents, and food coloring. This section is especially important for people who know they have allergies to food coloring or other chemicals.

7. **Questions or comments:** A toll-free number is provided to address any questions or comments you may have about the medicine.

How to Get the Most from Your Medicine

OTC medicines can help you feel better. But if they are taken the wrong way, they can actually make you feel worse. To use OTC medicines correctly, follow these guidelines.

Talk to Your Family Doctor

If there is something you don't understand about a medicine you're taking or are planning to take, ask your doctor or pharmacist. If you still don't understand, ask him or her to explain things more clearly. If you are taking more than one medicine, be sure to ask how the medicines will work together in your body. Sometimes medicines cause problems when they are taken together (called a drug interaction).

Following is a list of questions you can ask your doctor to learn how to use each medicine correctly and safely:

- What does the medicine do?
- When and how should I take the medicine?
- What are the possible side effects (reactions your body may have to the medicine)?
- Will the medicine react to any other medicines, foods, or drinks?
- Should I avoid any activities while I'm taking the medicine?
- How will I know if the medicine is working?

Know about the Medicine You Take

You should know the following things about each medicine you take:

- Name (generic name and brand name)
- Reason for taking it

- How much to take and how often to take it
- Possible side effects and what to do if you experience them
- How long to continue taking the medicine
- Special instructions (taking it at bedtime or with meals, and so forth)

Know What to Avoid While Taking the Medicine

Some foods can cause side effects, such as stomach upset, if you are taking medicine. Drinking alcohol is generally not a good idea while you are taking medicine. Some medicines cause reactions such as sun sensitivity (getting a sunburn or sun rash), so you may have to limit your outdoor activities or protect your skin from the sun.

Read the label to see what to avoid while you are taking an over-the-counter medicine. Follow the instructions just as you would with a prescription medicine. If you have questions, ask your doctor or pharmacist.

Follow these dos and don'ts:

- Do read the label carefully.
- Do take your medicine exactly as your doctor tells you to.
- Do make sure that each of your doctors (if you see more than one) has a list of all of the medicines you're currently taking.
- Do make sure everyone you live with knows what medicine you're taking and when you're supposed to take it.
- Don't combine prescription medicines and OTC medicines unless your doctor says it's okay.
- Don't stop taking a medicine, change how much you take, or how often you take it without first talking to your doctor.
- Don't take someone else's medicine.
- Don't use medicine after its expiration date.
- Don't crush, break, or chew tablets or capsules unless your doctor tells you to. Some medicines won't work right unless they are swallowed whole.

Understand Generic Versus Brand Name

Just like foods, some medicines come in both brand names and generics. Generic medicines are generally cheaper. Compare the list of ingredients. If the generic has the same ingredients as the brand name, you may want to consider using it. But be careful: the generic may contain different amounts of certain medicines. Ask your doctor or pharmacist if you have questions about which medicine to choose.

Follow these tips for choosing medicines:

- If you have questions, ask your doctor or pharmacist.
- Although it can seem overwhelming, take the time to look at all the choices.
- Read the label carefully and note what symptoms the medicine will treat.
- Look for a medicine that will treat only the symptoms you have. For example, if you only have a runny nose, don't pick a medicine that also treats coughs and headaches.
- Note how much medicine you should take, and what side effects it may cause.
- Note what medicines or foods you should not take with the medicine.
- Check to see if the medicine causes problems for people with certain health problems (such as asthma or hypertension).

Know When to Call Your Doctor

If you're taking an OTC medicine and it doesn't seem to be working, call your doctor. Your symptoms can get much worse if you wait too long to get treated by your doctor.

You should also call if you have side effects or any concerns about the medicine you're taking.

Potential Side Effects of OTC Medicines in Adults

While OTC medicines have a low risk of side effects when used occasionally by healthy adults, they can pose risks for very young children, the elderly, people with kidney problems, and people taking more than one medicine. These people have an increased risk of side effects when they take OTC medicines. Potential side effects are described here.

Aspirin and NSAIDs

The main side effect associated with aspirin and other NSAIDs is gastrointestinal (GI) problems. These problems can range from upset stomach to GI bleeding, a serious event that is most likely to occur in older people. The chances of experiencing GI problems from NSAIDs or aspirin increase the larger the dose you take and the longer you take them.

NSAIDs can cause a variety of side effects related to kidney function. These side effects range from reversible inflammation to permanent kidney damage.

Aspirin and NSAIDs may make high blood pressure worse or interfere with blood pressure medicines.

High doses of aspirin pose a risk of liver damage for people who have liver disease, juvenile arthritis, or rheumatic fever.

Acetaminophen

Although safe in the majority of users, long-term use of high doses of acetaminophen, especially in products that also contain caffeine (such as Excedrin) or codeine (such as Tylenol with Codeine), has been shown to cause a form of kidney disease called analgesic nephropathy. This serious condition may develop after years or decades of daily use.

Antihistamines

Antihistamines can cause sedation or drowsiness and, therefore, can significantly impair a person's ability to drive or operate machinery. The sedative effects of antihistamines may increase the risk of falling. Antihistamines can also cause temporary dry mouth or eyes.

Decongestants

Pseudoephedrine can temporarily cause nervousness, dizziness, and sleeplessness. It can make you lose your appetite or retain urine. It can also cause heart palpitations, high blood pressure, or high blood sugar levels.

Cough Medicines

Codeine, when used as a cough suppressant, can temporarily cause nausea, sedation, and constipation. Dextromethorphan, the medicine in Drixoral, Pertussin CS, and Robitussin, has a lower risk of sedation and GI side effects. It can, however, cause feelings of confusion, agitation, nervousness, or irritability.

Drug-Drug Interactions

The body processes (metabolizes) every drug differently. If drugs are used together, their metabolism and effect on the body can change. When this happens, the chance that you will have side effects for each drug may become greater.

Alcohol and OTC Medicines

Pain Relievers

If you drink more than one alcoholic beverage per week and use NSAIDs, including aspirin, you may be at increased risk of GI bleeding. People who consume three or more alcoholic beverages each day should consult their physician before using any pain reliever.

Acetaminophen is much less likely than NSAIDs to be associated with GI problems, including bleeding. But to minimize the risk of serious liver injury, you should never take more than the recommended daily dose (four grams per day).

Antihistamines, Decongestants, and Cough Medicines

The combination of OTC antihistamines and alcohol can increase drowsiness, especially in elderly people. In addition, alcohol makes the drowsiness, sedation, and impaired motor skills associated with the cough suppressants dextromethorphan (in products such as Drixoral, Robitussin) and codeine worse.

Special Groups

Some groups of people may be more likely to experience the side effects associated with OTC medicines. The sections below include tips for using OTC medicines in the following special populations:

- Children
- Older adults
- Pregnant or breastfeeding women
- Other groups

Children

When used properly, OTC medications pose little risk to children. However, children metabolize drugs differently than adults. You should know how OTC drugs will affect your children before you use them. Talk with your family doctor if you have any questions about giving your child OTC medicines.

- Acetaminophen is generally considered the treatment of choice for children's pain relief.

- Do not give ibuprofen to a child younger than six months of age.

- Do not give aspirin to children under the age of 18 because of the risk of Reye syndrome (a drug reaction that can lead to permanent brain injury).

- Do not use nasal decongestants, cough medicines and cold medicines in young children, especially those under two years of age. These medicines can produce dangerous side effects. In addition, cough and cold medicines are not effective in treating young children.

It can be helpful for parents and other caregivers to keep track of the medicine a child is taking. One way to do that is with a medication log. Using a log can help avoid giving too much medicine or giving it too often. It can also provide important information to your family doctor if there is a problem.

Medicine and Your Child: How to Give the Right Dose

Here are some tips on giving the right dose:

- When your doctor says to give the medicine "every six hours" that generally means the medicine is taken four times a day (for example, at breakfast, lunch, supper and bed time). It doesn't generally mean to wake the child up in the night to take medicine. And "take every eight hours" generally means the medicine should be taken three times a day.

- Pay close attention to the dosage given on the label. Labels for liquid medicines give measurements in both teaspoons (tsp) and in milliliters (mL). Your pharmacist can give you a measuring device (a spoon that's made especially for measuring medicine, a syringe or a cup) that's labeled with both tsp and mL. Your pharmacist should also show you how to use it. One tsp is not the same as one mL. Read the label carefully and make sure you give the right amount of medicine to your child. An ordinary kitchen teaspoon may not hold the correct amount of medicine.

- Measure the medicine carefully. If you're using a measuring cup, set it on a level surface such as a countertop and then pour the medicine in it.

- "If a little medicine is good, a lot is better (or will work quicker)" is wrong. Giving too much medicine can be harmful. Be sure you only give the recommended dose of each medicine.

- If you use a syringe-type measuring device to give liquid medicine to your child, first throw away the small cap of the syringe. Children can choke on these caps.

- If your child has a bad reaction to a medicine or is allergic to a medicine, tell your doctor right away. Also, keep a record of the following information at home: the name of the medicine, the dosage directions, the illness the medicine was used for, and the side effects the medicine caused.

Older Adults

The elderly use a number of medications at the same time and therefore need to pay careful attention to drug-drug interactions between OTC medications and prescription medications. Older adults should talk with their doctor about the medicines they take and potential interactions with OTC medicines.

- There is a relatively high risk of kidney disease and GI bleeding in elderly patients who use NSAIDs. Discuss this risk with your family doctor.

- Pseudoephedrine can increase blood pressure and the pressure in your eye that can lead to glaucoma. It can also make existing blockages in the urinary tract worse. Pseudoephedrine interacts negatively with many other drugs such as beta-blockers, antidepressants, insulin, and some medications that treat low blood sugar.

- If you use a monoamine oxidase inhibitor (MAOI), a type of prescription antidepressant, or take any medication for a seizure disorder, you should avoid using pseudoephedrine. Pseudoephedrine can change the way these drugs work in your system. Some common MAOIs include Marplan (generic: isocarboxazid), Nardil (generic: phenelzine sulfate), and Parnate (generic: tranylcypromine sulfate).

- If you use a MAOI, you should not use dextromethorphan. Dextromethorphan interferes with the way MAOIs work.

Pregnant or Breastfeeding Women

Pregnant or breastfeeding women should talk with their doctor before using any medicine. Some can affect your baby. The following are some general guidelines.

Pregnancy

- Acetaminophen is generally considered safe for short-term pain relief during pregnancy.
- Avoid using aspirin during pregnancy. It can cause birth defects or problems during delivery.
- Avoid using other NSAIDs, especially during the third trimester of pregnancy. They can cause heart defects in the baby.

Breastfeeding

- Acetaminophen and NSAIDs such as ibuprofen provide safe pain relief for women who are breastfeeding.
- Avoid using aspirin because it is excreted in breast milk and can cause rashes and bleeding problems in nursing infants.
- Limit long-term use of antihistamines. Antihistamines are excreted in breast milk, and may cause side effects such as sedation, irritability, crying, and sleep disturbances in nursing infants. Antihistamines may also interfere with the production of milk.

General Tips

These steps can help minimize the risk of side effects during pregnancy and breastfeeding:

- Talk to your doctor about possible alternatives to medicine.
- Avoid the use of medicines during the first trimester.
- Take oral medicines after nursing or before the infant's longest sleep period.
- Avoid the use of extra-strength, maximum-strength, or long-acting medicines.
- Avoid combination products.
- Watch your infant for possible side effects, such as a rash, difficulty breathing, headache, or other symptoms that your

child didn't have before you took the medicine and then breastfed.

Other Groups

People with health problems such as kidney disease, heart disease, diabetes, asthma, blood clotting disorders, or gout may be at increased risk of side effects associated with OTC medicines.

Section 60.2

Kids Are Not Just Small Adults: Tips on Giving OTC Medicine to Children

"Kids Aren't Just Small Adults–Medicines, Children and the Care Every Child Deserves," U.S. Food and Drug Administration (FDA), April 30, 2009.

Use care when giving any medicine to an infant or a child. Even over-the-counter (OTC) medicines that you buy are serious medicines. The following is advice for giving OTC medicine to your child, from the U.S. Food and Drug Administration (FDA) and the makers of OTC medicines:

1. Always read and follow the Drug Facts label on your OTC medicine. This is important for choosing and safely using all OTC medicines. Read the label every time, before you give the medicine. Be sure you clearly understand how much medicine to give and when the medicine can be taken again.

2. Know the active ingredient in your child's medicine. This is what makes the medicine work and is always listed at the top of the Drug Facts label. Sometimes an active ingredient can treat more than one medical condition. For that reason, the same active ingredient can be found in many different medicines that are used to treat different symptoms. For example, a medicine for a cold and a medicine for a headache could

each contain the same active ingredient. So, if you're treating a cold and a headache with two medicines and both have the same active ingredient, you could be giving two-times the normal dose. If you're confused about your child's medicines, check with a doctor, nurse, or pharmacist.

3. Give the right medicine, in the right amount, to your child. Not all medicines are right for an infant or a child. Medicines with the same brand name can be sold in different strengths, such as infant, child, and adult formulas. The amount and directions are also different for children of different ages or weights. Always use the right medicine and follow the directions exactly. Never use more medicine than directed, even if your child seems sicker than the last time.

4. Talk to your doctor, pharmacist, or nurse to find out what mixes well and what doesn't. Medicines, vitamins, supplements, foods, and beverages don't always mix well with each other. Your health care professional can help.

5. Use the dosing tool that comes with the medicine, such as a dropper or a dosing cup. A different dosing tool, or a kitchen spoon, could hold the wrong amount of medicine.

6. Know the difference between a tablespoon (tbsp.) and a teaspoon (tsp.) Do not confuse them. A tablespoon holds three times as much medicine as a teaspoon. On measuring tools, a teaspoon (tsp.) is equal to "5 cc" or "5 ml."

7. Know your child's weight. Directions on some OTC medicines are based on weight. Never guess the amount of medicine to give to your child or try to figure it out from the adult dose instructions. If a dose is not listed for your child's age or weight, call your doctor or other members of your health care team.

8. Prevent a poison emergency by always using a child-resistant cap. Re-lock the cap after each use. Be especially careful with any products that contain iron; they are the leading cause of poisoning deaths in young children.

9. Store all medicines in a safe place. Today's medicines are tasty, colorful, and many can be chewed. Kids may think that these products are candy. To prevent an overdose or poisoning emergency, store all medicines and vitamins in a safe place out of your child's (and even your pet's) sight and reach. If your

child takes too much, call the Poison Center Hotline at 800-222-1222 (open 24 hours every day) or call 9-1-1.

10. Check the medicine three times. First, check the outside packaging for such things as cuts, slices, or tears. Second, once you are at home, check the label on the inside package to be sure you have the right medicine. Make sure the lid and seal are not broken. Third, check the color, shape, size, and smell of the medicine. If you notice anything different or unusual, talk to a pharmacist or another health care professional.

Section 60.3

Nonprescription Cough and Cold Medicine Use in Children

"Using Over-the-Counter Cough and Cold Products in Children," U.S. Food and Drug Administration (FDA), October 22, 2008.

On Oct. 8, 2008, the Food and Drug Administration (FDA) released a statement that supports recent voluntary actions by many drug manufacturers regarding the use of nonprescription, over-the-counter (OTC) cough and cold products in children.

The voluntary actions announced by the Consumer Healthcare Products Association (CHPA) are intended to help prevent and reduce the misuse of these products in children and to better inform consumers about their safe and effective use. CHPA represents most of the manufacturers of these products.

Members of CHPA have volunteered to modify the product labels of OTC cough and cold medicines to state "do not use" in children under four years of age. (Many of the products currently state "do not use" in children under two years of age.) Additionally, the manufacturers are introducing new child-resistant packaging and new measuring devices for use with the products.

CHPA's voluntary actions will not affect the availability of the medicines, but will result in a transition period where the instructions for using some OTC cough and cold medicines in children will be different from others. Some product instructions will state "do not use" in children under four years of age, while others will instruct not to use in children under two years of age.

FDA does not typically request that OTC products with previous labeling be removed from the shelves during a voluntary label change such as this one. The agency recommends following the dosage instructions and warnings on the label that accompanies the medication if you have or buy a product that does not have the voluntarily modified labeling.

Recent FDA Actions

- FDA has held two public meetings on the safe use of nonprescription OTC cough and cold medicines in children. The meeting on Oct. 2, 2008, focused on labeling of these products.

- FDA issued a nationwide Public Health Advisory in January 2008 recommending that these products not be used in children under the age of two because of the risk of serious and potentially life-threatening side effects.

- FDA continues to reach out to other public health agencies, consumer and patient groups, drug manufacturers, CHPA, and the scientific community. As it obtains more up-to-date information and scientific data about the safety and effectiveness of these products in children, FDA can take the appropriate regulatory steps moving forward.

Tips for Parents and Caregivers

1. Do not give children medications labeled only for adults.

2. Talk to your health care professional, such as your doctor or pharmacist, if you have any questions about using cough or cold medicines in children.

3. Choose OTC cough and cold medicines with child-resistant safety caps, when available. After each use, make sure to close the cap tightly and store the medicines out of the sight and reach of children.

4. Check the "active ingredients" section of the "Drug Facts" label of the medicines that you choose. This section will help you understand what symptoms the active ingredients in the medicine are intended to treat. Cough and cold medicines often

have more than one active ingredient, such as an antihistamine, a decongestant, a cough suppressant, an expectorant, or a pain reliever, and fever reducer.

5. Be very careful if you are giving more than one medicine to a child. Make sure the medicines do not have the same type of active ingredients. For example, do not give a child more than one medicine that has a decongestant. If you use two medicines that have the same or similar active ingredients, your child could be harmed by getting too much of an ingredient.

6. Carefully follow the directions for how to use the medicine in the "Drug Facts" part of the label. These directions tell you how much medicine to give and how often you can give it. If you have a question about how to use the medicine, ask your pharmacist or other health care professional. Overuse or misuse of these products can lead to serious and potentially life-threatening side effects, such as rapid heartbeat, drowsiness, breathing problems, and seizures.

7. Only use measuring devices that come with the medicine or those specially made for measuring drugs. Do not use household spoons to measure medicines for children because household spoons come in different sizes and are not meant for measuring medicines.

8. Understand that using OTC cough and cold medicines does not cure the cold or cough. These medicines only treat your child's symptoms, such as runny nose, congestion, fever, and aches. They do not shorten the length of time your child is sick.

Chapter 61

Avoid Drug Interactions

People often combine foods. For example, chocolate and peanut butter might be considered a tasty combination. But eating chocolate and taking certain drugs might carry risks. In fact, eating chocolate and taking monoamine oxidase (MAO) inhibitors, such as Nardil (phenelzine) or Parnate (tranylcypromine) could be dangerous. MAO inhibitors treat depression. Someone who eats an excessive amount of chocolate after taking an MAO inhibitor may experience a sharp rise in blood pressure. Other foods that should be avoided when taking MAO inhibitors: aged cheese, sausage, bologna, pepperoni, and salami. These foods can also cause elevated blood pressure when taken with these medications.

There are three main types of drug interactions:

- Drugs with food and beverages
- Drugs with dietary supplements
- Drugs with other drugs

"Consumers should learn about the warnings for their medications and talk with their health care professionals about how to lower the risk of interactions," says Shiew-Mei Huang, PhD, deputy director of the Office of Clinical Pharmacology in FDA's Center for Drug Evaluation and Research (CDER).

"Avoiding Drug Interactions," U.S. Food and Drug Administration (FDA), November 28, 2008.

Drugs with Food and Beverages

Consequences of drug interactions with food and beverages may include delayed, decreased, or enhanced absorption of a medication. Food can affect the bioavailability (the degree and rate at which a drug is absorbed into someone's system), metabolism, and excretion of certain medications.

Examples of Drug Interactions with Food and Beverages

Alcohol: If you are taking any sort of medication, it's recommended that you avoid alcohol, which can increase or decrease the effect of many drugs.

Grapefruit juice: Grapefruit juice is often mentioned as a product that can interact negatively with drugs, but the actual number of drugs the juice can interact with is less well-known. Grapefruit juice shouldn't be taken with certain blood pressure-lowering drugs or cyclosporine for the prevention of organ transplant rejection. That's because grapefruit juice can cause higher levels of those medicines in your body, making it more likely that you will have side effects from the medicine. The juice can also interact to cause higher blood levels of the anti-anxiety medicine BuSpar (buspirone); the anti-malaria drugs Quinora or Quinate (quinine); and Halcion (triazolam), a medication used to treat insomnia.

Licorice: This would appear to be a fairly harmless snack food. However, for someone taking Lanoxin (digoxin), some forms of licorice may increase the risk for Lanoxin toxicity. Lanoxin is used to treat congestive heart failure and abnormal heart rhythms. Licorice may also reduce the effects of blood pressure drugs or diuretic (urine-producing) drugs, including HydroDIURIL (hydrochlorothiazide) and Aldactone (spironolactone).

Chocolate: MAO inhibitors are just one category of drugs that shouldn't be consumed with excessive amounts of chocolate. The caffeine in chocolate can also interact with stimulant drugs such as Ritalin (methylphenidate), increasing their effect, or by decreasing the effect of sedative-hypnotics such as Ambien (zolpidem).

Drugs with Dietary Supplements

Research has shown that 50 percent or more of American adults use dietary supplements on a regular basis, according to congressional testimony by the Office of Dietary Supplements in the National Institutes of Health. The law defines dietary supplements in part as products taken by mouth that contain a "dietary ingredient." Dietary ingredients include vitamins, minerals, amino acids, and herbs or botanicals, as well as other substances that can be used to supplement the diet.

Examples of Drug Interactions with Dietary Supplements

St. John's Wort (*Hypericum perforatum*): This herb is considered an inducer of liver enzymes, which means it can reduce the concentration of medications in the blood. St. John's Wort can reduce the blood level of medications such as Lanoxin, the cholesterol-lowering drugs Mevacor and Altocor (lovastatin), and the erectile dysfunction drug Viagra (sildenafil).

Vitamin E: Taking vitamin E with a blood-thinning medication such as Coumadin can increase anti-clotting activity and may cause an increased risk of bleeding.

Ginseng: This herb can interfere with the bleeding effects of Coumadin. In addition, ginseng can enhance the bleeding effects of heparin, aspirin, and nonsteroidal anti-inflammatory drugs such as ibuprofen, naproxen, and ketoprofen. Combining ginseng with MAO inhibitors such as Nardil or Parnate may cause headache, trouble sleeping, nervousness, and hyperactivity.

Ginkgo biloba: High doses of the herb Ginkgo biloba could decrease the effectiveness of anticonvulsant therapy in patients taking the following medications to control seizures: Tegretol, Equetro or Carbatrol (carbamazepine), and Depakote (valproic acid).

Drugs with Other Drugs

Two out of every three patients who visit a doctor leave with at least one prescription for medication, according to a 2007 report on medication safety issued by the Institute for Safe Medication Practices. Close to 40 percent of the U.S. population receive prescriptions for four or more medications. And the rate of adverse drug reactions increases dramatically after a patient is on four or more medications.

Drug-drug interactions have led to adverse events and withdrawals of drugs from the market, according to an article on drug interactions co-authored by Shiew-Mei Huang, PhD, deputy director of FDA's

Office of Clinical Pharmacology. The paper was published in the June 2008 issue of the *Journal of Clinical Pharmacology.*

However, market withdrawal of a drug is a fairly drastic measure. More often, FDA will issue an alert warning the public and health care providers about risks as the result of drug interactions.

Examples of Drug Interactions with Other Drugs

Cordarone (amiodarone): FDA issued an alert in August 2008, warning patients about taking Cordarone to correct abnormal rhythms of the heart and the cholesterol-lowering drug Zocor (simvastatin). Patients taking Zocor in doses higher than 20 milligram (mg) while also taking Cordarone run the risk of developing a rare condition of muscle injury called rhabdomyolysis, which can lead to kidney failure or death. "Cordarone also can inhibit or reduce the effect of the blood thinner Coumadin (warfarin)," said Huang. "So if you're using Cordarone, you may need to reduce the amount of Coumadin you're taking."

Lanoxin (digoxin): "Lanoxin has a narrow therapeutic range. So other drugs, such as Norvir (ritonavir), can elevate the level of Lanoxin," says Huang. "And an increased level of Lanoxin can cause irregular heart rhythms." Norvir is a protease inhibitor used to treat human immunodeficiency virus (HIV), the virus that causes acquired immunodeficiency syndrome (AIDS).

Antihistamines: Over-the-counter (OTC) antihistamines are drugs that temporarily relieve a runny nose, or reduce sneezing, itching of the nose or throat, and itchy watery eyes. If you are taking sedatives, tranquilizers, or a prescription drug for high blood pressure or depression, you should check with a doctor or pharmacist before you start using antihistamines. Some antihistamines can increase the depressant effects (such as sleepiness) of a sedative or tranquilizer. The sedating effect of some antihistamines combined with a sedating antidepressant could strongly affect your concentration level. Operating a car or any other machinery could be particularly dangerous if your ability to focus is impaired. Antihistamines taken in conjunction with blood pressure medication may cause a person's blood pressure to increase and may also speed up the heart rate.

Tips to Avoid Problems

There are lots of things you can do to take prescription or over-the-counter (OTC) medications in a safe and responsible manner.

- Always read drug labels carefully.

- Learn about the warnings for all the drugs you take.

- Keep medications in their original containers so that you can easily identify them.

- Ask your doctor what you need to avoid when you are prescribed a new medication. Ask about food, beverages, dietary supplements, and other drugs.

- Check with your doctor or pharmacist before taking an OTC drug if you are taking any prescription medications.

- Use one pharmacy for all of your drug needs.

- Keep all of your health care professionals informed about everything that you take.

- Keep a record of all prescription drugs, OTC drugs, and dietary supplements (including herbs) that you take. Try to keep this list with you at all times, but especially when you go on any medical appointment.

Chapter 62

Complementary and Alternative Medicine (CAM) for Contagious Diseases

Chapter Contents

411

Section 62.1

Discuss CAM Use with Your Health Care Providers

Text in this section is excerpted from "Time to Talk," National Center for Complementary and Alternative Medicine (NCCAM), 2006.

Why Talk?

To ensure safe, coordinated care among all conventional and complementary and alternative medicine (CAM) therapies, it's time to talk. Talking not only allows fully integrated care, but it also minimizes risks of interactions with a patient's conventional treatments. When patients tell their providers about their CAM use, they can better stay in control and more effectively manage their health. When providers ask their patients about CAM use, they can ensure that they are fully informed and can help patients make wise health care decisions.

CAM is defined as a group of diverse medical and health care systems, practices, and products that are not presently considered to be part of conventional medicine. CAM includes products and practices such as herbal supplements, meditation, chiropractic care, and acupuncture.

In a nationwide government survey, nearly 50 percent of all adults age 18 or older reported using some form of CAM (excluding prayer) during their lifetime, and 36 percent of adults reported CAM use in the past year; people age 50 to 59 were among the most likely to report using CAM.[1] However, in a survey of people age 50 or older, less than one-third of those who reported using CAM have discussed it with their physicians.[2]

The National Center for Complementary and Alternative Medicine (NCCAM) and the AARP (formerly the American Association of Retired Persons) partnered on a consumer telephone survey to measure and understand communication practices between patients age 50 or older and their physicians. The survey confirms that patients and physicians often do not discuss the use of CAM. The primary reasons are that patients do not know that they should tell their providers about their CAM use, and physicians do not ask their patients about CAM use.

Responses to the NCCAM/AARP Survey

CAM Use

- Nearly two-thirds of the respondents (63%) have used one or more CAM therapy.

Communication with Providers about CAM Use

- Of those age 50 or older who use CAM, more than two-thirds (69%) did not talk to their physicians about it.

- The most common reasons cited by respondents who had seen physicians but had not discussed CAM with them were that the physician never asked (42%), they did not know they should (30%), and there was not enough time during the office visit (19%).

- More than one-half of respondents (56%) who had talked about CAM with their physician said they—not their physician—had initiated the CAM discussion.

Topics Discussed with Providers

- For respondents who talked with their providers about CAM, the topics most frequently discussed were the effectiveness of a CAM therapy (67%), what to use (64%), how a CAM therapy might interact with other medications or treatments they receive (60%), advice on whether or not to pursue a CAM therapy (60%), and the safety of a CAM therapy (57%).

Reasons for Using CAM

- Of those who have used CAM, two-thirds did so to treat a specific condition (66%) and for overall wellness (65%).

Use of Conventional Medicine

- Nearly three-fourths of respondents (74%) said they take one or more prescription medicines, and more than one-half (59%) said they take one or more over-the-counter medicines. Twenty percent of respondents reported currently taking more than five prescription medicines.

Demographic Differences

- Women were more likely than men to discuss "what to use" with their physicians (26% versus 16%).

- Men were more likely than women not to have discussed CAM because their physician never asked (46% versus 38%).

- Non-Hispanic White respondents were more likely to say their physician never asked (44%) compared with non-Hispanic Black respondents (25%).

- Respondents in younger age groups (50–54 and 55–64) were more likely to say they had not discussed CAM with their physician because their physician never asked (50% and 44%, respectively) compared with those 65 and older (36%).

Patient Tips for Discussing CAM with Providers

- When completing patient history forms, be sure to include all therapies and treatments you use. Make a list in advance.

- Tell your health care providers about all therapies or treatments—including over-the-counter and prescription medicines, as well as herbal and dietary supplements.

- Take control. Don't wait for your providers to ask about your CAM use.

- If you are considering a new CAM therapy, ask your health care providers about its safety, effectiveness, and possible interactions with medications (both prescription and over-the-counter).

Provider Tips for Discussing CAM with Patients

- Include a question about CAM use on medical history forms.

- Ask your patients to bring a list of all therapies they use, including prescription, over-the-counter, and herbal therapies, and other CAM practices.

- Have your medical staff initiate the conversation.

References

1. Barnes PM, Powell-Griner E, McFann K, Nahin RL. *Complementary and alternative medicine use among adults: United States, 2002.* CDC Advance Data Report #343. 2004.

2. AARP, NCCAM. *Complementary and Alternative Medicine: What People 50 and Older Are Using and Discussing with Their Physicians.* Consumer Survey Report; January 18, 2007.

Section 62.2

Getting to Know
"Friendly Bacteria"—Probiotics

Text in this section is from "Getting to Know 'Friendly Bacteria',"
National Center for Complementary and Alternative Medicine
(NCCAM), March 2008.

If you go to the supermarket, or look at a health magazine or commercial website, chances are you will find products with "probiotics"—certain types of bacteria that are also called "friendly bacteria" or "good bacteria." Probiotics are available as conventional foods and dietary supplements (for example, capsules, tablets, and powders), and in some other forms as well. While some probiotic foods date back to ancient times (fermented foods and cultured milk products), recent interest in probiotics in general has been growing. Americans' spending on probiotic supplements, for example, nearly tripled from 1994 to 2003.

What Are Probiotics?

Experts have debated how to define probiotics more specifically. One widely used definition, developed by the United Nations Food and Agricultural Organization and the World Health Organization, calls probiotics "live microorganisms, which, when administered in adequate amounts, confer a health benefit on the host." (Microorganisms are tiny living organisms—such as bacteria, viruses, and fungi—that can be seen only under a microscope.) Probiotics are not the same thing as prebiotics—nondigestible food ingredients that selectively stimulate the growth and/or activity of bacterial species already in people's colons. When probiotics and prebiotics are mixed together, they form something else, a synbiotic.

Some conventional foods containing probiotics are yogurt, fermented and unfermented milk, miso, tempeh, and some juices and soy beverages. In those foods, and in probiotic supplements, the bacteria may have been present originally or added during preparation. Most often, they come from two groups of bacteria, *Lactobacillus* or *Bifidobacterium*.

415

Within each group, there are different species (for example, *Lactobacillus acidophilus* and *Bifidobacterium bifidus*), and within each species, different strains (or varieties).

A Balance of Bacteria

Why this interest in probiotics? It starts on a universal scale; the world is full of microorganisms (including bacteria), and so are people's bodies—in and on the skin, in the gut, and in other orifices. They take up residence in babies soon after birth. Friendly bacteria are vital to proper development of the immune system, to protection against agents that could cause disease, and to the digestion and absorption of food and nutrients. Each person's mix of bacteria varies. Interactions between a person and the microorganisms in his body, and between the microorganisms themselves, can be crucial to the person's health and well-being.

This bacterial "balancing act" can be thrown off in two major ways:

1. By antibiotics, when they kill friendly bacteria in the gut along with unfriendly bacteria. Some people use probiotics to try to offset side effects from antibiotics like gas, cramping, or diarrhea. Similarly, some use them with the intent to ease symptoms of lactose intolerance, a condition in which the gut cannot digest significant amounts of lactose, the major sugar in milk.

2. "Unfriendly" microorganisms such as disease-causing bacteria, yeasts, fungi, and parasites can also upset the balance. Researchers are exploring whether probiotics could halt these unfriendly agents in the first place and/or suppress their growth and activity in conditions like these:

   • Traveler's diarrhea

   • Irritable bowel syndrome

   • Inflammatory bowel disease (ulcerative colitis and Crohn disease)

   • Infection with *Helicobacter pylori* (*H. pylori*) , a bacterium that causes most ulcers and many types of chronic stomach inflammation

   • Tooth decay and periodontal disease

   • Vaginal infections

- Stomach and respiratory infections that children acquire in daycare
- Skin infections

Do Probiotics Work?

According to the conference report, some uses for which there is some encouraging evidence from study of specific probiotic formulations are as follows:

- To treat diarrhea (this is the strongest area of evidence, especially for diarrhea from rotavirus)
- To prevent and treat infections of the urinary or reproductive systems, such as urinary tract infections and bacterial vaginosis
- To treat irritable bowel syndrome
- To reduce recurrence of bladder cancer
- To shorten how long an intestinal infection that is caused by a bacterium called *Clostridium difficile* lasts
- To prevent and treat pouchitis (a condition that can follow surgery to remove the colon)
- To prevent and manage atopic dermatitis (eczema) in children

Advice to Consumers

If you are a consumer who is thinking about using a probiotic product as complementary and alternative medicine (CAM), consult your health care provider first. No CAM therapy should be used in place of conventional medical care or to delay seeking that care. Also, if you use a probiotic product and experience an effect that concerns you, contact your provider. Keep in mind that effects from one strain of probiotics do not necessarily hold true for other strains, or even for other preparations of the same strain.

In sum, there is limited evidence supporting some uses of probiotics. Better scientific understanding these tiny forms of life and their effects on people is needed.

Section 62.3

Herbal Supplements

This section includes text from the following National Center for Complementary and Alternative Medicine (NCCAM) documents: "Using Dietary Supplements Wisely," February 2009; "Herbs at a Glance: Echinacea," March 2008; "Herbs at a Glance: Goldenseal," May 2008; and "Herbs at a Glance: Licorice Root," June 2008.

Using Herbal Supplements Wisely

Be aware that an herbal supplement may contain dozens of compounds and that its active ingredients may not be known. Researchers are studying many of these products in an effort to identify active ingredients and understand their effects in the body. Also consider the possibility that what's on the label may not be what's in the bottle. Analyses of dietary supplements sometimes find differences between labeled and actual ingredients. For example:

- An herbal supplement may not contain the correct plant species.

- The amount of the active ingredient may be lower or higher than the label states. That means you may be taking less, or more, of the dietary supplement than you realize.

- The dietary supplement may be contaminated with other herbs, pesticides, or metals, or even adulterated with unlabeled ingredients such as prescription drugs.

Echinacea

There are nine known species of echinacea, all of which are native to the United States and southern Canada. The most commonly used, *Echinacea purpurea*, is believed to be the most potent.

Common names: echinacea, purple coneflower, coneflower, American coneflower

Latin names: *Echinacea purpurea, Echinacea angustifolia, Echinacea pallida*

What Echinacea Is Used For

- Echinacea has traditionally been used to treat or prevent colds, flu, and other infections.

- Echinacea is believed to stimulate the immune system to help fight infections.

- Less commonly, echinacea has been used for wounds and skin problems, such as acne or boils.

How It Is Used

The aboveground parts of the plant and roots of echinacea are used fresh or dried to make teas, squeezed (expressed) juice, extracts, or preparations for external use.

What the Science Says

- Study results are mixed on whether echinacea effectively treats colds or flu. For example, two NCCAM-funded studies did not find a benefit from echinacea, either as *Echinacea purpurea* fresh-pressed juice for treating colds in children, or as an unrefined mixture of *Echinacea angustifolia* root and *Echinacea purpurea* root and herb in adults. However, other studies have shown that echinacea may be beneficial in treating upper respiratory infections.

- Most studies to date indicate that echinacea does not appear to prevent colds or other infections.

- NCCAM is continuing to support the study of echinacea for the treatment of upper respiratory infections. NCCAM is also studying echinacea for its potential effects on the immune system.

Side Effects and Cautions

- When taken by mouth, echinacea usually does not cause side effects. However, some people experience allergic reactions, including rashes, increased asthma, and anaphylaxis (a life-threatening allergic reaction). In clinical trials, gastrointestinal side effects were most common.

- People are more likely to experience allergic reactions to echinacea if they are allergic to related plants in the daisy family, which includes ragweed, chrysanthemums, marigolds, and daisies. Also, people with asthma or atopy (a genetic tendency toward allergic reactions) may be more likely to have an allergic reaction when taking echinacea.

• Tell your health care providers about any complementary and alternative practices you use. Give them a full picture of what you do to manage your health. This will help ensure coordinated and safe care.

Goldenseal

Goldenseal is a plant that grows wild in parts of the United States but has become endangered by overharvesting. With natural supplies dwindling, goldenseal is now grown commercially across the United States, especially in the Blue Ridge Mountains.

Common names: goldenseal, yellow root

Latin name: *Hydrastis canadensis*

What Goldenseal Is Used For

• Historically, Native Americans have used goldenseal for various health conditions such as skin diseases, ulcers, and gonorrhea.

• Now, goldenseal is used for colds and other respiratory tract infections, infectious diarrhea, eye infections, and vaginitis (inflammation or infection of the vagina). It is occasionally used to treat cancer.

• It is also applied to wounds and canker sores, and is used as a mouthwash for sore gums, mouth, and throat.

How It Is Used

• The underground stems or roots of goldenseal are dried and used to make teas, liquid extracts, and solid extracts that may be made into tablets and capsules.

• Goldenseal is often combined with echinacea in preparations that are intended to be used for colds.

What the Science Says

• Few studies have been published on goldenseal's safety and effectiveness, and there is little scientific evidence to support using it for any health problem.

- Clinical studies on a compound found in goldenseal, berberine, suggest that the compound may be beneficial for certain infections—such as those that cause some types of diarrhea, as well as some eye infections. However, goldenseal preparations contain only a small amount of berberine, so it is difficult to extend the evidence about the effectiveness of berberine to goldenseal.

- NCCAM is funding research on berberine, including a study to understand the mechanism by which it may act against tumors.

Side Effects and Cautions

- Goldenseal is considered safe for short-term use in adults at recommended dosages. Rare side effects may include nausea and vomiting.

- There is little information about the safety of high dosages or the long-term use of goldenseal.

- Although drug interactions have not been reported, goldenseal may cause changes in the way the body processes drugs, and could potentially increase the levels of many drugs. However, a study of goldenseal and indinavir, a drug used to treat human immunodeficiency virus (HIV) infection, found no interaction.

- Other herbs containing berberine, including Chinese goldthread (*Coptis trifolia*) and Oregon grape (*Mahonia aquifolium*), are sometimes substituted for goldenseal. These herbs may have different effects, side effects, and drug interactions than goldenseal.

- Women who are pregnant or breastfeeding should avoid using goldenseal. The berberine in the herb may cause the uterus to contract, increasing the risk of premature labor or miscarriage. Berberine may also be transferred through breast milk, causing life-threatening liver problems in nursing infants.

- Goldenseal should not be given to infants and young children.

- Tell your health care providers about any complementary and alternative practices you use. Give them a full picture of what you do to manage your health. This will help ensure coordinated and safe care.

Licorice Root

Most licorice is grown in Greece, Turkey, and Asia. Licorice contains a compound called glycyrrhizin (or glycyrrhizic acid). Licorice has a long history of medicinal use in both Eastern and Western systems of medicine.

Common names: licorice root, licorice, liquorice, sweet root, gan zao (Chinese licorice)

Latin names: *Glycyrrhiza glabra*, *Glycyrrhiza uralensis* (Chinese licorice)

What Licorice Root Is Used For

Licorice root has been used as a dietary supplement for stomach ulcers, bronchitis, and sore throat, as well as infections caused by viruses, such as hepatitis.

How It Is Used

- Peeled licorice root is available in dried and powdered forms.
- Licorice root is available as capsules, tablets, and liquid extracts.
- Licorice can be found with glycyrrhizin removed; the product is called DGL (for deglycyrrhizinated licorice).

What the Science Says

- A review of several clinical trials found that glycyrrhizin might reduce complications from hepatitis C in some patients. However, there is not enough evidence to confirm that glycyrrhizin has this effect.
- There are not enough reliable data to determine whether licorice is effective for stomach ulcers.

Side Effects and Cautions

- In large amounts, licorice containing glycyrrhizin can cause high blood pressure, salt and water retention, and low potassium levels, which could lead to heart problems. DGL products are thought to cause fewer side effects.
- The safety of using licorice as a supplement for more than 4–6 weeks has not been thoroughly studied.
- Taking licorice together with diuretics (water pills) or other medicines that reduce the body's potassium levels could cause dangerously low potassium levels.

- People with heart disease or high blood pressure should be cautious about using licorice.

- When taken in large amounts, licorice can affect the body's levels of a hormone called cortisol and related steroid drugs, such as prednisone.

- Pregnant women should avoid using licorice as a supplement or consuming large amounts of licorice as food, as some research suggests it could increase the risk of preterm labor.

Section 62.4

Dietary Supplements

Text in this section is excerpted from "Using Dietary Supplements Wisely," National Center for Complementary and Alternative Medicine (NCCAM), February 2009; and "Colloidal Silver Products," NCCAM, July 2009.

Wise Use of Dietary Supplements

Many people take dietary supplements in an effort to be well and stay healthy. With so many dietary supplements available and so many claims made about their health benefits, how can a consumer decide what's safe and effective?

Key Points

- Federal regulations for dietary supplements are very different from those for prescription and over-the-counter drugs. For example, a dietary supplement manufacturer does not have to prove a product's safety and effectiveness before it is marketed.

- If you are thinking about using a dietary supplement, first get information on it from reliable sources. Keep in mind that dietary supplements may interact with medications or other dietary supplements and may contain ingredients not listed on the label.

- Tell your health care providers about any complementary and alternative practices you use, including dietary supplements. Give them a full picture of what you do to manage your health. This will help ensure coordinated and safe care.

About Dietary Supplements

Dietary supplements were defined in a law passed by Congress in 1994 called the Dietary Supplement Health and Education Act (DSHEA). According to DSHEA, a dietary supplement is a product that:

- is intended to supplement the diet;
- contains one or more dietary ingredients (including vitamins, minerals, herbs or other botanicals, amino acids, and certain other substances) or their constituents;
- is intended to be taken by mouth, in forms such as tablet, capsule, powder, softgel, gelcap, or liquid; and
- is labeled as being a dietary supplement.

Herbal supplements are one type of dietary supplement. An herb is a plant or plant part (such as leaves, flowers, or seeds) that is used for its flavor, scent, and/or therapeutic properties. "Botanical" is often used as a synonym for "herb." An herbal supplement may contain a single herb or mixtures of herbs.

Research has shown that some uses of dietary supplements are effective in preventing or treating diseases. For example, scientists have found that folic acid (a vitamin) prevents certain birth defects, and a regimen of vitamins and zinc can slow the progression of the age-related eye disease macular degeneration. Also, calcium and vitamin D supplements can be helpful in preventing and treating bone loss and osteoporosis (thinning of bone tissue).

Research has also produced some promising results suggesting that other dietary supplements may be helpful for other health conditions (for example, omega-3 fatty acids for coronary disease), but in most cases, additional research is needed before firm conclusions can be drawn.

Dietary Supplement Use in the United States

A national survey conducted in 2007 found that 17.7 percent of American adults had used "natural products" (dietary supplements other than vitamins and minerals) in the past 12 months. The most popular products used by adults for health reasons in the past 30 days were fish oil/omega 3/DHA (37.4%), glucosamine (19.9%), echinacea

(19.8%), flaxseed oil or pills (15.9%), and ginseng (14.1%). In another, earlier national survey covering all types of dietary supplements, approximately 52 percent of adult respondents said they had used some type of supplement in the last 30 days; the most commonly reported were multivitamins/multiminerals (35 percent), vitamins E and C (12–13 percent), calcium (10 percent), and B-complex vitamins (5 percent).

Federal Regulation of Dietary Supplements

The federal government regulates dietary supplements through the U.S. Food and Drug Administration (FDA). The regulations for dietary supplements are not the same as those for prescription or over-the-counter drugs. In general, the regulations for dietary supplements are less strict.

- A manufacturer does not have to prove the safety and effectiveness of a dietary supplement before it is marketed.
- Manufacturers are expected to follow certain "good manufacturing practices" (GMPs) to ensure that dietary supplements are processed consistently and meet quality standards. Requirements for GMPs went into effect in 2008 for large manufacturers and are being phased in for small manufacturers through 2010.
- Once a dietary supplement is on the market, the FDA monitors safety.

Also, once a dietary supplement is on the market, the FDA monitors product information, such as label claims and package inserts. The Federal Trade Commission (FTC) is responsible for regulating product advertising; it requires that all information be truthful and not misleading.

The federal government has taken legal action against a number of dietary supplement promoters or websites that promote or sell dietary supplements because they have made false or deceptive statements about their products or because marketed products have proven to be unsafe.

Safety Considerations

If you are thinking about or are using a dietary supplement, here are some points to keep in mind. Tell your health care providers about any complementary and alternative practices you use, including dietary supplements. Give them a full picture of what you do to manage your health. This will help ensure coordinated and safe care. It is especially important to talk to your health care provider if you are:

- Thinking about replacing your regular medication with one or more dietary supplements.

- Taking any medications (whether prescription or over-the-counter), as some dietary supplements have been found to interact with medications.

- Planning to have surgery. Certain dietary supplements may increase the risk of bleeding or affect the response to anesthesia.

- Pregnant or nursing a baby, or are considering giving a child a dietary supplement. Most dietary supplements have not been tested in pregnant women, nursing mothers, or children.

If you are taking a dietary supplement, read the label instructions. Talk to your health care provider if you have any questions, particularly about the best dosage for you to take. If you experience any side effects that concern you, stop taking the dietary supplement, and contact your health care provider. You can also report your experience to the FDA's MedWatch program. Consumer safety reports on dietary supplements are an important source of information for the FDA.

Keep in mind that although many dietary supplements (and some prescription drugs) come from natural sources, natural does not always mean safe. For example, the herbs comfrey and kava can cause serious harm to the liver. Also, a manufacturer's use of the term standardized (or verified or certified) does not necessarily guarantee product quality or consistency.

Colloidal Silver

Colloidal silver consists of tiny silver particles suspended in liquid. Usually marketed as dietary supplements, colloidal silver products have been used for a variety of health purposes—although there is no scientific evidence to support their safety or effectiveness.

Key Points

- The U.S. Food and Drug Administration (FDA) does not consider colloidal silver to be safe or effective for treating any disease or condition.

- The FDA and the Federal Trade Commission (FTC) have taken action against a number of colloidal silver companies (including some companies that sell products over the internet) for making drug-like claims about their products.

- Colloidal silver can cause many side effects. One example is argyria, a bluish-gray discoloration of the body, which is not treatable or reversible.

Background

Silver is a metallic element. Its many uses include making jewelry, silverware, electronic equipment, and dental fillings; processing photographs; and disinfecting water. People are exposed to silver, usually in tiny amounts, through the air, drinking water, and food, and possibly in certain activities, such as work or hobbies.

Silver has had some medicinal uses going back for centuries. However, modern drugs have eliminated most of those uses. A few prescription drugs containing silver are still available. For example, silver nitrate can be used to prevent the eye condition conjunctivitis in newborn babies and to treat certain skin conditions, such as corns and warts. Another drug, silver sulfadiazine, can be used to treat burns. These drugs are applied to the body (they are not taken internally), and they can have negative side effects.

Colloidal silver products consist of tiny silver particles suspended in a liquid base. The products are usually taken by mouth. Other forms of colloidal silver may be sprayed, applied directly to the skin, or injected into a vein.

Marketing Claims for Colloidal Silver

Colloidal silver products are often marketed as dietary supplements with various unproven health-related claims. For example, advertisements may claim that the products benefit the immune system; kill disease-causing agents such as bacteria, viruses, and fungi; serve as an alternative to prescription antibiotics; or treat diseases such as cancer, human immunodeficiency virus/acquired immunodeficiency syndrome (HIV/AIDS), diabetes, tuberculosis, syphilis, scarlet fever, shingles, herpes, pneumonia, and prostatitis (inflammation of the prostate).

Scientific Evidence

Reviews of the scientific literature on colloidal silver products found the following:

- Silver has no known function in the body.

- Silver is not an essential mineral supplement or a cure-all and should not be promoted as such.

- Claims that there can be a "deficiency" of silver in the body and that such a deficiency can lead to disease are unfounded.

- Claims made about the effectiveness of colloidal silver products for numerous diseases are unsupported scientifically.

- Colloidal silver products can have serious side effects.

- Laboratory analysis has shown that the amounts of silver in supplements vary greatly, which can pose risks to the consumer.

Side Effects and Risks

Animal studies have shown that silver builds up in the tissues of the body. In humans, buildup of silver from colloidal silver can lead to a side effect called argyria, which causes a bluish-gray discoloration of the skin, other organs, deep tissues, nails, and gums. Argyria is permanent and cannot be treated or reversed. Other side effects from using colloidal silver products may include neurologic problems (such as seizures), kidney damage, stomach distress, headaches, fatigue, and skin irritation. Colloidal silver may interfere with the body's absorption of some drugs, such as penicillamine, quinolones, tetracyclines, and thyroxine.

If You Are Thinking about Using Colloidal Silver Products

- There is a lack of evidence for effectiveness and a risk for serious side effects from colloidal silver products. The FDA does not consider colloidal silver to be safe or effective for treating any disease or condition.

- Do not use any dietary supplement as a replacement for conventional care, or as a reason to postpone seeing a doctor about a medical problem.

- If you are pregnant or nursing a child, or if you are considering giving a child a dietary supplement, it is especially important to consult your health care provider. Supplements can act like drugs in the body, and many have not been tested in pregnant women, nursing mothers, or children.

- Tell all your health care providers about any complementary and alternative practices you use. Give them a full picture of what you do to manage your health. This will help ensure coordinated and safe care.

Section 62.5

CAM and Hepatitis C

Text in this section is from "CAM and Hepatitis C: A Focus on Herbal Supplements," National Center for Complementary and Alternative Medicine (NCCAM), October 2008.

Introduction

Hepatitis C, a liver disease caused by a virus, is usually chronic (long-lasting), with symptoms ranging from mild (or even none) to severe. Conventional medical treatments are available for hepatitis C; however, some people also try complementary and alternative medicine (CAM) therapies, especially herbal supplements.

Key Points

- No CAM treatment has yet been proven effective for treating hepatitis C or its complications.

- It is important not to replace conventional medical therapy for hepatitis C with an unproven CAM therapy.

- Tell your health care providers about any complementary and alternative practices you use. Give them a full picture of what you do to manage your health. This will help ensure coordinated and safe care.

About Hepatitis C

Hepatitis C, a communicable (contagious) disease of the liver, is caused by the hepatitis C virus (HCV). The term hepatitis means inflammation of the liver; HCV is one of several viruses in the hepatitis family. If the liver becomes inflamed, it cannot function properly and remove harmful material from the blood or convert food into energy.

Use of Herbal Supplements for Hepatitis C

A number of herbal products claim to be beneficial for the liver, and hepatitis C patients who do not respond to conventional drug therapy, cannot tolerate its side effects, or simply want to support their body's fight against the disease may try these products. For example, a recent survey of 1,145 participants in the HALT-C (Hepatitis C Antiviral Long-Term Treatment against Cirrhosis) trial, a study supported by the National Institutes of Health (NIH), found that 23 percent were using herbal products at the time of enrollment. Although participants reported using many different herbal products, silymarin (milk thistle) was by far the most common.

What the Science Says

A review of the scientific evidence on CAM and hepatitis C found the following:

- No CAM treatment has been scientifically proven to successfully treat hepatitis C.

- A 2003 analysis of results from 13 clinical trials testing the effects of various medicinal herbs on hepatitis C concluded that there is not enough evidence to support using herbs to treat the disease.

- Two other reviews that covered a variety of CAM modalities for hepatitis C concluded that conventional therapies are the only scientifically proven treatments for the disease.

- In a 2002 NIH consensus statement on the management of hepatitis C, a panel of medical and scientific experts concluded that "alternative and nontraditional medicines" should be studied. Participants in a 2001 NIH research workshop on the benefits and risks of CAM therapies for chronic liver disease recommended research support for related laboratory and clinical studies.

Other CAM Products Used by People with Hepatitis C

Milk thistle (scientific name *Silybum marianum*) is a plant from the aster family. Silymarin, the active extract of milk thistle, is believed to be responsible for the herb's medicinal qualities. Milk thistle has been used in Europe as a treatment for liver disease and jaundice since the 16th century. In the United States, silymarin is the most popular CAM product taken by people with liver disease.

Laboratory studies suggest that milk thistle may benefit the liver by protecting and promoting the growth of liver cells, fighting oxidation (a chemical process that can damage cells), and inhibiting inflammation. Study results from small clinical trials on milk thistle for liver diseases have been mixed; however, most of these studies have not been rigorously designed, or they have looked at various types of liver diseases—not just hepatitis C. High-quality, well-designed clinical trials have not proven that milk thistle or silymarin is beneficial for treating hepatitis C. The HALT-C study found that silymarin use by hepatitis C patients was associated with fewer and milder symptoms of liver disease and somewhat better quality of life, but there was no change in virus activity or liver inflammation. The researchers emphasize that this was a retrospective study, not a controlled clinical trial. More research on milk thistle for hepatitis C is needed before a recommendation can be made.

Milk thistle is generally well tolerated and has shown few side effects in clinical trials involving patients with liver disease. It may cause a laxative effect, nausea, diarrhea, abdominal bloating, fullness, and pain, and it can produce allergic reactions (especially among people who are allergic to plants in the same family, such as ragweed, chrysanthemum, marigold, and daisy).

Other supplements are also being studied for hepatitis C. For example:

- Ginseng has shown some beneficial effects on the liver in laboratory studies but has not yet shown effects in people.

- Thymus extract and colloidal silver are sometimes marketed for the treatment of hepatitis C, but there is currently no research to support their use for this purpose. Colloidal silver products can cause serious side effects.

- People with chronic liver disease sometimes use licorice root or its extract glycyrrhizin. Some studies, reported from outside the United States, have looked at glycyrrhizin administered intravenously for hepatitis C. Preliminary evidence from these studies suggests that glycyrrhizin may have beneficial effects against hepatitis C. However, additional research is needed before reaching any conclusions.

- Preliminary studies conducted primarily outside the United States have examined the potential of the following herbal products for treating chronic hepatitis C: lactoferrin, TJ-108 (a mixture of herbs used in Japanese Kampo medicine), schisandra, and oxymatrine (an extract from the sophora root). More research is needed before the safety and effectiveness of these products can be fully evaluated.

If You Have Hepatitis C and Are Thinking about Using an Herbal Supplement

- Do not replace proven conventional treatments for hepatitis C with CAM treatments that are unproven.

- Be aware that some herbal products may damage the liver. For example, the herbs kava and comfrey have been linked to serious liver damage.

- Also be aware that the label on a supplement bottle may not accurately reflect what is inside. For example, some tests of dietary supplements have found that the contents did not match the dosage on the label, and some herbal supplements have been found to be contaminated.

- Tell your health care providers about any complementary and alternative practices you use. Give them a full picture of what you do to manage your health. This will help ensure coordinated and safe care. If you are pregnant or nursing a child, or if you are considering giving a child a dietary supplement, it is especially important to consult your health care provider. Supplements can act like drugs, and many have not been tested in pregnant women, nursing mothers, or children.

Part Four

Medical Diagnosis and Treatment of Contagious Diseases

Chapter 63

Diagnostic Tests for Contagious Diseases

Chapter Contents

Section 63.1

Medical Tests That Diagnose Infection

A Directory of Medical Tests

Taking a medical history and performing a physical examination usually provide the information a doctor needs to evaluate a child's health or to understand what's causing an illness. But sometimes, doctors need to order tests to find out more.

Here are some common tests and what they involve:

Blood Tests

Blood tests usually can be done in a doctor's office or in a lab where technicians are trained to take blood. When only a small amount of blood is needed, the sample can sometimes be taken from a baby by sticking a heel and from an older child by sticking a finger with a small needle.

If a larger blood sample is needed, the technician drawing the blood will clean the skin, insert a needle into a vein (usually in the arm or hand), and withdraw blood. In kids, it sometimes takes more than one try. A bandage and a cotton swab will help dry any blood left when the needle is removed.

Blood tests can be scary for kids, so try to be a calming presence during the procedure. Holding your child's hand or offering a stuffed animal or other comforting object can help. Tell your child that it may pinch a little, but that it will be over soon. With younger kids, try singing a song, saying the alphabet, or counting together while the blood is being drawn.

Common blood tests include:

- **Complete blood count (CBC):** A CBC measures the levels of different types of blood cells. By determining if there are too many or not enough of each blood cell type, a CBC can help to detect a wide variety of illnesses or signs of infection.

- **Blood chemistry test:** Basic blood chemistry tests measure the levels of certain electrolytes, such as sodium and potassium, in the blood. Doctors typically order them to look for any sign of kidney dysfunction, diabetes, metabolic disorders, and tissue damage.

- **Blood culture:** A blood culture may be ordered when a child has symptoms of an infection—such as a high fever or chills—and the doctor suspects bacteria may have spread into the blood. A blood culture shows what type of germ is causing an infection, which will determine how it should be treated.

- **Lead test:** The American Academy of Pediatrics (AAP) recommends that all toddlers get tested for lead in the blood at one and two years of age since young kids are at risk for lead poisoning if they eat or inhale particles of lead-based paint. High lead levels can cause stomach problems and headaches and also have been linked to some developmental problems.

- **Liver function test:** Liver function tests check to see how the liver is working and look for any sort of liver damage or inflammation. Doctors typically order one when looking for signs of a viral infection (like mononucleosis or viral hepatitis) or liver damage from other health problems.

Pregnancy and Newborns Tests

State requirements differ regarding tests for newborns and pregnant women, and recommendations by medical experts are often updated. So talk with the doctor if you have questions about what's right for you.

- **Prenatal tests:** From ultrasounds to amniocentesis, a wide array of prenatal tests can help keep pregnant women informed. These tests can help identify—and then treat—health problems that could endanger both mother and baby. Some tests are done routinely for all pregnancies. Others are done if the pregnancy is considered high-risk (for example, when a woman is 35 or older, is younger than 15, is overweight or underweight, or has a history of pregnancy complications).

- **Multiple marker test:** Most pregnant women are offered a blood-screening test between weeks 15–20. Also known as a "triple marker" or quadruple screen, this blood test can reveal conditions like spina bifida or Down syndrome by measuring certain hormones and protein levels in the mother's blood. Keep in mind that these are screening tests and only show the possibility of a problem existing—they don't provide definitive diagnoses. However, if results show a potential problem, a doctor will recommend other diagnostic tests.

- **Newborn screening tests:** These tests are done soon after a child is born to detect conditions that often can't be found before delivery, like sickle cell anemia or cystic fibrosis. Blood is drawn (usually from a needle stick on the heel) and spots are placed on special paper, which is then sent to a lab for analysis. Different states test for different diseases in infants.

- **Bilirubin level:** Bilirubin is a substance in the blood that can build up in babies and cause their skin to appear jaundiced (yellow). Usually jaundice is a harmless condition, but if the level of bilirubin gets too high, it can lead to brain damage. A baby who appears jaundiced may have a bilirubin level check, which is done with an instrument placed on the skin or by blood tests.

- **Hearing screen:** The American Academy of Pediatrics (AAP) recommends that all babies have a hearing screen done before discharge from the hospital, and most states have universal screening programs. It's important to pick up hearing deficits early so that they can be treated as soon as possible. Hearing screens take 5–10 minutes and are painless. Sometimes they involve putting small probes in the ears; other times, they're done with electrodes.

Radiology Tests

- **X-rays:** X-rays can help doctors find a variety of conditions, including broken bones and lung infections. X-rays aren't painful, and typically involve just having the child stand, sit, or lie on a table while the x-ray machine takes a picture of the area the doctor is concerned about. The child is sometimes given a special gown or covering to help protect other areas of the body from radiation.

- **Ultrasound:** Though they're typically associated with pregnancy, doctors order ultrasounds in lots of different cases. For example, ultrasounds can be used to look for collections of fluid in the body, for problems with the kidneys, or to look at a baby's brain. An ultrasound is painless and uses high-frequency sound waves to bounce off organs and create a picture. A special jelly is applied to the skin, and a handheld device is moved over the skin. The sound waves that come back produce an image on a screen. The images seen on most ultrasounds are difficult for the untrained eye to decipher, so a doctor will view the image and interpret it.

- **Computed tomography (CAT scan or CT-Scan):** CAT scans are a kind of x-ray, and typically are ordered to look for things such as appendicitis, internal bleeding, or abnormal growths. A scan is not painful, but sometimes can be scary for young kids. A child is asked to lie on a narrow table, which slides into a scanner. A scan may require the use of a contrast material (a dye or other substance) to improve the visibility of certain tissues or blood vessels. The contrast material may be swallowed or given intravenously (IV).

- **Magnetic resonance imaging (MRI):** MRIs use radio waves and magnetic fields to produce an image. MRIs are often used to look at bones, joints, and the brain. The child is asked to lie on a narrow table and it slides in to the middle of an MRI machine. While MRIs are not painful, they can be noisy and long, making them scary to kids. Often, children need to be sedated for MRIs. Contrast material is sometimes given through an IV in order to get a better picture of certain structures.

- **Upper gastrointestinal imaging (upper GI):** An upper GI is a study that involves swallowing contrast material while X-rays are taken of the top part of the digestive system. This allows the doctor to see how a child swallows. Upper GI studies are used to evaluate things like difficulty swallowing and gastroesophageal reflux (GERD). An upper GI isn't painful, but some kids don't like to drink the contrast material, which sometimes can be flavored to make it more appealing.

- **Voiding cystourethrogram (VCUG):** A VCUG involves putting dye into the bladder and then watching with continuous x-rays to see where the dye goes. Doctors typically order a VCUG when they are concerned about urinary reflux, which can sometimes lead to kidney damage later. A catheter is inserted through the urethra, into the bladder, which can be uncomfortable and scary for a child, but usually is not painful. The bladder is then filled with contrast material that is put in through the catheter. Images are taken while the bladder is filling and then while the child is urinating, to see where the dye and the urine go.

Other Tests

- **Throat culture (strep screen):** Doctors often order throat cultures to test for the germs that cause strep throat, which are known as group A streptococcus, or strep. The cultures are done in the doctor's office and aren't painful, but can be uncomfortable for a few seconds. The doctor or medical assistant wipes the back of the throat with a long cotton swab. This tickles the back of the throat and can cause a child to gag, but will be over very quickly, especially if your child stays still.

- **Stool test:** Stool (or feces or poop) can provide doctors with valuable information about what's wrong when your child has a problem in the stomach, intestines, or another part of the gastrointestinal system. The doctor may order stool tests if there is suspicion of something like an allergy, an infection, or digestive problems. Sometimes it is collected at home by a parent in a special container that the doctor provides. The doctor will also provide instructions on how to get the most useful sample for analysis.

- **Urine test:** Doctors order urine tests to make sure that the kidneys are functioning properly or when they suspect an infection in the kidneys or bladder. It can be taken in the doctor's office or at home. It's easy for toilet-trained kids to give a urine sample since they can go in a cup. In other cases, the doctor or nurse will insert a catheter (a narrow, soft tube) through the urinary tract opening into the bladder to get the urine sample. While this can be uncomfortable and scary for kids, it's typically not painful.

- **Lumbar puncture (spinal tap):** During a lumbar puncture a small amount of the fluid that surrounds the brain and spinal cord, the cerebrospinal fluid, is removed and examined. In kids, a lumbar puncture is often done to look for meningitis, an infection of the meninges (the membrane covering the brain and spinal cord). Other reasons to do lumbar punctures include: to remove fluid and relieve pressure with certain types of headaches, to look for other diseases in the central nervous system, or to place chemotherapy medications into the spinal fluid. Spinal taps, which can be done on an inpatient or outpatient basis, might be uncomfortable but shouldn't be too painful. Depending on a child's age, maturity, and size, the test may be done while the child is sedated.

- **Electroencephalography (EEG):** EEGs often are used to detect conditions that affect brain function, such as epilepsy, seizure disorders, and brain injury. Brain cells communicate by electrical impulses and an EEG measures and records these impulses to detect anything abnormal. The procedure isn't painful but kids often don't like the electrodes being applied to their heads. A technician arranges several electrodes at specific sites on the head, fixing them in place with sticky paste. The patient must remain still and lie down while the EEG is done.

- **Electrocardiography (EKG):** EKGs measure the heart's electrical activity to help evaluate its function and identify any problems. The EKG can help determine the rate and rhythm of heartbeats, the size and position of the heart's chambers, and whether there is any damage present. EKGs can detect abnormal heart rhythms, some congenital heart defects, and heart tissue that isn't getting enough oxygen. It's not a painful procedure—the child must lie down and a series of small electrodes are fixed on the skin with sticky papers on the chest, wrists, and ankles. The patient must sit still and may be asked to hold his or her breath briefly while the heartbeats are recorded.

- **Electromyography (EMG):** An EMG measures the response of muscles and nerves to electrical activity. It's used to help determine muscle conditions that might be causing muscle weakness, including muscular dystrophy and nerve disorders. A needle electrode is inserted into the muscle (the insertion might feel similar to a pinch) and the signal from the muscle is transmitted from the electrode through a wire to a receiver/amplifier, which is connected to a device that displays a readout. EMGs can be uncomfortable and scary to kids, but aren't usually painful. Occasionally kids are sedated while they're done.

- **Biopsies:** Biopsies are samples of body tissues taken to look for things such as cancer, inflammation, celiac disease, or the presence or absence of certain cells. Biopsies can be taken from almost anywhere, including lymph nodes, bone marrow, or kidneys. Doctors examine the removed tissue under a microscope to make a diagnosis. Kids are usually sedated for a biopsy.

Section 63.2

Rapid Strep Test

This chapter includes "Strep Throat: Test Sample, The Test, and Common Questions," © American Association for Clinical Chemistry. Reprinted with permission. For additional information about clinical lab testing, visit the Lab Tests Online website at www.labtestsonline.org.

The Test Sample

What is being tested?

This test identifies the presence of the bacteria *Streptococcus pyogenes*, also known as group A beta-hemolytic streptococcus and group A streptococcus (GAS). Group A streptococci can infect the back of the throat and cause strep throat, the most common bacterial cause of inflammation and soreness of the back of the throat (pharyngitis).

While most sore throats are caused by a virus and will resolve without treatment within a few days, 5–15% of adults and 15–30% of children have bacterial infections caused by this bacteria. It is important that these strep infections be promptly identified and treated with antibiotics. Strep throat is contagious and can spread to close contacts. If the infection is not treated, secondary complications may develop, such as rheumatic fever which can damage the heart, and glomerulonephritis which affects the kidneys. Because streptococcal infections are routinely diagnosed and treated, these complications have become much rarer in the United States, but they do still occur.

How is the sample collected for testing?

A doctor, nurse, or other health care professional uses a tongue depressor to hold down your tongue and then inserts a special swab into your mouth and rubs it against the back of the throat and tonsils. The swab may be used to do a rapid strep test in a doctor's office or clinic, or it may be sent to a laboratory. A second swab may be collected along with the first one. This extra sample is used to perform a throat culture as a follow-up test when necessary.

Is any test preparation needed to ensure the quality of the sample?

No test preparation is needed. The test should be performed before antibiotics are prescribed.

The Test

How is it used?

A rapid strep test is used to determine whether a person with a sore throat (pharyngitis) has a group A streptococcal infection.

If the results of the rapid test, which takes 10–20 minutes, are positive, further testing is not needed. If the rapid strep test is negative, a throat culture should be performed to grow the bacteria in the laboratory and confirm the results. A throat culture is more accurate than the rapid strep test, but it may take several days to get results.

When is it ordered?

A doctor will typically order this test when a person has a sore throat and other symptoms that suggest strep throat. He will have a higher suspicion of strep when the affected person is a child and/or if the person has been in close contact with someone who has been diagnosed with strep throat. Symptoms of strep throat vary and may include:

- sore throat,
- fever,
- headache,
- reddened (inflamed) throat with or without white or yellow spots,
- a swollen, tender neck,
- weakness,
- loss of appetite.

What does the test result mean?

A positive rapid strep test indicates the presence of group A streptococci, the bacteria that cause strep throat. A negative rapid test indicates that the affected person probably does not have strep throat, but the possibility cannot be ruled out until the laboratory performs a throat culture. If the throat culture is positive for group A streptococci, then the person tested does have strep throat. If it is negative, then it is most likely that the sore throat is due to a viral infection that will resolve on its own.

Is there anything else I should know?

Strep throat spreads from person-to-person through contact with respiratory secretions that contain the streptococcal bacteria. During influenza season, the early symptoms of influenza, such as fever, chills, headache, sore throat, muscle pain, may mimic strep throat. Very rarely, these same symptoms may be due to a more serious acute illness, septicemia. To differentiate between strep and influenza, a rapid strep test and a rapid influenza test may both be done. If both tests are negative and the clinical signs warrant it, a complete blood count (CBC) may be ordered to evaluate the person's white blood cells and, rarely, blood cultures may be drawn to rule out sepsis. The treatment for each of these infections differs greatly and making a prompt diagnosis is imperative to starting the correct therapy.

Most people with streptococcal pharyngitis would eventually recover without antibiotic treatment, but they will be contagious for a longer period of time and are at a greater risk of developing secondary complications.

Strep throat is most common in 5- to 10-year olds. Up to 20% of school children may be carriers, persons who have the bacteria but who have no symptoms. Carriers can still spread the infection to others.

Recent antibiotic therapy or gargling with some mouthwashes may affect the rapid strep test results.

Common Questions

How long does treatment for strep throat usually last?

Ten to 14 days, depending on the antibiotic prescribed.

How long should I stay away from other people if I have a positive test result?

You should complete at least 24 hours of antibiotics before close contact with others.

When can my child go back to school?

Usually after one full day of therapy and absence of significant fever.

If one child in my family has strep throat, is everyone going to get sick?

Other family members, including adults, can be infected by the bacteria. The doctor will usually test all family members who have sore throats and may, in some instances, want to test the whole family for strep throat. Although antibodies may protect those who have had previous strep infections, there are so many different strains of this organism that being immune to all of them is unlikely. Therefore, someone could potentially get strep throat again and again. The best way to decrease the risk of transmission of the bacteria to others is to cover coughs and sneezes by coughing and/or sneezing into the bend of your arm or shoulder. After sneezing or coughing into a tissue or handkerchief, wash hands thoroughly with soap and water or alcohol-based hand scrub.

What is an ASO test and how is it used to detect a strep infection?

Antistreptolysin O (ASO) is a blood test used to help diagnose a current or past infection with group A strep (*Streptococcus pyogenes*). It detects antibodies to streptolysin O, one of the many strep antigens. This test is rarely ordered now compared to thirty years ago. For an acute strep throat infection, the ASO test is not helpful; the rapid strep test or throat culture should be used. However, if a doctor is trying to find out if someone had a recent strep infection that may not have been diagnosed, this test could be helpful. In addition, it may be used to help diagnose rheumatic fever or glomerulonephritis, which occurs weeks after a strep throat infection when the rapid strep and throat culture would no longer be positive.

Do other group A streptococcus infections occur?

Group A streptococcus can also cause infections that occur separately from strep throat, such as impetigo and, rarely, more invasive conditions such as toxic shock syndrome or necrotizing fasciitis (the so-called flesh-eating bacteria).

Section 63.3

Testing for Influenza, Respiratory Infections, and Drug-Resistant Staph Infections

Text in this section is from "Rapid Diagnostic Testing for Influenza," Centers for Disease Control and Prevention (CDC), January 22, 2009; "FDA Clears First Quick Test for Drug-Resistant Staph Infections," U.S. Food and Drug Administration (FDA), January 2, 2008; and "FDA Clears for Marketing Real-Time Test for Respiratory Viruses," FDA, January 16, 2008.

Rapid Diagnostic Testing for Influenza

The availability and use of commercial influenza rapid diagnostic tests by laboratories and clinics have substantially increased in recent years.

- Influenza rapid diagnostic tests are screening tests for influenza virus infection.
- They can provide results within 15 minutes.
- More than ten rapid influenza tests have been approved by the U.S. Food and Drug Administration (FDA).
- Rapid tests differ in some important respects:
  - Some can identify influenza A and B viruses and distinguish between them.
  - Some can identify influenza A and B viruses but cannot distinguish between them.
  - Some tests are waived from requirements under the Clinical Laboratory Improvement Amendments of 1988 (CLIA).
  - Most tests can be used with a variety of specimen types, but the accuracy of the tests can vary based on the type of specimen collected (for example throat swab versus nasal swab).
- FDA approval is based upon specific specimen types.
- Specimens to be used with rapid tests generally should be collected as close as is possible to the start of symptoms and usually no more than 4–5 days later in adults. In very young children, influenza

viruses can be shed for longer periods; therefore, in some instances, testing for a few days after this period may still be useful.

When is use of rapid diagnostic tests beneficial?

- Testing during an outbreak of acute respiratory disease can determine if influenza is the cause.

- During influenza season, testing of selected patients presenting with respiratory illnesses compatible with influenza can help establish whether influenza is present in a specific patient population and help health-care providers determine how to use their clinical judgment for diagnosing and treating respiratory illness. (Testing need not be done for all patients.)

- Otherwise, rapid tests do not address the public health need for influenza virus isolated that can only be obtained through the collection of specimens for viral culture. Influenza virus isolates are essential for determining the match between circulating influenza viruses and those viruses contained in the vaccine and for aiding in the selection of new vaccine strains.

FDA Clears First Quick Test for Drug-Resistant Staph Infections

Test Identifies Methicillin-Resistant Staphylococcus aureus (MRSA) Bacterium in Two Hours

The U.S. Food and Drug Administration (FDA) has cleared for marketing the first rapid blood test for the drug-resistant staph bacterium known as MRSA (methicillin-resistant *Staphylococcus aureus*), which can cause potentially deadly infections.

Methicillin is an antibiotic that has been used successfully to treat infections from the *Staphylococcus aureus* bacterium. Over the years, the staph bacterium mutated and spawned MRSA, a strain of staph bacterium that is resistant to methicillin and which has a higher rate of being fatal.

The BD GeneOhm StaphSR Assay uses molecular methods to identify whether a blood sample contains genetic material from the MRSA bacterium or the more common, less dangerous staph bacterium that can still be treated with methicillin.

"The BD GeneOhm test is good news for the public health community. Rather than waiting more than two days for test results, health care personnel will be able to identify the source of a staph infection in only two hours, allowing for more effective diagnosis and treatment," said Daniel G. Schultz, MD, director, FDA's Center for Devices and Radiological Health.

Staph infections occur most frequently among persons in hospitals and health care facilities (such as nursing homes and dialysis centers) who have weakened immune systems. Both types of bacteria also can infect healthy people.

Distinguishing between the two sources of infection is critical to successful treatment. The more common, less dangerous strain of staph results in infections that are generally mild and affect the skin with pimples or boils that can be swollen, painful, and drain pus. However, the MRSA staph bacterium is difficult to treat with ordinary antibiotics. It can cause potentially life-threatening conditions such as blood stream infections, surgical site infections or pneumonia.

FDA cleared the BD GeneOhm StaphSR assay based on the results of a clinical trial at five locations. The new assay identified 100 percent of the MRSA-positive specimens and more than 98 percent of the more common, less dangerous staph specimens.

In order to preserve the integrity of positive test results, this test should be used only in patients suspected of a staph infection. The test should not be used to monitor treatment for staph infections because it cannot quantify a patient's response to treatment. Test results should not be used as the sole basis for diagnosis as they may reflect the bacteria's presence in patients who have been successfully treated for staph infections. Also, the test will not rule out other complicating conditions or infections.

The BD GeneOhm StaphSR test is manufactured by BD Diagnostics, a subsidiary of BD of Franklin Lakes, New Jersey.

FDA Clears for Marketing Real-Time Test for Respiratory Viruses

The U.S. Food and Drug Administration (FDA) has cleared for marketing a test that simultaneously detects four common respiratory viruses, including the flu, in a patient's respiratory secretions. The ProFlu+ test provides results in as few as three hours. Other diagnostic tests for respiratory viruses are fast but not as accurate or are accurate but not as rapid.

The real-time test employs a multiplex platform that allows several tests to be processed using the same sample to detect influenza A virus, influenza B virus, and respiratory syncytial virus A and B (RSV). These viruses can cause influenza, an infection of the airways called bronchiolitis, and pneumonia. All are among the leading causes of lower respiratory tract infections.

"Antiviral drugs are most effective when initiated within the first two days of symptoms," said Daniel Schultz, MD, director of FDA's Center for Devices and Radiological Health. "This new test, which is part of the new era of molecular medicine, can help the medical community quickly determine whether a respiratory illness is caused by one of these four viruses and initiate the appropriate treatment."

ProFlu+ uses a molecular biology process to isolate and amplify viral genetic material present in secretions taken from the back of the throat in patients.

While ProFlu+ is faster than conventional tests, it is specific to the four viruses, and is more accurate when used with other diagnostics, such as patient data, bacterial, or viral cultures, and x-rays, in diagnosing a patient. Positive results do not rule out other infection or co-infection and the virus detected may not be the specific cause of the disease or patient symptoms.

ProFlu+ is manufactured by Prodesse, Inc. of Milwaukee, Wisconsin.

Section 63.4

Rapid and Home Tests for Human Immunodeficiency Virus (HIV)

This section includes text from "Rapid HIV Test Distribution–United States, 2003–2005," *MMWR Weekly*, June 23, 2006, 55(24); 673–676, Centers for Disease Control and Prevention (CDC); and from "Vital Facts about HIV Home Test Kits," U.S. Food and Drug Administration (FDA), January 29, 2008.

Rapid Human Immunodeficiency Virus (HIV) Test Distribution in the United States, 2003–2005

At the end of 2003, an estimated one million persons in the United States were living with human immunodeficiency virus (HIV) infection, including those with acquired immunodeficiency syndrome (AIDS); approximately one-fourth of these persons had not had their infections diagnosed. In 2003, the Centers for Disease Control and Prevention (CDC) implemented a new initiative, Advancing HIV Prevention (AHP), focused, in part, on reducing the prevalence of undiagnosed HIV infection by expanding HIV testing and taking advantage of rapid HIV tests that enable persons to receive results within 30 minutes, instead of the two weeks typically associated with conventional tests.

In support of AHP strategies, during September 2003–December 2005, CDC purchased and distributed rapid HIV tests to expand testing and assess the feasibility of using rapid tests in new environments (for example, outreach settings or emergency departments). CDC distributed tests to 230 organizations in the United States and identified 4,650 (1.2%) HIV infections among 372,960 rapid tests administered. The results suggest that the rapid HIV-test distribution program (RTDP) helped scale up rapid HIV-testing programs in the United States and enabled diagnosis of HIV in persons who might not have had their infections diagnosed otherwise.

The findings in this report suggest that HIV testing might be increased by using rapid tests and that RTDP might have enabled diagnosis of HIV infection in persons who would not have known their HIV status otherwise. Although follow-up client data were not collected on the 4,650 confirmed HIV-positive test results, previous research has indicated that the majority of persons who learn they are infected with HIV take steps to prevent transmission to others and obtain health care that can prolong the quality and duration of their lives. Previous research also has suggested that many providers and clients prefer rapid HIV tests, which allow clients to receive test results in less than 30 minutes, eliminating for those with negative results the two-week waiting period typically associated with conventional tests. Rapid tests also are simple to use and accurate. For example, the sensitivity of the OraQuick Advance test is 99.3% using oral fluid specimens and 99.6% using whole blood specimens; the specificity is 99.8% and 100.0%, respectively.

Despite obstacles associated with implementing a new diagnostic technology, RTDP has helped initiate rapid HIV testing at sites throughout the United States. CDC will continue to work with federal, state, and local partners to increase the efficient use of rapid HIV tests, providing more access to HIV testing in settings and communities in which many HIV infections are undiagnosed.

Vital Facts about HIV Home Test Kits

Privacy and confidentiality are main factors that lead people to choose home testing kits to find out if they are infected with human immunodeficiency virus (HIV), which causes acquired immunodeficiency syndrome (AIDS).

It is important that consumers know there is only one product currently approved by FDA and legally sold in the United States as a home testing system for HIV. This product is a kit marketed as either "The Home Access HIV-1 Test System" or "The Home Access Express HIV-1 Test System." The kit is a home collection-test system that requires users to collect a blood specimen, and then mail it to a laboratory for professional testing. No test kits allow consumers to interpret the results at home.

Beware of False Claims

Numerous HIV home test systems that have not been approved by FDA are currently being marketed online and in newspapers and magazines. Manufacturers of unapproved systems have falsely claimed that their products can detect antibodies to HIV in blood or saliva samples, and that they can provide results in the home in 15 minutes or less. Some have even claimed that their systems are approved by FDA or are manufactured in a facility that is registered with FDA. FDA takes appropriate action against people or firms that sell unapproved and ineffective tests.

About the Approved Product

The FDA-approved Home Access System kits allow people to collect a blood sample. Using a personal identification number (PIN), they then mail the sample anonymously to a laboratory for testing. The PIN can then be used to obtain results.

The kits, manufactured by Illinois-based Home Access Health Corp., can be purchased at pharmacies, by mail order, or online. They only allow testing for the presence of antibodies of the virus known as HIV-1. They do not provide the ability to test for HIV-2, a less common cause of AIDS.

The Home Access System offers users pre- and post-test, anonymous and confidential counseling through both printed material and telephone interaction. It also provides the user with an interpretation of the test result.

Checking for Antibodies to HIV

Like most HIV tests, the approved Home Access testing system checks for the presence of antibodies to HIV that are produced once the virus enters the body. The rate at which individuals infected with HIV produce these antibodies differs. There's a window period between the time someone is infected with HIV and the time the body produces enough antibodies to be detected through testing. During this time, an HIV-infected person will still get a negative test result.

According to FDA's Center for Biologics and Research (CBER), which regulates all HIV tests, detectable antibodies usually develop within two to eight weeks. The average is about 22 days. Still, some people take longer to develop detectable antibodies. Most will develop antibodies within three months following infection. In very rare cases, it can take up to six months to develop detectable antibodies to HIV.

Rapid Tests: A Clinical Option

Consumers do have the option of taking a rapid test, some of which test for both HIV-1 and HIV-2. These tests are run where the sample is collected, and produce results within 20 minutes. Because HIV testing requires interpretation and confirmation, rapid antibody tests are only approved and available in a professional health care setting, such as doctors' offices, clinics and outreach testing sites.

According to the Centers for Disease Control and Prevention (CDC), there are tests that look for HIV's genetic material directly, but these are not in widespread use. Tests using saliva or urine are also available, although not for at-home use. If you are unsure whether a certain type of HIV test is FDA-approved, look for the test on the agency's list of screening tests for infectious agents.

Chapter 64

Prescription Medicines That Treat Contagious Disease

What are antibiotics?

Antibiotics are medicines that help your body fight bacteria and viruses, either by directly killing the offending bugs or by weakening them so that your own immune system can fight and kill them more easily. The vast majority of antibiotics are bacteria fighters; although there are millions of viruses, we only have antivirals for half-a-dozen or so of them. Bacteria, on the other hand, are more complex (while viruses must live in a host (us), bacteria can live independently) and so are easier to kill.

Antibiotic Resistance

Bacteria (and viruses) aren't particularly intelligent. However, it is possible—and unfortunately all too common—for bacteria and some viruses to learn how to survive even with antibiotics around.

There are several ways that bacteria can become resistant. All of them involve changes in the bacteria's genes.

- Bacterial genes mutate (change), just like the genes of larger organisms (including humans) mutate. Some of these changes happen because of chemical or radiation exposure; some just

Excerpted from "Antibiotics, Bacteria, and (usually not) Viruses," http://www .drreddy.com/antibx.html. © 2008 Vinay N. Reddy, MD. Reprinted with permission.

453

happen randomly, and no one is sure quite why. If bacteria with a changed gene is less susceptible to an antibiotic, and that antibiotic is around, the less susceptible (and more resistant) version of the bacteria is more likely to survive the antibiotic and continue to multiply. This is particularly likely to happen if the amount of antibiotic around isn't quite enough to kill all of the bacteria quickly—as can happen if you don't take enough of the antibiotic to keep its level in your body high, or if you stop taking the antibiotic too early. This is why when you are prescribed an antibiotic you must take it exactly as prescribed, and for as long as it was prescribed: you may feel better after only a short time, but you may still have some bacteria left in you—not enough to make you feel bad, but enough to come back—and those bacteria left include the ones that are partly resistant to the antibiotic already and likely to become more resistant. It's also why we don't (or shouldn't) give you an antibiotic for an illness like a cold that isn't likely to be bacterial: the antibiotic will kill off susceptible bacteria, leaving bacteria that are resistant to that antibiotic and which can cause a later infection—and one that won't respond to the previous antibiotic.

• Although there are many different species of bacteria, some bacteria can trade genes with other bacteria. If you have a relatively harmless bacteria in you—say, in your mouth or your intestines (both places are chock full of bacteria)—and you've used (or overused or misused) antibiotics some of those harmless bacteria will become resistant to the antibiotics you've overused or misused. They can then give the resistance genes they have developed to other, harmful bacteria.

• There are viruses around that attack bacteria rather than plants, animals, or people. Most of these viruses just kill the bacteria, but sometimes the viruses can copy genes—like the antibiotic resistance genes—from one kind of bacteria to another.

Human and animal viruses can also develop resistance to antiviral antibiotics, usually through mutation. This isn't a big issue, since there aren't a lot of antiviral antibiotics. However, antiviral resistance has become a major problem in human immunodeficiency virus /acquired immunodeficiency syndrome (HIV/AIDS) therapy, where the virus rapidly becomes resistant to the first-line antivirals such as azidothymidine (AZT). Resistance develops particularly fast in patients who do not take their medicines properly, and in those whose immune systems can't help clean up after the antibiotics. This is one reason why tuberculosis (which is caused by a bacterium that multiplies very slowly and that is specifically fought by the part of the immune system that HIV disables) has reemerged since the appearance of AIDS.

Kinds of Antibiotics

Penicillins and Cephalosporins

In the early 20th century, Alexander Fleming discovered that a mold called *Penicillium* (the cells are pencil-shaped when you look at them under a microscope) produces chemicals which kill most of the bacteria nearby. (The mold is green when it grows in large amounts, and is often found on bread. This, however, does not mean that eating moldy bread will cure your earache—or anything else. There are other things produced by molds.) He was able to isolate these chemicals, which are now known as penicillins. Sometime later, another mold was found which produced a bacteria-killing chemical, and this chemical's molecule was found to be very similar to the penicillin molecule; this chemical and its cousins were called cephalosporins after the mold it came from. The vast majority of antibiotics are either penicillins or cephalosporins; chemical changes have been made to the molecules over the years to improve their bacteria-fighting abilities and to help them overcome breakdown and immunity of resistant bacteria.

Most bacterial cells have double layers on their outside. The outermost layer—the cell wall—is similar to the outer layer of plant cells, but is missing in human and animal cells. This wall must grow along with the cell, or the growing cell will eventually become too big for the wall and burst and die. Penicillins and cephalosporins kill bacteria by messing up the wall-building system. Since we don't have cell walls, and plants have a different wall-building system, neither we, nor animals, nor plants are affected by the medicine.

There are a very few bacteria that don't have cell walls, either. These bugs are immune to penicillins and cephalosporins for the same reasons we are. Most bacteria do have cell walls, but many have changed their wall-building systems so that penicillins can't interfere, or have come up with ways to break down the medicines before the medicines can work. When we first started using penicillin in the 1940s and 1950s, most bacteria could be killed by plain penicillin. Now, because we have used penicillins and cephalosporins so often (and, in many cases, when we really shouldn't have), there are many bacteria that can't be killed any more by plain penicillin or even by the super-penicillins and super-cephalosporins.

Penicillins and cephalosporins usually don't cause many problems for a patient. Like all antibiotics, they can cause mild side effects like diarrhea. Less common side effects include rashes (which may or may not imply a true allergy) and hives (which usually means you're allergic to the medicine). The rarest—and scariest—side effect is anaphylactic allergy, in which your airway swells up when you take a dose of the medicine, sometimes to the point where you can't breathe. Although the reaction can be treated if you are close to help, the safest thing if you are that allergic to the medicine is never to take it at all. (In cases where you have an anaphylactic allergy to penicillin or cephalosporins and must have it to treat an infection, doctors can desensitize you temporarily, using very small doses that are given frequently and in increasing amounts. That is almost always done in a hospital.)

Macrolides (Erythromycin and Its Relatives)

Erythromycin is another antibacterial produced by a mold. There are a couple of new relatives of erythromycin (azithromycin and clarithromycin) that work the same way, but kill more bugs and have slightly fewer side effects. The erythromycin-like antibiotics are also known as macrolides.

Erythromycin works by blocking the bacterial cell's machinery for making new proteins. Since proteins both make up much of the cell's structure and make the enzymes that direct all the cell's chemical reactions, blocking protein manufacturing makes the cell unable to function. Erythromycin in low doses will stop bacteria from growing and multiplying, but you need a higher concentration to kill the bacteria. However, if you can stop growth until your immune system kicks in, that will help you get rid of the infection.

Since all protein making is affected, erythromycin can slow down or kill any bacteria, even those without cell walls. Because of this, we use the erythromycins for several diseases, including bacterial bronchitis, chlamydia, and whooping cough, which penicillins and cephalosporins can't touch.

Erythromycin and its cousins don't have anything like the allergy problems we see with the penicillins and cephalosporins, although there are rare people who have reactions to it. The biggest problem with these medicines is that they can irritate the stomach. I have seen one patient who ended up with bleeding stomach ulcers after taking

erythromycin; this irritation seems to happen most often when someone tries to take the medicine on an empty stomach. Always take
erythromycin with food or milk. (The same goes for clarithromycin.
Azithromycin doesn't irritate the stomach nearly as much as the others.) Another problem with erythromycin—but not with azithromycin—
is that it may cause enlargement of the pylorus, the muscle that serves
as the valve at the outlet of the stomach—in infants. This condition is
known as pyloric stenosis, and is a surgical emergency if it occurs since
nothing can leave the stomach properly. In the past we treated infants
with erythromycin if they developed whooping cough. We now use
azithromycin, which works just as well as erythromycin but doesn't
affect the pylorus (and needs to be given for only five days; you need
14 days of erythromycin for complete treatment of whooping cough).

Sulfas

The sulfas (more properly sulfanilamide or sulfonamides) were the
first antibiotics to be developed; they are actually completely man-made.
They interfere with certain manufacturing systems in the bacterial cell,
including ones that bacteria use to produce new deoxyribonucleic acid
(DNA) for new bacteria. Sulfas can stop bacteria from growing, but they
cannot actually kill the bacteria.

When they were first used, sulfas worked against many kinds of
bacteria. Unfortunately, as with penicillin, the more we used the sulfas
the more bacteria became resistant to it. Sulfas also have a tendency
to produce allergic reactions—different than those we see with the
penicillins, for the most part, but including some that are rare but
life-threatening. Because of this we don't use sulfas nearly as much
we used to, and most often when we use sulfas it's in combination with
another drug which attacks a different part of the bacteria (an attack
on two fronts is usually better than an attack on one). The drugs we
usually combine with sulfas are either erythromycin or trimethoprim;
these combinations usually can kill bacteria rather than just slow-
ing them down. One frequent use of plain sulfas is in antibiotic
eyedrops used for conjunctivitis (pink eye).

Trimethoprim-Sulfamethoxazole

Trimethoprim (TMP) is another man-made antibiotic. Like the
sulfas, trimethoprim blocks an important step in the bacteria's system
for making new DNA—but it's a different step. By itself, TMP can kill
bacteria, but very slowly. Usually, though, we use TMP in combination

with sulfamethoxazole (SMX), and the combination of TMP and a sulfa kills bugs better. In fact, bacteria that are partly resistant to either TMP or SMX can still be killed by the combination of the two. The side effects of the combination are the same as those of the two separate components.

Other Medicines

Nitrofurantoin

Nitrofurantoin is another synthetic antibiotic, used mainly for urinary tract infections (UTI). (Since it is excreted in the urine, it concentrates in the bladder very nicely.) Nitrofurantoin stops bacteria from growing, and can kill bacteria with a high enough level, by blocking the bacteria's ability to use energy it makes by digesting nutrients like sugar, and by blocking other chemical reactions that use the same system. It is not usually used for infections other than UTIs, and there are several side effects (ranging from stomach upset to [very rarely] malfunctioning nerves) which limit its use.

Aminoglycosides

The aminoglycosides are drugs which stop bacteria from making proteins; they work by attaching permanently to the protein machinery. Since they attach permanently, the bacterial cell will die if it gets enough of the drug. They can be used by themselves, or along with penicillins or cephalosporins to give a two-pronged attack on the bacteria.

Aminoglycosides work quite well, but bacteria can become resistant to them. The drawbacks are large, though. Since aminoglycosides are broken down easily in the stomach, they can't be given by mouth and must be injected or given intravenously (IV) (although we can use them as eyedrops for pink eye). When injected, their side effects include possible damage (temporary or permanent) to the ears and to the kidneys; this can be minimized by checking the amount of the drug in the blood and adjusting the dose so that there is enough drug to kill bacteria but not too much of it. Generally, aminoglycosides are given for short time periods, and in the hospital where we can check both the drug levels and the bacteria's sensitivity easily.

Quinolones

The quinolones, of which the best known is ciprofloxacin (Cipro®), interfere with an enzyme called DNA gyrase that is essential for duplication of bacterial DNA. (Bacteria have only one long chromosome [DNA molecule]; the chromosome gets twisted during replication, like a telephone cord, and, again like the telephone cord, the chromosome can become so twisted that nothing more can be done with it. DNA gyrase is the untwisting enzyme.) This interference is completely different from the interference of other antibiotics with bacterial machinery, and so bacteria that are resistant to other antibiotics may be sensitive to the quinolones.

However, bacteria can develop resistance to the quinolones, too. Also, researchers have noticed that young animals given quinolones can have damage to their cartilage (the hard but slippery material that connects some bones and covers the sliding surfaces of joints). In the past, we have avoided using quinolones in children because of this finding, but we sometimes have to give some children quinolones when there is no alternative antibiotic available.

Polymyxin B

Polymyxin B is an antibacterial that is produced by another bacteria. (We usually take our antibiotics wherever we can find them.) It kills bacteria by damaging the cell wall chemically—just the way soap does. It can't be taken internally, but it's very useful for skin infections (it's part of Polysporin) and for conjunctivitis (pink eye).

Tetracyclines

Tetracyclines are yet another family of antibiotics originally found in bacteria. They also block the protein-making machinery of certain bacteria. One of the tetracyclines, doxycycline, is often used to treat certain sexually transmitted diseases (such as chlamydia and gonorrhea) in older patients. One known side effect of the tetracyclines is that they affect development of bone and of tooth enamel in young children, and because of this we do not usually give tetracyclines to children under age eight years. However, tetracycline may be the best antibiotic for some life-threatening infections, such as cholera and anthrax, and in such cases we may use tetracycline to treat a young child (tetracycline often leaves a permanent brown stain on developing teeth, but that's better than death).

Antifungals

Some microorganisms, known as fungi (fungus in the singular), are cells that are biologically more similar to animal cells than to bacteria.

Since many of the antibacterial antibiotics take advantage of the difference between bacterial cells and animal cells, the fungi's similarity to animal cells makes them immune to the antibacterial antibiotics. However, there are antifungals available for fungi such as *Candida.* These include nystatin, the azoles (including fluconazole, ketoconazole, and similar antibiotics), and amphotericin B. These work by disrupting the fungal cells' machinery. Some of these antibiotics may be applied to the skin or taken by mouth, while others must be given intravenously (by IV).

Antivirals

Since viruses can't live outside the person or animal they infect, they are much harder to kill off. Our immune system can find and kill many of the viruses that attack us, but sometimes a virus can multiply and overwhelm the immune system before the immune system comes up to full speed. We immunize or vaccinate people against diseases—mostly viral, but some bacterial—so that their immune systems do have that head start. That seems to be the most successful way to kill viruses permanently. An example is smallpox, which has been eradicated due mainly to the use of vaccines against it—without which the virus killed thousands, if not millions, in epidemics. Some viruses, such as HIV (which specifically attacks the immune system), are very hard to become immune to, but a great deal of research is being aimed at producing a working vaccine for those diseases.

Unfortunately, since viruses are completely dormant outside a host (an infected human or animal), they can't be attacked biologically unless they infect someone. The immune system can't go after the virus unless it's in the body, and all of the antiviral medicines we have work only when the virus is trying to reproduce in the body. We can destroy viruses in the environment if we know they are there (an example is using household bleach to kill HIV that might be on equipment contaminated with body fluids—but bleach won't kill HIV in the body, even if we could get it into the body safely). Once the virus is in the body, however, all we can do is let the immune system do its work, and in very rare cases (perhaps half-a-dozen viruses at most) give drugs that slow down the infection so that the body can clear it out more easily.

Acyclovir

One often-used antiviral medicine is acyclovir; ganciclovir and valacyclovir are similar to acyclovir. These medicines slow down infections with viruses of a certain family, which include both varicella (chickenpox and shingles) and the herpes viruses. Acyclovir slows down the virus' multiplication and therefore slows down the infection. The problem is that the varicella and herpes viruses are never actually eradicated—they stay in the body forever, and reactivate later (sometimes years later). The recurrent sores of herpes, and the appearance of shingles years after you have chickenpox, are examples of reactivation, and although acyclovir can help you get over the reactivation infection, it can't actually get rid of the viruses.

Azidothymidine (AZT) and other Reverse-Transcriptase Inhibitors

Another very well-known antiviral is triazidothymidine, better known as zidovudine or AZT. This drug and others like it, are used to inhibit an enzyme called reverse transcriptase which HIV uses to copy its own genes into the genes of the cells it infects. Once the HIV genes are copied, the infected cell and all of its offspring can produce more HIV. (This is why an AIDS patient cannot actually get rid of the entire virus once infected: the virus may lie dormant as inactive genes for months or years, and the anti-AIDS drugs cannot get to the gene copies.) Like bacteria, viruses can mutate, changing their structure so that drugs that used to work no longer help; this explains why AZT and other reverse-transcriptase inhibitors eventually lose their effectiveness in many patients.

Protease Inhibitors

A newer class of anti-AIDS drugs, the protease inhibitors, work by blocking a different HIV enzyme. HIV uses reverse transcriptase to copy its genes into the cell it's infecting; it uses protease (an enzyme that breaks down protein) to get into the cell in the first place. Many people with AIDS have been able to eliminate the virus from their bloodstream—or almost eliminate it—by using both reverse-transcriptase inhibitors and protease inhibitors at the same time. However, since the virus has copied itself into cells where neither kind of drug can attack it, a patient must keep taking the drugs forever to keep the virus from reactivating.

Note that the antiviral drugs, even more than the antibacterials, are tailored to the kind of viruses they are intended to attack. AZT won't do anything for a cold, and neither will acyclovir. In fact, there are—so far—no antivirals that will do anything for the common cold.

And, since there are many different viruses in several different families that can cause colds, we are not likely to have any anti-common-cold drugs in the near future.

The Common Cold

Since most colds are due to viruses attacking the mucus membranes of the nose and throat, the only way to get over the cold is to wait for your immune system to get rid of the virus, and for your body to produce a new, virus-free mucus membrane surface. Resurfacing the mucus membranes takes 3–4 days (you automatically resurface the membranes every 3–4 days), but getting rid of the virus takes a week or two, and until the virus is gone the new membranes will keep getting infected. Since we have no medicines that will slow down the cold viruses, we can't do anything to speed up this process. Antibacterial antibiotics will do nothing to help get rid of the virus, and giving antibacterial antibiotics when there is a viral cold will likely do nothing except help the bacteria in the nose and throat become resistant—which makes the next bacterial infection much harder to treat. I never give antibiotics to someone who has only a cold, unless there seems to me to be a very good chance that he or she may develop a bacterial infection on top of the cold—or unless there is clearly a bacterial infection already.

Chapter 65

Antibiotic Safety

What are antibiotics?

Antibiotics are powerful medicines that help stop bacterial infections. They are used to kill germs that cause certain illnesses. Protect yourself and your family by learning how to take them correctly. Learn when you should and should not take antibiotics.

What germs cause most infections?

Viruses and bacteria are the two types of germs that cause infections. It is very important to know that antibiotics cannot kill virus germs but can kill bacteria germs.

Viral infections should not be treated with antibiotics. Some examples of viral illnesses include the following:

- Common cold—stuffy nose, sore throat, sneezing, cough, headache
- Influenza (flu)—fever, chills, body aches, headache, sore throat, dry cough
- Most coughs
- Acute bronchitis (cough, fever)—almost always caused by viruses

- Pharyngitis (sore throat)—most sore throats are caused by viruses and are not effectively treated with an antibiotic
- Viral gastroenteritis

Bacterial infections should be treated with antibiotics. Some examples of bacterial infections include these:

- Ear infections—(Antibiotics are used for most, but not all ear infections.)
- Severe sinus infections—lasting two or more weeks
- Strep throat
- Bladder infection

What should I ask my doctor?

If your doctor prescribes antibiotics, you should ask the following questions:

1. Why do I need the antibiotic?
2. What is the antibiotic suppose to do?
3. What are the side effects of the antibiotic?
4. Is there anything that can prevent the side effects?
5. Should the drug be taken at a special time? With or without food?
6. Does the antibiotic interfere with the effectiveness of other medications such as birth control pills?
7. Are there any possible adverse reactions if the antibiotic is taken with other medications, food, or alcohol?

Also, be sure to tell your doctor about any of the following:

- Previous drug reactions
- Special diet
- Allergies to drugs or foods
- Health problems
- Chance of pregnancy
- Medicines you are currently taking
- Herbal supplements you are currently using

Always keep your doctor's phone number nearby in case of an emergency. If you have any questions or problems regarding your antibiotic treatment or your illness, don't hesitate to call your doctor, nurse, or health care provider.

How do I take antibiotics safely and effectively?

Over half of the people who use medications don't use them as prescribed. Here are some tips to avoid misuse and/or overuse of antibiotics:

- Do not demand that your doctor give you antibiotics for a viral infection. Antibiotics kill bacteria, not viruses.

- Take all of your prescribed antibiotic, even if you start to feel better. Do not save some of your antibiotic for the next time you get sick.

- Do not take an antibiotic that has been prescribed for someone else. Do not let anyone take your antibiotic, even if the symptoms are the same.

- Keep a written record of each time antibiotics are taken, including the name, strength, how often and how long the antibiotic was taken and any side effects experienced. Share this information with your doctor each time antibiotics are prescribed in order to assist your doctor in determining which antibiotic is best for you.

- Ask your doctor or pharmacist what to do if you should forget or miss a dose.

Tips to help you protect yourself from infections:

- Wash your hands properly to reduce the chance of getting sick and spreading infection. Alternatively, use an alcohol based hand rub if soap and water are not available.

- Wash fruits and vegetables thoroughly; avoid raw eggs and undercooked meat to help prevent foodborne infection.

- When caring for an ill person whose defenses are weakened, antibacterial soaps or products are helpful, but should be used as directed.

- Make sure you are current on all of your vaccinations. Ask your doctor if you have all of the vaccinations you need to protect yourself from illness. Getting vaccinated will help prevent having to take more medications.

Can antibiotics sometimes be harmful?

Antibiotics are generally safe and very helpful in fighting disease, but there are certain cases where antibiotics can actually be harmful. These are some things to watch for while taking antibiotics:

Side effects of the antibiotics: Some common side effects of antibiotics include nausea, diarrhea, and stomach pain. Sometimes these symptoms can lead to dehydration and other problems. Be sure that your doctor has told you about side effects. It is very important to notify your doctor if you have any side effects from your antibiotics.

Allergic reaction: Some people may experience an allergic reaction characterized by rash, itching, and in severe cases, difficulty breathing. Tell your doctor about any drug allergies you have had in the past.

Antibiotic resistance: Antibiotic resistance has become a very big problem in the world today. Resistance may result when antibiotics are used too often or inappropriately for viral infections. When resistance develops, the antibiotic is not able to kill the germs causing the infection. Your infection may last longer, and instead of getting better you get worse. Every time you take an antibiotic when you really don't need it or if you take it incorrectly, you increase your chance of getting an illness someday that is resistant to antibiotics.

Antibiotic Issues Specific to Women

Antibiotics can lead to vaginal yeast infections. This happens because antibiotics kill the normal bacteria in the vagina and this causes yeast to grow rapidly. Symptoms of a yeast infection include one or all of the following symptoms: itching, burning, pain during sex, and vaginal discharge. Antibiotics may cause birth control pills to be less effective. Another method of birth control may be needed during antibiotic treatment. Some antibiotics may be passed on to a fetus and cause harm. Because of this, it is important to let your doctor know if you are pregnant or nursing.

Chapter 66

Antiviral Drugs for Seasonal Flu

While getting a flu vaccine each year is the best way to protect you from the flu, there also are drugs that can fight against influenza viruses, offering a second line of defense against the flu. These are called influenza antiviral drugs and they must be prescribed by a health care professional. These drugs can be used to treat the flu or to prevent infection with flu viruses. Influenza antiviral drugs only work against influenza viruses—they will not help treat or prevent symptoms caused by infection from other viruses that can cause symptoms similar to the flu. Antiviral drugs are used in different settings and circumstances to treat the flu and to prevent people from getting the flu:

- Antiviral drugs are used to help control flu outbreaks in places where a lot of people at high risk of serious flu complications live in close contact with each other, like nursing homes or hospital wards, for example.

- Antiviral drugs are used in the community setting to treat people with the flu to reduce severity of symptoms and reduce the number of days that people are sick.

- Antiviral drugs are used to prevent the flu:

  - for people who have been close to someone with the flu; or

---

Text in this chapter is from "Key Facts about Antiviral Drugs and Influenza (Flu)," Centers for Disease Control and Prevention (CDC), April 7, 2009.

- for people that need protection from the flu but they either don't get protection after vaccination, or the vaccine is unavailable or they can't get the vaccine because of allergies, for example.

While most healthy people recover from the flu and don't have serious complications, some people—such as older people, young children, and people with certain health conditions (such as asthma, diabetes, or heart disease)—are at higher risk for serious flu-related complications. It's especially important that these people are protected from the flu. A flu vaccine is the first and best defense against the flu, but antiviral drugs can be an important second line of defense to treat the flu or prevent flu infection.

Antiviral Drugs

There are four flu antiviral drugs approved for use in the United States. The Centers for Disease Control and Protection (CDC) issued interim guidance on which antiviral drugs to use during the 2008-09 flu season including the following antiviral drugs:

- Oseltamivir (brand name Tamiflu®) is approved to both treat and prevent influenza A and B virus infection in people one year of age and older.

- Zanamivir (brand name Relenza®) is approved to treat influenza A and B virus infection in people seven years and older and to prevent influenza A and B virus infection in people five years and older.

- Amantadine (Symmetrel®, generic) is approved to treat and prevent only influenza A viruses in people older than one year.

- Rimantadine (Flumadine®, generic) is approved to prevent only influenza A virus infection among people older than one year. It is approved to treat only influenza A virus infections in people 13 and older.

Antiviral drugs differ in terms of who can take them, how they are given, their dose (which can vary depending on a person's age or medical conditions), and side effects. Your doctor can help decide whether you should take an antiviral drug this flu season and which one you should use.

Use of Antiviral Drugs for Treatment

For treatment, influenza antiviral drugs should be started within two days after becoming sick. When used this way, these drugs can reduce flu symptoms and shorten the time you are sick by 1–2 days.

If you become sick with flu-like symptoms this season, your doctor will consider the likelihood of influenza being the cause of your illness, the number of days you have been sick, side effects of the medication, and so forth, before making a recommendation about using antiviral drugs. He or she may test you for influenza, but testing is not required in order for a health care provider to recommend influenza antiviral medications for you.

Use of Antiviral Drugs for Prevention

Influenza antiviral drugs also can be used to prevent influenza when they are given to a person who is not ill, but who has been or may be near a person with influenza. When used to prevent the flu, antiviral drugs are about 70% to 90% effective. It's important to remember that flu antiviral drugs are not a substitute for getting a flu vaccine. When used for prevention, the number of days that they should be used will vary depending on a person's particular situation.

In some instances, your doctor may choose to prescribe antiviral drugs to you as a preventive measure, especially if you are at high risk for serious flu complications and either did not get the flu vaccine or may still be at risk of illness even after vaccination. Also, if you are in close contact with someone who is considered at high risk for complications, you may be given antiviral drugs to reduce the chances of catching the flu and passing it on to the high-risk person.

Who Should Get Antiviral Drugs?

In general, antiviral drugs can be offered to anyone one year of age or older who wants to avoid and/or treat the flu. People who are at high risk of serious complications from the flu may benefit most from these drugs. Antiviral drugs can also be used to prevent influenza among people with weak immune systems who may not be protected after getting a flu vaccine or who haven't been vaccinated.

Remember: Flu vaccine is the first and best defense against seasonal flu, but antiviral drugs can be an important second line of defense to treat the flu or prevent flu infection.

Chapter 67

Antimicrobial (Drug) Resistance

Antimicrobial (Drug) Resistance Is a Growing Health Issue

The emergence of drug-resistant microbes is not new or unexpected. Both natural causes and societal pressures drive bacteria, viruses, parasites, and other microbes to continually change in an effort to evade the drugs developed to kill them.

Natural causes: Like all organisms, microbes undergo random genetic mutations, and these changes can enhance drug resistance. Resistance to a drug arising by chance in just a few organisms can quickly spread through rapid reproduction to entire populations of a microbe.

Societal pressures: Antimicrobial resistance is fostered by the overuse and misuse of antimicrobial drugs in people as well as animals; a lack of diagnostic tests to rapidly identify infectious agents; and poor hand hygiene and infection control in health care and community settings.

Text in this chapter is from "Antimicrobial (Drug) Resistance: A Growing Health Issue," National Institute of Allergy and Infectious Diseases (NIAID), March 4, 2008; and "Antimicrobial (Drug) Resistance: Quick Facts, Definitions, History, Causes, Diagnosis, Treatment, Prevention," NIAID, updated July, 2009.

Together, these forces contribute to the problem of drug-resistant infections that are increasingly difficult and costly to treat.

Drug-Resistant Microbes of Concern Today

Methicillin-resistant *Staphylococcus aureus* (MRSA): MRSA bacteria, increasingly seen not only in hospitals and health care settings (hospital acquired or HA-MRSA) but also in the wider community, especially among people in close contact such as athletes (community associated or CA-MRSA).

Vancomycin-resistant *Enterococci* (VRE): VRE bacteria are resistant to vancomycin, an antibiotic regarded as a drug of last resort.

Other microbes that are increasingly resistant to drugs include the following:

- Food-borne bacteria such as *E. coli*, *Salmonella*, and *Campylobacter* that can cause diarrhea and gastroenteritis
- Sexually transmitted bacteria that cause gonorrhea
- Penicillin-resistant *Streptococci* responsible for pneumonia
- Tuberculosis
- Influenza
- Human immunodeficiency virus (HIV)
- Malaria

Quick Facts about Antimicrobial (Drug) Resistance

- Increasing use of antimicrobials in humans, animals, and agriculture has resulted in many microbes developing resistance to these powerful drugs.
- Many infectious diseases are increasingly difficult to treat because of antimicrobial-resistant organisms, including HIV infection, staphylococcal infection, tuberculosis, influenza, gonorrhea, candida infection, and malaria.
- Between 5–10 percent of all hospital patients develop an infection, leading to an increase of about $5 billion in annual U.S. health care costs.

- About 90,000 of these patients die each year as a result of their infection, up from 13,300 patient deaths in 1992.

- People infected with antimicrobial-resistant organisms are more likely to have longer hospital stays and may require more complicated treatment.

Definitions

Antimicrobial

Antimicrobial is a general term given to substances including medicines that kill or slow the growth of microbes. Microbe is a collective name given to bacteria (*Staphylococcus aureus*), viruses (influenza, which causes the flu), fungi (for example, *Candida albicans*, which causes some yeast infections), and parasites (for example, *Plasmodium falciparum*, which causes malaria).

Examples of antimicrobial agents:

- Tetracycline (one antibiotic used to treat urinary tract infections)

- Oseltamivir or Tamiflu (antiviral that treats the flu)

- Terbinafine or Lamisil (antifungal that treats athlete's foot)

Antibiotic

An antibiotic is a medicine designed to kill or slow the growth of bacteria and some fungi. Antibiotics are commonly used to fight bacterial infections, but cannot fight against infections caused by viruses.

Examples of an antibiotic:

- Azithromycin or Zithromax (Z-Pak)

- Vancomycin is the last line of defense for certain MRSA infections.

Antibacterial

Antibacterial is the term given to substances that kill or slow the growth of bacteria when treating human and environmental surfaces. These include substances that aid in proper hygiene.

Examples of antibacterial-containing commercial products:

- Hand soaps, gels, foams

- Dishwashing detergents
- Mattresses

MRSA and VRE

Examples of antimicrobial (drug) resistance:

- Methicillin-resistant *Staphylococcus aureus* (MRSA)
- Vancomycin-resistant *Enterococci* (VRE)

The History of Antimicrobial (Drug) Resistance

In 1928 while working with *Staphylococcus* bacteria, Scottish scientist Alexander Fleming noticed that a type of mold growing by accident on a laboratory plate was protected from, and even repelled, the bacteria. The active substance, which Fleming called penicillin, was literally an antibiotic—it killed living organisms.

Thus began the age of using natural and, later, synthetic drugs to treat people with bacterial infections. Though not widely popular until the 1940s, antibiotics and other antimicrobials (medicines that kill or slow growth of a microbe) have saved countless lives and blunted serious complications of many feared diseases and infections. The success of antimicrobials against disease-causing microbes is among modern medicine's great achievements.

The Problem

After more than 50 years of widespread use, evolution of disease-causing microbes has resulted in many antimicrobials losing their effectiveness. As microbes evolve, they adapt to their environment. If something stops them from growing and spreading—such as an antimicrobial—they evolve new mechanisms to resist the antimicrobials by changing their genetic structure. Changing the genetic structure ensures that the offspring of the resistant microbes are also resistant.

Antimicrobial resistance makes it harder to eliminate infections from the body. As a result of a microbe's ability to survive in spite of antimicrobials, some infectious diseases are now more difficult to treat than they were just a few decades ago. In fact, antimicrobials have helped people so effectively that humans are hurting the protective value of medicines through overuse and misuse. More prudent use of antimicrobials will help to slow the development of resistance.

Causes

Microbes, such as bacteria, viruses, fungi, and parasites, are living organisms that evolve over time. Their primary function is to reproduce, thrive, and spread, quickly and efficiently. Therefore, microbes adapt to their environment and change in ways that ensure their survival. If something stops their ability to spread, such as an antimicrobial, genetic changes can occur that enable the microbe to survive. There are several ways this happens.

Natural (Biological) Causes

Mutation: Microbes reproduce by dividing every few hours, allowing them to evolve rapidly and adapt quickly to new environmental conditions. With each replication, mutations arise, and some of these mutations may help an individual microbe survive exposure to an antimicrobial.

Gene transfer: Microbes may also acquire genes from each other, including genes that make the microbe drug resistant.

Selective pressure: In the presence of an antimicrobial, microbes are either killed or, if they carry resistance genes, survive. These survivors will replicate and their progeny will quickly become the dominant type throughout the microbial population.

Societal Pressures

The use of antibiotics, even when used appropriately, creates a selective pressure for resistant organisms. However, there are additional societal pressures that act to accelerate the increase of antimicrobial resistance.

Inappropriate use: Selection of resistant microorganisms is exacerbated by inappropriate use of antimicrobials. Sometimes physicians will prescribe inappropriate antimicrobials wishing to placate an insistent patient who has a viral infection or an as-yet undiagnosed condition.

Inadequate diagnostics: More often, physicians must use incomplete or imperfect information to diagnose an infection and thus prescribe an antimicrobial just-in-case or prescribe a broad-spectrum antimicrobial when a specific antibiotic might be better. These situations contribute to selective pressure and accelerate antimicrobial resistance.

Hospital use: Critically ill patients are more susceptible to infections and, thus, often require the aid of antimicrobials. However, the heavier use of antimicrobials in these patients can worsen the problem by selecting for antimicrobial-resistant microorganisms. The extensive use of antimicrobials and close contact among sick patients creates a fertile environment for the spread of antimicrobial-resistant germs.

Agricultural use: Scientists also believe that the practice of adding antibiotics to agricultural feed promotes drug resistance. More than half of the antibiotics produced in the United States are used for agricultural purposes. However, there is still much debate about whether drug-resistant microbes in animals pose a significant public health burden.

Diagnosis

Diagnostic tests are designed to determine which microbe is causing infection and to which antimicrobials the microbe might be resistant. This information would be used by a health care provider to choose an appropriate antimicrobial. However, current diagnostic tests often take a few days to give results. Oftentimes, health care providers need to make treatment decisions before the results are known. While waiting for test results, health care providers may prescribe a broad-spectrum antimicrobial when a more specific treatment might be better. The common practice of treating unknown infections with broad-spectrum antimicrobials is another factor in the emergence of antimicrobial resistance

Treatment

If you think you have an infection of any type—bacterial, viral, or fungal—talk with your health care provider. Some infections will resolve without medical intervention. Others will not and can become extremely serious. Ear infections are a good example: Some middle ear infections are caused by a virus and will get better without treatment; while other middle ear infections caused by bacteria can cause perforated eardrums, or worse, if left untreated.

The decision to use antimicrobials should be left to your health care provider. In some cases, antimicrobials will not shorten the course of the disease, but they might reduce your chance of transmitting it to others, as is the case with pertussis (whooping cough).

Antibiotics cannot fight against infections caused by viruses. Antibiotics are appropriate to use when:

- there is a known bacterial infection; or
- if the cause is unknown, then the consequences of not treating a condition could be devastating (for example, in early meningitis).

Of note, the color of your sputum (saliva) does not indicate whether antibiotics are required. Most cases of bronchitis are caused by viruses; therefore, a change in sputum color does not indicate a bacterial infection.

Prevention

To prevent antimicrobial resistance, you and your health care provider should discuss the appropriate medication for your illness and avoid overusing or misusing medicines. Strictly follow prescription medication directions and never share or take medicine that was prescribed for someone else. Communicate effectively with your health care provider, so that he or she has a clear understanding of your symptoms and can determine whether an antimicrobial drug, such as an antibiotic, is appropriate. Do not save your antibiotic for the next time you get sick; take all of the medication as prescribed by your health care provider. If the health care provider has prescribed more than the required dose, discard leftover medications once you have completed the prescribed course of treatment. Do not share your medication with another person.

Healthy lifestyle habits always go far in preventing illness, including proper diet, exercise, sleeping patterns, and good hygiene, such as frequent hand washing.

Chapter 68

Surveillance of Antimicrobial Resistance Patterns and Rates

Surveillance

Surveillance for resistant microorganisms and antimicrobial agent use remains a priority at Centers for Disease Control and Prevention (CDC), U.S. Food and Drug Administration (FDA), U.S. Department of Agriculture (USDA), and other federal agencies. Data on patterns and rates of antimicrobial resistance are collected for a variety of microorganisms including over 15 species of bacteria, *Mycobacterium tuberculosis*, yeasts and moulds, viruses, and selected parasites through a series of ongoing surveillance systems.

Methicillin-Resistant Staphylococcus Aureus

According to CDC's Active Bacterial Core Surveillance (ABCs) system, there are approximately 94,000 new cases of invasive methicillin-resistant *Staphylococcus aureus* (MRSA) infection reported annually in the United States, resulting in over 19,000 deaths. In contrast, data from the National Healthcare Safety Network (NHSN) indicate that the incidence of central line-associated bloodstream infections per 1,000 central line days in 2006 decreased by 49.6% compared to 2005 data, while the incidence of central line-associated methicillin-susceptible *S. aureus* (MSSA) infections decreased even more substantially, by 70.1%. Data

Excerpted from "Antimicrobial Resistance Interagency Task Force 2007 Annual Report: Executive Summary," Centers for Disease Control and Prevention (CDC), June 2008.

on invasive MRSA infections from the ABC's system for 2005–2006 also show a decrease in hospital-onset and healthcare-associated MRSA infections, confirming this downward trend. Although community onset infections of MRSA did not decrease significantly, there was a downward trend.

Streptococcus Pneumoniae

ABC's data through 2006 show that invasive pneumococcal disease (IPD) caused by antimicrobial-resistant *S. pneumoniae* isolates covered by the conjugate vaccine (designated PCV7) remain low; however, infections caused by multidrug resistant serotype 19A strains are increasing. Development of a 13-valent pneumococcal conjugate vaccine is in progress. Data from ABC will help document the vaccine's impact on invasive infections caused by drug-resistant pneumococci.

Tuberculosis

A pilot exercise was initiated in 2007 to provide additional surveillance data for tuberculosis (TB) cases reported as multi-drug resistant (MDR) or extensively drug resistant (XDR) from four geographic areas, which provide about 55% of the reported MDR-TB cases in the United States. The results of this pilot will provide important information on the burden and impact of MDR-TB and inform CDC on how a nationwide supplemental registry for MDR/XDR TB would assist public health efforts.

Drug-resistant tuberculosis continued to spread internationally and is now approaching critical proportions. A focus on providing care in low resource, high burden areas is critical for preventing the transmission of drug-resistant TB in health care settings, especially among human immunodeficiency virus (HIV)-infected persons. In November 2006, a federal TB task force convened to discuss the possible U.S. government response to the global threat of XDR-TB. In 2007, an action plan was developed, which is currently undergoing review.

Sexually Transmitted Diseases

The Gonococcal Isolate Surveillance Project (GISP) provides national antimicrobial susceptibility data to guide recommendations for treating gonorrhea in the United States. Data from GISP showed increases in fluoroquinolone resistance in all regions of the country prompting

CDC to revise its sexually transmitted disease (STD) Treatment Guidelines in 2007. CDC no longer recommends fluoroquinolones for the treatment of gonorrhea. As a result, CDC recommends only one class of antibiotics, the cephalosporins, for the treatment of gonococcal infections. Continued monitoring for the emergence of cephalosporin resistance will remain a critical CDC activity.

CDC is working with the World Health Organization to expand its sentinel surveillance system for monitoring antimicrobial resistance of *Neisseria gonorrhoeae* in the Western Pacific Region. CDC launched a sentinel surveillance project to monitor azithromycin-resistant syphilis in the United States. Residual clinical specimens and demographic data are submitted to CDC from STD clinics in 11 cities for screening.

Influenza

In 2007, surveillance for resistance to both classes of licensed anti-influenza drugs, M2 blockers (amantadine and rimantadine) and neuraminidase inhibitors (NI) (oseltamivir and zanamivir) in seasonal influenza viruses was expanded. Over 3,500 influenza A and B viruses isolated in 46 states and 73 foreign countries (Africa, North America, South America, Asia, Europe, and Oceania) were tested for antiviral resistance. Resistance to M2 blockers among influenza A (H3N2) viruses continued to be very high worldwide especially in South Asia (essentially 100% in China). A rise of M2-blocker resistance was also detected among A (H1N1) viruses circulated in the United States. Resistance to the licensed NI was low (less than 1%) among influenza A and B viruses circulating during several previous seasons. Therefore, the use of NI rather than M2 blockers has been recommended by CDC and public health agencies in other countries.

In the early 2007–2008 influenza season, a small (5.5%), but noticeable, increase in resistance to oseltamivir was detected among influenza A (H1N1) viruses circulating in the United States. Around the same time, a very high frequency of oseltamivir resistance was reported for A (H1N1) viruses circulating in Norway (up to 66%) and some other countries in Europe. All oseltamivir-resistant A (H1N1) viruses shared the same mutation (H274Y) in the neuraminidase gene. They all were susceptible to M2 blockers and to another licensed NI, zanamivir. The alarming increase of resistance to oseltamivir among influenza A (H1N1) viruses prompted the Influenza Division of CDC to enhance surveillance efforts within the United States and to develop new methods for drug resistance detection.

Also, testing of available, highly pathogenic avian A (H5N1) viruses for their susceptibility to M2 blockers and NI was expanded.

Antimicrobial Agent Use

The National Hospital Ambulatory Medical Care Survey (NHAMCS) is an annual national survey that collects data on the utilization of ambulatory medical care services provided by hospital emergency and outpatient departments in the United States. Findings are based on a sample of visits to emergency departments and outpatient clinics. NHAMCS monitors trends in prescription of antimicrobial drugs in hospital emergency and outpatient departments. Antimicrobial prescribing in ambulatory care settings decreased from 154 antimicrobials per 1,000 visits in 1993–94 to 123 antimicrobials per 1,000 visits in 2005–06 (down by 20%). This decline was observed in all age groups, except for persons 15–24 years of age. Among children and adolescents less than 15 years of age, decreasing trends in antimicrobial prescribing rates were found in the physician office and emergency department (ED) settings, but not in the hospital outpatient department (OPD). For persons 15 years of age and over, antimicrobial prescribing rates increased by 29% in the OPD and 15% in the ED; no change was observed in physician offices.

Chapter 69

Influenza Antiviral Drug Resistance

What is antiviral resistance?

Antiviral resistance means that a virus has changed in such a way that the antiviral drug is less effective in treating or preventing illnesses caused by the virus. In the United States, four antiviral drugs are U.S. Food and Drug Administration (FDA)–approved for use against influenza: amantadine, rimantadine, zanamivir and oseltamivir. Amantadine and rimantadine are approved for influenza A while the neuraminidase inhibitor drugs zanamivir and oseltamivir are approved for influenza A and influenza B.

How does antiviral resistance happen?

Influenza viruses constantly change as the virus makes copies of itself (replicates). The ability to constantly change is a hallmark of influenza viruses. Flu viruses often change from one season to the next, or they can even change within the course of one flu season. Some changes can result in the viruses being resistant to one or more of the antiviral drugs that are used to treat or prevent influenza.

How is antiviral resistance detected?

Samples of viruses collected from around the United States and worldwide are studied to determine if they are resistant to any of the

"Influenza Antiviral Drug Resistance," Centers for Disease Control and Prevention (CDC), December 19, 2008.

four FDA-approved influenza antiviral drugs. The Centers for Disease Control and Prevention (CDC) routinely collects viruses through a domestic and global surveillance system to monitor for changes in influenza viruses.

What has CDC done to improve monitoring of influenza viruses for antiviral resistance?

In the last two years, CDC has improved the ability to rapidly detect and monitor for resistant viruses.

How is this surveillance information used?

Enhanced surveillance efforts have provided CDC with the capability to detect resistant strains more quickly, and enabled CDC to monitor for changing trends overtime. Virus surveillance information is helpful in making recommendations for how to treat or prevent flu.

How did influenza antiviral resistance patterns change during the 2007-08 influenza season?

During the 2007–08 influenza season, the CDC influenza laboratory and other influenza laboratories around the world showed a significant increase in the prevalence of resistance to oseltamivir among A (H1N1) viruses. In the U.S., about 13% of H1N1 viruses were found to be resistant to oseltamivir, whereas prior to 2007–08, less than 1% of viruses were resistant. Additionally, laboratory surveillance indicated continued high resistance to amantadine and rimantadine among influenza A (H3N2) influenza viruses in the United States and about 11% among influenza A (H1N1) viruses.

What have we seen during the 2008–2009 season in terms of antiviral resistance monitoring in the United States?

As a result of low U.S. flu activity early during this period, few viruses have been available to CDC for antiviral resistance testing. However, among viruses tested, a high proportion of the few influenza A (H1N1) viruses analyzed by CDC have been resistant to oseltamivir (Tamiflu®). CDC continues to track this information and updated antiviral resistance figures are published in the weekly U.S. Influenza Surveillance Report.

Is CDC recommending any changes to the current guidance on the use of antivirals for the 2008–09 influenza season?

Recommendations regarding the use of antiviral medications have been reviewed given:

- surveillance data that indicates all influenza A (H3N2) and influenza B viruses remain susceptible to oseltamivir;
- an increase in the number of, and geographic spread of, oseltamivir-resistance influenza A (H1N1) viruses in the United States has been detected;
- all influenza A (H1N1), H3N2, and influenza B viruses remain susceptible to zanamivir; and
- the high levels of resistance to amantadine and rimantadine among H3N2 viruses.

Different options for antiviral treatment in the setting of increased circulation of oseltamivir-resistant H1N1 viruses have been considered. These options, such as dual therapy with oseltamivir and rimantadine or use of zanamivir, were outlined in the 2008 influenza recommendations and can be found on the CDC website at http://www.cdc.gov/flu/professionals/antivirals/resistance.htm

On December 19, 2008 CDC issued interim guidance on the use of influenza antiviral medications in the United States for the 2008–09 season which is based on the 2008 Advisory Committee on Immunization Practices (ACIP) recommendations.

What is CDC doing to monitor antiviral resistance in the United States?

CDC will continue ongoing surveillance and testing of influenza viruses. Additionally, CDC is working with the state public health departments and the World Health Organization to collect additional information on oseltamivir resistance in the U.S. and worldwide. The information collected will assist in making informed public health policy recommendations.

What implications does antiviral resistance have for the U.S. antiviral stockpile that was created as part of the United States pandemic plan?

The U.S. antiviral drug stockpile contains both neuraminidase inhibitor agents, oseltamivir and zanamivir. These medications are to be used in the event that a novel influenza A subtype virus, such as avian influenza A (H5N1) virus, emerges and spreads easily among humans. Current pandemic antiviral drug use strategies include containment of an initial pandemic outbreak and treatment of persons with pandemic disease.

The stockpile is for the control of pandemic influenza, and is not for seasonal influenza use. And, resistance among seasonal strains does not predict resistance among pandemic influenza viruses. Antiviral drugs, such as oseltamivir are one component of a multi-faceted approach to pandemic preparedness planning and response. The effectiveness of any drug during a pandemic is difficult to predict, as it is not possible to know which virus will cause the next pandemic.

Oseltamivir remains the drug recommended by the World Health Organization as the first-line influenza antiviral drug for the treatment of patients infected with influenza A (H5N1). A very small number of patients infected with avian influenza A (H5N1) virus had evidence of oseltamivir resistance in viruses that were isolated from them. These influenza A (H5N1) viruses did not spread to others

CDC will continue ongoing surveillance and testing of influenza viruses for antiviral resistance among seasonal and novel influenza viruses such as H5N1 viruses.

Chapter 70

Combating Antibiotic Resistance

Antibiotics are drugs used for treating infections caused by bacteria. Also known as antimicrobial drugs, antibiotics have saved countless lives. Misuse and overuse of these drugs, however, have contributed to a phenomenon known as antibiotic resistance. This resistance develops when potentially harmful bacteria change in a way that reduces or eliminates the effectiveness of antibiotics.

A Public Health Issue

Antibiotic resistance is a growing public health concern worldwide. When a person is infected with an antibiotic-resistant bacterium, not only is treatment of that patient more difficult, but the antibiotic-resistant bacterium may spread to other people.

When antibiotics don't work, the result can be:

- longer illnesses,

- more complicated illnesses,

- more doctor visits,

- the use of stronger and more expensive drugs,

- more deaths caused by bacterial infections.

"Combating Antibiotic Resistance," U.S. Food and Drug Administration (FDA), May, 1, 2008.

Examples of the types of bacteria that have become resistant to antibiotics include the species that cause skin infections, meningitis, sexually transmitted diseases, and respiratory tract infections such as pneumonia.

In cooperation with other government agencies, the Food and Drug Administration (FDA) has launched several initiatives to address antibiotic resistance. The agency has issued drug labeling regulations, emphasizing the prudent use of antibiotics. The regulations encourage health care professionals to prescribe antibiotics only when clinically necessary, and to counsel patients about the proper use of such drugs and the importance of taking them as directed. FDA has also encouraged the development of new drugs, vaccines, and improved tests for infectious diseases.

Antibiotics Fight Bacteria, Not Viruses

Antibiotics are meant to be used against bacterial infections. For example, they are used to treat strep throat, which is caused by streptococcal bacteria, and skin infections caused by staphylococcal bacteria. Although antibiotics kill bacteria, they are not effective against viruses. Therefore, they will not be effective against viral infections such as colds, most coughs, many types of sore throat, and influenza (flu).

Using antibiotics against viral infections:

- will not cure the infection;

- will not keep other individuals from catching the virus;

- will not help a person feel better;

- may cause unnecessary, harmful side effects; and

- may contribute to the development of antibiotic-resistant bacteria.

Patients and health care professionals alike can play an important role in combating antibiotic resistance. Patients should not demand antibiotics when a health care professional says the drugs are not needed. Health care professionals should prescribe antibiotics only for infections they believe to be caused by bacteria.

As a patient, your best approach is to ask your health care professional whether an antibiotic is likely to be effective for your condition. Also, ask what else you can do to relieve your symptoms.

Follow Directions for Proper Use

When you are prescribed an antibiotic to treat a bacterial infection, it's important to take the medication exactly as directed. Here are more tips to promote proper use of antibiotics:

- Complete the full course of the drug. It's important to take all of the medication, even if you are feeling better. If treatment stops too soon, the drug may not kill all the bacteria. You may become sick again, and the remaining bacteria may become resistant to the antibiotic that you've taken.

- Do not skip doses. Antibiotics are most effective when they are taken regularly.

- Do not save antibiotics. You might think that you can save an antibiotic for the next time you get sick, but an antibiotic is meant for your particular infection at the time. Never take leftover medicine. Taking the wrong medicine can delay getting the appropriate treatment and may allow your condition to worsen.

- Do not take antibiotics prescribed for someone else. These may not be appropriate for your illness, may delay correct treatment, and may allow your condition to worsen.

- Talk with your health care professional. Ask questions, especially if you are uncertain about when an antibiotic is appropriate or how to take it.

It's important that you let your health care professional know of any troublesome side effects. Consumers and health care professionals can also report adverse events to FDA's MedWatch program at 800-332-1088 or online at MedWatch http://www.fda.gov/Safety/MedWatch/default.htm.

What FDA Is Doing

Efforts to combat antibiotic resistance include agency-wide cooperation and development of an FDA Task Force on Antimicrobial Resistance. FDA activities include the following:

- Labeling regulations addressing proper use of antibiotics. Antibiotic labeling contains required statements in several places advising health care professionals that these drugs should be used only to treat infections that are believed to be caused by bacteria.

Labeling also encourages health care professionals to counsel patients about proper use.

- Partnering to promote public awareness. FDA is partnering with the Centers for Disease Control and Prevention (CDC) on "Get Smart: Know When Antibiotics Work," a campaign that offers web pages, brochures, fact sheets, and other information sources aimed at helping the public learn about preventing antibiotic-resistant infections.

- Encouraging the development of new antibiotics. FDA is actively engaged in developing guidance for industry on the types of clinical studies that could be performed to evaluate how an antibacterial drug works for the treatment of different types of infections.

Part Five

Preventing Contagious Diseases

Chapter 71

Handwashing Prevents the Spread of Germs

Frequent and Proper Hand Hygiene Can Stop Germs and Illness in Their Tracks

Many cases of colds, flu, and foodborne illness are spread by unclean hands, and these diseases are responsible for billions of dollars each year in health care expenditures and productivity losses in the United States. Worldwide, infectious diseases remain the leading cause of illness and death and the third-leading cause of death in the United States. Good hand hygiene will also reduce the risk of spreading germs that have become resistant to antibiotics, such as methicillin-resistant *Staphylococcus aureus*, or MRSA. Some viruses and bacteria can live two hours or longer on surfaces like tables, doorknobs, and telephones. These disease causing germs can enter your body when your unwashed hands touch your nose, mouth, eyes, or open wounds. Simple handwashing with soap and water can in some cases reduce infections by more than 50 percent. (Source: Didier Pittet, "Clean hands reduce the burden of disease," *The Lancet*, www.thelancet.com, Vol. 366, July 16 2005, pp. 185–187.)

Hand Hygiene Products

Hand hygiene has been an important practice for centuries. And, since its establishment in 1926, The Soap and Detergent Association (SDA) has been a leader in educating the public about hand hygiene and its impact on preventing illness. According to the World Health Organization, "Hand hygiene is the primary measure to reduce infections." Just imagine what life would be like if we didn't clean our hands:

It's Monday morning: You catch the early train to work. Taking public transportation is a great way to meet a lot of new, interesting people, but opening a door or holding that handrail can also put you in touch with many of their germs.

You arrive at your office: To your pleasant surprise, the company tech person is installing your new e-mail program. The only thing is she has a cold. After a couple of sniffles, coughs, and keystrokes, she hands you your keyboard and says, "Log in please." Instead of you've got mail, you've got germs.

Later on, your boss treats you to lunch to celebrate your big promotion: He sneezes just before shaking your hand—ka-ching turns into ka-choo.

After work, you remember you have to pick up the chicken for dinner: You stop at the local market, and grab the handle of the first shopping cart in sight. Then, squish—your hands are covered in baby drool, a surprise left over from the previous little customer. Having second thoughts about that chicken dinner?

As you can see, there's plenty of opportunity for germs to sneak up on us when we least expect them. But, frequent and proper hand hygiene can stop germs and illness in their tracks. Read on to find out how hand cleaning products can help.

Products

Hand hygiene products come in many forms—each having its own benefits. Look for easy, convenient, portable, and refillable packaging options. Select the form that best suits your needs.

- **Bar soaps:** Designed to clean the skin by removing dirt and oils.

- **Hand sanitizer:** Designed to kill germs on hands that are not visibly dirty, without the need for water or towels.

- **Liquid or foaming hand soaps:** Designed to dispense a single dose for cleaning hands.

- **Wipes:** Designed to wipe away dirt from hands.

Remember to read the label. Product labels may contain information about ingredients, proper use, and other useful information, such as how to contact the product manufacturer with questions.

Ingredients

Ingredients may be listed on product packaging. The following are common ingredients used in many hand hygiene products. Not all products contain all ingredients.

- **Cleaning agents/surfactants:** Lift dirt and soil and help remove germs from hands.

- **Moisturizers:** Leave hands feeling soft and smooth.

- **Fragrances:** Give consumers a choice of pleasing scents.

- **Antibacterial/germ-killing agents:** Help kill germs that may cause odors or illness. Some of the more frequently used ingredients are:
  - triclocarban—used in bar soaps;
  - triclosan—used in bar and liquid soaps;
  - alcohol—used in hand sanitizer and hand wipes;
  - benzalkonium chloride—used in hand sanitizer and hand wipes; and
  - benzethonium chloride—used in hand sanitizer and hand wipes.

Safety First

- Always read and follow instructions on all products before using.

- Avoid contact with eyes. In case of eye contact, flush with water.

- Hand hygiene products are intended for external use only. If swallowed, get medical help or call the number on the product label or the U.S. Poison Control Center's toll-free hotline at 800-222-1222. To locate a provincial Poison Control Center in Canada, visit www.healthycleaning101.org/english/safety.html.

Clean Hands Report Card®

The Soap and Detergent Association (SDA) posed the following questions to four distinct groups—American parents, teachers, students, and school nurses/health care professionals—as part of a survey on hand hygiene knowledge and behavior

Table 71.1. What do you think is the number one way to prevent colds and flu?

	Teachers	School Nurses/ Health Professionals	Students	Parents
Clean hands regularly	97.9%	99.7%	87.2%	50.0%
Healthy diet	1.5%	0.3%	3.0%	25.9%
Immunization	0.0%	0.0%	3.6%	9.4%
Proper sleep	0.4%	0.0%	4.6%	7.1%
Stress reduction	0.2%	0.0%	0.3%	1.8%
No prevention	0.0%	0.0%	0.3%	0.0%
Don't know	0.0%	0.0%	1.0$	5.8%

Insight: The Centers for Disease Control and Prevention (CDC) says that cleaning your hands is the single most important thing we can do to keep from getting sick and spreading illness to others. Yet just half of American parents know this simple fact. More education is needed as the country faces the potential of its worst cold and flu season.

Table 71.2. Approximately how many times do you wash your hands on an average day?

	Teachers	School Nurses/ Health Professionals	Students	Parents
1 to 2 times	1.0%	0.9%	3.7%	50.0%
3 to 4 times	8.2%	2.2%	20.6%	25.9%
5 to 6 times	23.1%	8.4%	31.6%	9.4%
7 to 10 times	32.3%	24.0%	22.7%	7.1%
More than 10 times	34.9%	64.2%	16.6%	1.8%
I don't wash my hands	0.0%	0.3%	0.0%	0.0%
Don't know	0.6%	0.0%	4.9%	5.8%

Table 71.2. (*continued*)

Insight: Not surprisingly, school nurses and health professionals report being the most conscientious about frequent hand washing, while mothers were significantly more likely than fathers to wash their hands ten or more times per day—59% versus 36%. SDA reported last year that the number of Americans who wash their hands more than ten times per average day increased to 42%. In this most recent survey, parents and school nurses/health professionals make the grade but teachers and students have some catching up to do.

Table 71.3. When you wash your hands, how long do you typically lather them, or rub them with soap?

	Teachers	School Nurses/ Health Professionals	Students	Parents
Less than 10 seconds	9.5%	4.7%	12.0%	10.8%
10 to 15 seconds	36.0%	39.2%	39.1%	31.6%
15 to 20 seconds	34.4%	29.5%	29.8%	23.9%
More than 20 seconds	19.7%	26.3%	16.9%	32.2%
Don't know	0.4%	0.3%	2.2%	1.4%

Insight: Nearly one-third of parents say they regularly wash their hands with soap for at least 20 seconds. School nurses and health professionals look as though they could use a little more education.

Table 71.4. How often do you wash your hands after you cough or sneeze?

	Teachers	School Nurses/ Health Professionals	Students	Parents
Always	27.0%	32.8%	17.8%	30.1%
Frequently	56.4%	56.3%	38.7%	37.2%
Seldom	15.4%	10.6%	36.8%	21.8%
Never	0.8%	0.3%	4.6%	9.6%
Don't know	0.4%	0.0%	2.1%	1.2%

Insight: In a 2006 survey, SDA found that 36% of Americans seldom or never wash their hands after they cough or sneeze. Based on this new research, teachers and school nurses/health professionals go to the head of the class; parents are better than the national average; and students need a refresher course.

Table 71.5. How often do you wash your hands before eating lunch?

	Teachers	School Nurses/ Health Professionals	Students	Parents
Always	50.0%	69.0%	23.6%	76.4%
Frequently	43.3%	27.6%	44.8%	15.3%
Seldom	6.2%	3.4%	28.5%	6.3%
Never	0.2%	0.0%	2.5%	1.2%
Don't know	0.4%	0.0%	0.6%	0.8%

Insight: Germs jump from counters, money, desks, and door handles to hands and then lunches if they aren't stopped. Handwashing simply is not a priority for students; nearly one-third seldom or never wash their hands before eating lunch.

Table 71.6. How often do you wash your hands after going to the bathroom?

	Teachers	School Nurses/ Health Professionals	Students	Parents
Always	91.5%	96.9%	78.2%	93.7%
Frequently	7.9%	3.1%	20.9%	4.5%
Seldom	0.6%	0.0%	0.9%	0.5%
Never	0.0%	0.0%	0.0%	0.6%
Don't know	0.0%	0.0%	0.0%	0.8%

Insight: If you compare survey responses with observational studies, there's a major gap between what people say and what they do. A 2005 observational study commissioned by SDA and the American Society for Microbiology found that just 83% of people washed their hands after using a public restroom. If that's the case, imagine how many students are not always washing their hands after going to the bathroom.

Methodology

An omnibus survey of 664 parents/guardians (311 male and 353 female) of children in grades K–12 was conducted July 26 through August 5, 2007 on behalf of The Soap and Detergent Association (SDA), by International Communications Research (ICR). The survey has a margin of error of plus or minus 3.8 percent.

School nurses/health professionals, students, and teachers completed surveys at a series of conferences in June and July 2007. Those

Table 71.7. Did the survey find any significant gender difference?

	Mothers	Fathers
Cleaning hands regularly is the number one way to prevent colds and flu	7%	41%
Washing hands ten or more times per day	59%	36%
"Never" washing hands after coughing or sneezing	3%	17%
"Always" washing hands after coughing or sneezing	38%	21%
"Always" washing hands after going to the bathroom	97%	89%

Insight: Mothers practice significantly better hand hygiene than fathers, but in general, parents could use additional education on the role hand washing plays in preventing colds and flu.

conferences included the American Association of Family and Consumer Sciences (AAFCS), the National Association of School Nurses (NASN) and the Family, Career, and Community Leaders of America (FCCLA). Of the 1,190 surveys collected, 508 self-identified as teachers, 356 as health professionals (nearly nine out of ten were school nurses) and 326 as students.

Chapter 72

Vaccines: What They Are and How They Work

What is a vaccine?

Chances are you never had diphtheria. You probably don't know anyone who has suffered from this disease, either. In fact, you may not know what diphtheria is, exactly. Similarly, diseases like whooping cough (pertussis), measles, mumps, and German measles (rubella) may be unfamiliar to you. In the 19th and early 20th centuries, these illnesses struck hundreds of thousands of people in the United States each year, mostly children, and tens of thousands of people died. The names of these diseases were frightening household words. Today, they are all but forgotten. That change happened largely because of vaccines.

Chances are you've been vaccinated against diphtheria. You even may have been exposed to the bacterium that causes it, but the vaccine prepared your body to fight off the disease so quickly that you were unaware of the infection.

Vaccines take advantage of your body's natural ability to learn how to eliminate almost any disease-causing germ, or microbe, that attacks it. What's more, your body remembers how to protect itself from the microbes it has encountered before. Collectively, the parts of your body that recall and repel microbes are called the immune system. Without the immune system, the simplest illness—even the common cold—

Text in this chapter is excerpted from "Understanding Vaccines: What They Are, How They Work," National Institute of Allergy and Infectious Diseases (NIAID), NIH Publication No. 08–4219, January 2008. The complete document is available online at http://www3.niaid.nih.gov/topics/vaccines/PDF/undvacc.pdf.

could quickly turn deadly. On average, your immune system takes more than a week to learn how to fight off an unfamiliar microbe. Sometimes that isn't soon enough. Stronger microbes can spread through your body faster than the immune system can fend them off. Your body often gains the upper hand after a few weeks, but in the meantime you are sick. Certain microbes are so powerful, or virulent, that they can overwhelm or escape your body's natural defenses. In those situations, vaccines can make all the difference.

Traditional vaccines contain either parts of microbes or whole microbes that have been killed or weakened so that they don't cause disease. When your immune system confronts these harmless versions of the germs, it quickly clears them from your body. In other words, vaccines trick your immune system but at the same time teach your body important lessons about how to defeat its opponents.

How Vaccines Work

The Immune System

Your immune system is a complex network of cells and organs that evolved to fight off infectious microbes. Much of the immune system's work is carried out by an army of various specialized cells, each type designed to fight disease in a particular way. The invading viruses first run into the vanguard of this army, which includes big and tough patrolling white blood cells called macrophages (literally, big eaters). The macrophages grab onto and gobble up as many of the viruses as they can, engulfing them into their blob-like bodies.

How do the macrophages recognize the virus? All cells and microbes wear a uniform made up of molecules that cover their surfaces. Each of your cells displays marker molecules unique to you. The viruses display different marker molecules unique to them. The macrophages and other cells of your immune system use these markers to distinguish among the cells that are part of your body, harmless bacteria that reside in your body, and harmful invading microbes that need to be destroyed.

The molecules on a microbe that identify it as foreign and stimulate the immune system to attack it are called antigens. Every microbe carries its own unique set of antigens, and, as we will see, they are central to creating vaccines.

Antigens Sound the Alarm

The macrophages digest most parts of the viruses but save the antigens and carry them back to the immune system's base camps, also known as lymph nodes. Lymph nodes, bean-sized organs scattered throughout your body, are where immune system cells congregate. In these nodes, macrophages sound the alarm by regurgitating the antigens, displaying them on their surfaces so other cells can recognize them. In this particular case, the macrophages will show the virus antigens to specialized defensive white blood cells called lymphocytes, spurring them to swing into action.

Lymphocytes: T Cells and B Cells

There are two major kinds of lymphocytes, T cells and B cells, and they do their own jobs in fighting off a virus. T cells and B cells head up the two main divisions of the immune system army.

T Cells

T cells function either offensively or defensively. The offensive T cells don't attack the virus directly, but they use chemical weapons to eliminate the cells of your body already infected with the virus. Because they have been programmed by their exposure to the virus antigen, these cytotoxic T cells, also called killer T cells, can sense diseased cells that are harboring the virus. The killer T cells latch onto these cells and release chemicals that destroy the infected cells and the viruses inside. The defensive T cells, also called helper T cells, defend the body by secreting chemical signals that direct the activity of other immune system cells. Helper T cells assist in activating killer T cells, and helper T cells also stimulate and work closely with B cells. The work done by T cells is called your cellular or cell-mediated immune response.

B Cells

B cells are like weapons factories. They make and secrete extremely important molecular weapons called antibodies. Antibodies usually work by first grabbing onto the microbe's antigen, and then sticking to and coating the microbe. Antibodies and antigens fit together like pieces of a jigsaw puzzle—if their shapes are compatible, they bind to each other.

Each antibody can usually fit with only one antigen. So your immune system keeps a supply of millions and possibly billions of different antibodies on hand to be prepared for any foreign invader. Your immune system does this by constantly creating millions of new B cells. About 50 million B cells circulate in each teaspoonful of your blood, and almost every B cell—through random genetic shuffling—produces a unique antibody that it displays on its surface.

Before you contracted a virus, somewhere in your body B cells were probably circulating with antibodies that, purely by chance, matched antigens from the virus. When these B cells came into contact with their matching antigen, they were stimulated to divide into many larger cells called plasma cells that secreted mass quantities of antibodies to the virus.

Antibodies in Action

The antibodies secreted by B cells circulate throughout your body until they run into the virus. Antibodies attack the viruses that have not yet infected any cells but are lurking in the blood or the spaces between cells. When antibodies gather on the surface of a microbe, it is bad news for the microbe. The microbe becomes generally bogged down, gummed up, and unable to function. Antibodies also signal macrophages and other defensive cells to come eat the microbe. Antibodies are like big, bright signs stuck to a microbe saying, "Hey, get rid of this!" Antibodies also work with other defensive molecules that circulate in the blood, called complement proteins, to destroy microbes.

Your immune system is a complex network of cells and organs. Cells called macrophages gobble up the invading virus and sound the alarm by showing pieces of the invader to T cells and B cells. B cells produce defensive molecules called antibodies that stick to the virus.

The work of B cells is called the humoral immune response, or simply the antibody response. The goal of most vaccines is to stimulate this response. In fact, many infectious microbes can be defeated by antibodies alone, without any help from killer T cells.

Clearing the Infection: Memory Cells and Natural Immunity

While your immune system works to rid your body of the virus, you feel awful. You lie in bed, too dizzy and weak even to sit up. After about a week, your immune system gains the upper hand. Your T cells and antibodies begin to eliminate the virus faster than it can reproduce. Gradually, the virus disappears from your body, and you feel better. You get out of bed. Eventually, you go back to work. If you ever encounter that virus again, you won't get the disease again. You won't even feel slightly sick. You have become immune because of another kind of immune system cell: memory cells. After your body eliminated the disease, some of your virus-fighting B cells and T cells converted into memory cells. These cells will circulate through your body for the rest of your life, ever watchful for a return of their enemy. Memory B cells can quickly divide into plasma cells and make more antibody if needed. Memory T cells can divide and grow into a fighting army. If that virus shows up in your body again, your immune system will act swiftly to stop the infection.

How Vaccines Mimic Infection

Vaccines teach your immune system by mimicking a natural infection. To show how, let's jump ahead to the 21st century. Yellow fever is no longer a problem in the United States, but you are a relief worker stationed in a part of the world where the disease still occurs, and the Centers for Disease Control and Prevention (CDC) recommends vaccination prior to your departure.

The yellow fever vaccine, first widely used in 1938, contains a weakened form of the virus that doesn't cause disease or reproduce very well. This vaccine is injected into your arm. Your macrophages can't tell that the vaccine viruses are duds, so they gobble up the viruses as if they were dangerous, and in the lymph nodes, the macrophages present yellow fever antigen to T cells and B cells. The alarm is sounded, and your immune system swings into action. Yellow-fever-specific T cells rush out to meet the foe. B cells secrete yellow fever antibodies. But the battle is over quickly. The weakened viruses in the vaccine can't put up much of a fight. The mock infection is cleared, and you are left with a supply of memory T and B cells to protect you against yellow fever, should a mosquito carrying the virus ever bite you.

Chapter 73

Types of Vaccines and Vaccine Strategies

Live, Attenuated Vaccines

Live, attenuated vaccines contain a version of the living microbe that has been weakened in the lab so it cannot cause disease. This weakening of the organism is called attenuation. Because a live, attenuated vaccine is the closest thing to a natural infection, these vaccines are good teachers of the immune system: They elicit strong cellular and antibody responses, and often confer lifelong immunity with only one or two doses.

Despite the advantages of live, attenuated vaccines, there are some downsides. It is the nature of living things to change, or mutate, and the organisms used in live, attenuated vaccines are no different. The remote possibility exists that the attenuated bacteria in the vaccine could revert to a virulent form and cause disease. Also, not everyone can safely receive live, attenuated vaccines. For their own protection, people who have damaged or weakened immune systems—because they've undergone chemotherapy or have human immunodeficiency virus (HIV), for example—cannot be given live vaccines.

Another limitation is that live, attenuated vaccines usually need to be refrigerated to stay potent. If the vaccine needs to be shipped overseas and stored by health care workers in developing countries

Text in this chapter is excerpted from "Understanding Vaccines: What They Are, How They Work," National Institute of Allergy and Infectious Diseases (NIAID), NIH Publication No. 08–4219, January 2008. The complete document is available online at http://www3.niaid.nih.gov/topics/vaccines/PDF/undvacc.pdf.

507

that lack widespread refrigeration, a live vaccine may not be the best choice.

Live, attenuated vaccines are relatively easy to create for certain viruses. Vaccines against measles, mumps, and chickenpox, for example, are made by this method. Viruses are simple microbes containing a small number of genes, and scientists can therefore more readily control their characteristics. Viruses often are attenuated through a method of growing generations of them in cells in which they do not reproduce very well. This hostile environment takes the fight out of viruses: As they evolve to adapt to the new environment, they become weaker with respect to their natural host, human beings.

Live, attenuated vaccines are more difficult to create for bacteria. Bacteria have thousands of genes and thus are much harder to control. Scientists working on a live vaccine for bacterium, however, might be able to use recombinant DNA technology to remove several key genes from the bacterium. This approach has been used to create a vaccine against the bacterium that causes cholera, *Vibrio cholerae*, although the live cholera vaccine has not been licensed in the United States.

Inactivated Vaccines

An inactivated vaccine, or killed vaccine, might be better for bacterium. Scientists produce inactivated vaccines by killing the disease-causing microbe with chemicals, heat, or radiation. Such vaccines are more stable and safer than live vaccines: The dead microbes cannot mutate back to their disease-causing state. Inactivated vaccines usually do not require refrigeration, and they can be easily stored and transported in a freeze-dried form, which makes them accessible to people in developing countries.

Most inactivated vaccines, however, stimulate a weaker immune system response than do live vaccines. So it would likely take several additional doses, or booster shots, to maintain a person's immunity. This quality could be a drawback in areas where people do not have regular access to health care and cannot get booster shots on time.

Subunit Vaccines

Instead of the entire microbe, subunit vaccines include only the antigens that best stimulate the immune system. In some cases, these vaccines use epitopes—the very specific parts of the antigen that antibodies or T cells recognize and bind to. Because subunit vaccines contain only the essential antigens and not all the other molecules that make up the microbe, the chances of adverse reactions to the vaccine are lower.

Subunit vaccines can contain anywhere from 1–20 or more antigens. Of course, identifying which antigens best stimulate the immune system is a tricky, time-consuming process. Once scientists do that, however, they can make subunit vaccines in one of two ways. They could grow bacterium in the laboratory, and then use chemicals to break the bacteria apart and gather the important antigens. They also could manufacture the antigen molecules using recombinant deoxyribonucleic acid (DNA) technology. Vaccines produced this way are called recombinant subunit vaccines. Such a vaccine has been made for the hepatitis B virus. Scientists inserted hepatitis B genes that code for important antigens into common baker's yeast. The yeast then produced the antigens, which the scientists collected and purified for use in the vaccine. Research is also continuing on a recombinant subunit vaccine against hepatitis C virus.

Toxoid Vaccines

These vaccines are used when a bacterial toxin is the main cause of illness. Scientists have found they can inactivate toxins by treating them with formalin, a solution of formaldehyde and sterilized water. Such detoxified toxins, called toxoids, are safe for use in vaccines.

When the immune system receives a vaccine containing a harmless toxoid, it learns how to fight off the natural toxin. The immune system produces antibodies that lock onto and block the toxin. Vaccines against diphtheria and tetanus are examples of toxoid vaccines.

Conjugate Vaccines

Polysaccharide coatings disguise a bacterium's antigens so that the immature immune systems of infants and younger children cannot recognize or respond to them. Conjugate vaccines, a special type of subunit vaccine, get around this problem. When making a conjugate vaccine, scientists link antigens or toxoids from a microbe that an infant's immune system can recognize to the polysaccharides. The linkage helps the immature immune system react to polysaccharide coatings and defend against the disease-causing bacterium. The vaccine that protects against Hib is a conjugate vaccine.

DNA Vaccines

Still in the experimental stages, these vaccines show great promise, and several types are being tested in humans. DNA vaccines take immunization to a new technological level. These vaccines dispense with both the whole organism and its parts and get right down to the essentials: the microbe's genetic material. In particular, DNA vaccines use the genes that code for those all-important antigens.

Researchers have found that when the genes for a microbe's antigens are introduced into the body, some cells will take up that DNA. The DNA then instructs those cells to make the antigen molecules. The cells secrete the antigens and display them on their surfaces. In other words, the body's own cells become vaccine-making factories, creating the antigens necessary to stimulate the immune system. A DNA vaccine against would evoke a strong antibody response to the free-floating antigen secreted by cells, and the vaccine also would stimulate a strong cellular response against the antigens displayed on cell surfaces. The DNA vaccine could not cause the disease because it would not contain bacterium, just copies of a few of its genes. In addition, DNA vaccines are relatively easy and inexpensive to design and produce.

So-called naked DNA vaccines consist of DNA that is administered directly into the body. These vaccines can be administered with a needle and syringe or with a needle-less device that uses high-pressure gas to shoot microscopic gold particles coated with DNA directly into cells. Sometimes, the DNA is mixed with molecules that facilitate its uptake by the body's cells. Naked DNA vaccines being tested in humans include those against the viruses that cause influenza and herpes as well as HIV.

Recombinant Vector Vaccines

These experimental vaccines are similar to DNA vaccines, but they use an attenuated virus or bacterium to introduce microbial DNA to cells of the body. Vector refers to the virus or bacterium used as the carrier. In nature, viruses latch on to cells and inject their genetic material into them. The carrier viruses then ferry that microbial DNA to cells. Recombinant vector vaccines closely mimic a natural infection and therefore do a good job of stimulating the immune system.

Attenuated bacteria also can be used as vectors. In this case, the inserted genetic material causes the bacteria to display the antigens of other microbes on its surface. In effect, the harmless bacterium mimics a harmful microbe, provoking an immune response. Researchers are working on both bacterial and viral-based recombinant vector vaccines for HIV, rabies, and measles.

Vaccine Strategies

One promising, but still experimental, approach to vaccination is the prime-boost strategy. This strategy involves two vaccines. The first (frequently a DNA vaccine) is given to prepare (prime) the immune system. Next, this response is boosted through the administration of a second vaccine (such as a viral-based vector vaccine). Several prime-boost HIV vaccine candidates are being tested in humans.

Some vaccines come in combinations. You might be familiar with the DTP (diphtheria, tetanus, pertussis) and the MMR (measles, mumps, rubella) vaccines that children in the United States receive. Combination vaccines reduce visits to the doctor, saving time and money and sparing children extra needle sticks. Without combination vaccines, parents would have to bring their children in for each vaccination and all its boosters, and the chances would be greater that kids would miss their shots. Missed shots put children, as well as their communities, at risk.

Some people have wondered whether combination vaccines might overwhelm or weaken a child's immune system, but the immune system contains billions of circulating B and T cells capable of responding to millions of different antigens at once. Because the body constantly replenishes these cells, a healthy immune system cannot be used up or weakened by a vaccine. According to one published estimate, infants could easily handle 10,000 vaccines at once.

Adjuvants and Other Vaccine Ingredients

An adjuvant is an ingredient added to a vaccine to improve the immune response it produces. Currently, the only adjuvant licensed for human use in the United States is an alum adjuvant, which is composed of aluminum salts. Adjuvants do a variety of things; they can bind to the antigens in the vaccine, help keep antigens at the site of injection, and help deliver antigens to the lymph nodes, where immune responses to the antigens are initiated. The slowed release of antigens to tissue around the injection site and the improved delivery of antigens to the lymph nodes can produce a stronger antibody response than can the antigen alone. Alum adjuvants are also taken up by cells such as macrophages and help these cells better present antigens to lymphocytes.

Scientists are trying to develop new and better adjuvants. One oil-based adjuvant, MF59, has been used in seasonal influenza vaccines already available in Europe. Other adjuvants under study include tiny spheres made of fatty molecules that carry the vaccine's antigen, and inert nano-beads that can be coated with antigen. In addition to adjuvants, vaccines may contain antibiotics to prevent bacterial contamination during manufacturing, preservatives to keep multidose vials of vaccine sterile after they are opened, or stabilizers to maintain a vaccine's potency at less-than-optimal temperatures.

Chapter 74

Childhood Immunizations: Ten Vaccines for Fourteen Diseases

Some childhood vaccines have been used since the 1940s, others have been around for only a short time. Currently there are ten routinely used vaccines that protect children against fourteen diseases. All of them have done an excellent job of reducing the burden of those diseases to their lowest point in history. Because the diseases they prevent affect children, these vaccines are given during childhood. Contrary to a fairly common misperception, children have very robust immune systems, and can easily cope with multiple vaccines given on the same day.

Vaccine Side Effects

Editor's Note: For detailed information about side effects of the listed childhood vaccines, see "Problems with Vaccinations" in Chapter 78.

While vaccines are very safe, like any medicine they do sometimes cause reactions. Mostly, these are mild local reactions (soreness or redness where the shot is given) or a low-grade fever. They last a day or two and then go away. Sometimes more serious reactions are associated with vaccines. These are much less common. Some of them are clearly caused by the vaccine; some have been reported after vaccination but are so rare that it is impossible to tell if they were caused by the vaccine or would have happened anyway.

Text in this chapter is from "Parents' Guide to Childhood Immunizations: Part Three," Centers for Disease Control and Prevention (CDC), February 6, 2008.

Some children also have allergies, and occasionally a child will have a severe allergy to a substance that is component of a vaccine. There is a very small risk (estimated at around one in a million) that a vaccine could trigger a severe reaction in a child who has such an allergy. Should one of these allergic reactions occur, it would usually happen within several minutes to several hours after the vaccination, and would be characterized by hives, difficulty breathing, paleness, weakness, hoarseness or wheezing, a rapid heart beat, and dizziness. Doctors' offices are equipped to deal with these reactions. Always tell your provider if your child has any allergies that you know of.

Vaccine Precautions

A child who has had a severe (life-threatening) allergic reaction to a previous dose of any vaccine should not get another dose of that vaccine. A child with a known severe (life-threatening) allergy to any vaccine component should not get a vaccine containing that component.

If a child has any moderate or severe illness on the day any vaccine is scheduled, it should probably be delayed until the child has recovered. A mild illness or fever is usually not a reason to delay an immunization.

Diphtheria, Tetanus, and Pertussis (DTaP) Vaccine

DTaP combines vaccines against three diseases, diphtheria, tetanus, and pertussis into one shot. (The small "a" in the name stands for acellular, which means that the pertussis component of the vaccine contains only parts of the pertussis bacterium rather than the whole cell.) The diphtheria and tetanus components of the vaccine are not technically vaccines, but toxoids. In other words, they help the immune system develop protection against the toxins produced by the diseases rather than against the disease bacteria themselves. All three components of DTaP are inactivated (killed).

Children need five DTaP shots for maximum protection. The first three shots are given at 2, 4, and 6 months of age. The fourth (booster) shot is given between 15 and 18 months, and a fifth shot—another booster—is given when a child enters school, at 4–6 years. When it is given according to this schedule, DTaP protects most children from all three diseases (80%–85% from pertussis, 95% from diphtheria, nearly 100% from tetanus). Protection can fade with time, so booster doses (using Td or Tdap vaccine) are recommended every ten years.

These vaccines are also sometimes given when a person gets a serious wound that could contain tetanus bacteria.

DTaP vaccine precautions: In addition to the normal precautions for all vaccines, a child who developed encephalopathy (brain illness) within seven days after a dose of DTaP should not get another dose of pertussis-containing vaccine.

There are several other conditions that might cause a doctor to recommend not getting DTaP. These are: a temperature of 105° F, a collapse or shock-like state, or continuous crying for three or more hours, occurring within 48 hours of a previous dose; or convulsions occurring within three days after a previous dose. If your child had any of these conditions after a previous dose of DTaP, be sure to talk with your doctor before getting another dose of the vaccine. He or she might recommend getting a non-pertussis-containing vaccine.

Other Related Vaccines

- DT is a tetanus/diphtheria vaccine, which does not contain pertussis. It is used for children younger than seven years old who should not get pertussis vaccine (for example, because they have had a reaction to pertussis vaccine in the past).

- Td is similar to of DT, but is for children seven years old and older and for adults. It has a lower concentration of diphtheria toxoid than DT. It is used for routine 10-year boosters.

- Tdap was licensed in 2005. It contains a full concentration of tetanus and lower concentrations of both diphtheria and pertussis. It is the first pertussis-containing vaccine licensed in the United States for older children, adolescents, and adults. It is currently recommended as a once-only booster for adolescents.

Hepatitis A Vaccine

Hepatitis A vaccine is made from inactivated (killed) hepatitis A virus. It is 94%–100% effective in preventing hepatitis A. Because it has been available only since 1995, we don't know yet how long immunity will last, but mathematical modeling suggests that it should protect for 20 years or more. The vaccine is not licensed for children younger than one year of age.

As of 2005 hepatitis A vaccine has been routinely recommended for all children from 12 through 23 months of age. Two doses of hepatitis A vaccine are recommended, the second dose given at least six months after the first. For travelers who don't have time to get the second dose before their departure, one dose provides good short-term protection.

Hepatitis A vaccine precautions: Children who are known to have a severe allergy to alum should not get hepatitis A vaccine.

Hepatitis B Vaccine

Hepatitis B vaccine is an inactivated (killed) vaccine that is made from a small, non-infectious part of the hepatitis B virus, called hepatitis B surface antigen. The vaccine was licensed in 1986, and 98%–100% of children who get the vaccine develop immunity.

Some parents question why infants and young children should be vaccinated against hepatitis B when they don't have the risk factors (drug use, sexual activity, professional risk) that lead to many infections. Vaccinating only high-risk adolescents and adults has proved not to be a very effective way to control the disease. It was only after we began routine childhood vaccination that rates of disease began to drop significantly.

Three doses of hepatitis B vaccine are needed for full protection. The first dose is recommended at birth. This is particularly important for children whose mothers are chronically infected. The second dose is recommended at 1–4 months and the third at 6–18 months. These three doses should protect children for life. No additional booster doses are needed.

Hepatitis B vaccine precautions: Children who are known to have a severe allergy to yeast should not get hepatitis B vaccine.

Haemophilus Influenzae *Type B (Hib) Vaccine*

There are several brands of *Haemophilus influenzae* type b (Hib) vaccine used in the United States. They are all inactivated (killed) vaccines, made from a only a small part of the Hib bacterium. All brands work equally well, protecting 95%–100% of children from Hib disease. The first Hib vaccine was licensed in 1985, and several improved versions have become available since then.

Children should get either three or four doses of Hib vaccine, depending on which brand your doctor uses. The vaccine is recommended at 2, 4, 6, and 12–15 months of age. The six-month dose is not given with one brand of vaccine.

Influenza Vaccine

There are two types of influenza vaccine. The first is an inactivated (killed) vaccine given as a shot, which has been used for many years. It can be given to anyone six months of age and older. The second is a live, attenuated (weakened) vaccine, which is sprayed into the nose and was licensed in 2003. It is not licensed for children younger than two years old.

Because influenza viruses change from year to year, new vaccines must also be formulated each year, and annual vaccination is recommended. The inactivated influenza vaccine is 70%–90% effective in healthy children, and the live, intranasal vaccine is about 87% effective in healthy children 5–7 years of age.

One dose of vaccine (either type, depending on age) is recommended annually, beginning around October or November. For children younger than nine who are getting influenza vaccine for the first time, two doses are recommended, and should be given at least a month apart.

Influenza Vaccine Precautions

Inactivated vaccine: Children who are known to have a severe allergy to eggs should not get inactivated influenza vaccine.

Live, intranasal vaccine: Children who have a weakened immune system, who have chronic medical conditions such as asthma, reactive airways disease, diabetes, renal disease, or sickle cell disease, or who are receiving long-term therapy with aspirin or other salicylates should also not get this vaccine. The vaccine is not known to be harmful to these people, but it has not yet been thoroughly tested in them.

Measles, Mumps, Rubella (MMR) Vaccine

Measles, mumps, rubella (MMR) vaccine combines vaccines for all three into one shot. MMR has been around since 1971, although its three components were licensed separately during the 1960s. It is a live vaccine, containing measles, mumps, and rubella viruses that have been attenuated (weakened) so they won't cause disease. Most children who get the vaccine develop immunity to all three diseases (over 99% for measles and 95% for mumps and rubella). Protection is believed to be lifelong.

Two doses of vaccine are recommended, with the first dose given at 12–15 months of age. The second dose may be given four weeks after the first, but it is usually given at 4–6 years.

MMR vaccine precautions: Children who are known to have a severe allergy to gelatin or the antibiotic neomycin should not get MMR. A child who has a suppressed immune system, either because of a disease such as cancer or human immunodeficiency virus (HIV) infection or a medication such as steroids, should be evaluated by a doctor before getting MMR. A child who has recently gotten a transfusion or other blood product might have to wait up to several months before getting MMR.

Pneumococcal Vaccine

Pneumococcal conjugate vaccine was licensed in 2000. It is an inactivated (killed) vaccine, which gives immunity against the seven strains of the pneumococcal bacterium that have caused most of the serious infections in children. It is more than 90% effective against invasive disease (for example, blood infections and meningitis). Some ear infections are prevented by pneumococcal vaccine, but many are caused by other organisms, and the vaccine will not prevent these.

Four doses of pneumococcal vaccine are recommended, at 2, 4, 6, and 12–15 months of age. Children who are late starting the series may need fewer doses. Check with your doctor or clinic for the recommended schedule if your child starts late. This vaccine is usually not given to children five years old and older. But some older children (those with certain chronic diseases or damaged immune systems) still need pneumococcal vaccine. There is a different vaccine—called pneumococcal polysaccharide vaccine—that can be given to these children and to adults. Pneumococcal vaccine may be given at the same time as other childhood vaccines.

Polio Vaccine

The polio vaccine used in the United States contains three types of inactivated (killed) polio virus. It is sometimes called IPV (inactivated polio vaccine). The vaccine protects 99% of children who get at least three doses.

Children should get four doses of polio vaccine, the first three doses at 2, 4, and 6–18 months of age, and a booster dose at 4–6 years.

Polio vaccine precautions: A child who is known to have a severe allergy to the antibiotics neomycin, streptomycin, or polymyxin B should not get polio vaccine.

Rotavirus Vaccine

Rotavirus vaccine is a live vaccine, which is given orally rather than by injection. Children should get a total of three doses, one dose at 2, 4, and 6 months of age. The vaccine protects against five different strains of rotavirus, so even a child who has had a case of rotavirus disease should get the vaccine. The vaccine has been very effective in preventing rotavirus gastroenteritis (about 74%) and even more effective in preventing severe rotavirus gastroenteritis (about 98%).

Rotavirus vaccine precautions: A child who has a weakened immune system should be evaluated by a doctor before getting rotavirus vaccine. Suppression of the immune system can be caused by certain diseases such as cancer or HIV infection, or by medications such as steroids or chemotherapy. A child who has recently gotten a transfusion or other blood product might have to wait before getting rotavirus vaccine. Talk to your doctor if your child has any ongoing digestive problems or has ever had intussusception. Even though this vaccine hasn't been associated with intussusception, children who had this condition in the past may be at higher risk of getting it again.

Varicella Vaccine

Varicella vaccine is made with live, attenuated (weakened) varicella virus. It was licensed in the United States in 1995. It prevents chickenpox in 70%–90% of people who get it, and it prevents severe chickenpox in more than 95%. It is expected to provide life-long immunity.

Two doses of varicella vaccine are recommended for children. The first dose is recommended at 12–15 months of age. It is usually given at the same time as MMR vaccine. The second dose is recommended at 4–6 years, before entering kindergarten or first grade. It may be given sooner, as long as it is separated from the first dose by at least three months. Anyone who has had chickenpox does not need the vaccine.

Each year, about 1% of people who have gotten varicella vaccine develop chickenpox in spite of having responded to the vaccine. This is called breakthrough infection. Breakthrough infections are much milder than normal chickenpox. Patients generally have fewer than 50 lesions, which do not form blisters. They also do not get a fever and have no complications. We don't know why breakthrough infections occur.

519

Varicella vaccine precautions: Children who are known to have a severe allergy to gelatin or the antibiotic neomycin should not get varicella vaccine. A child who has a suppressed immune system, either because of a disease such as cancer or HIV infection, or a medication such as steroids, should be evaluated by a doctor before getting varicella vaccine. A child who has recently gotten a transfusion or other blood product might have to wait up to several months before getting varicella vaccine.

The manufacturer recommends not using aspirin or other salicylates for six weeks after varicella vaccine. This is because Reye syndrome has been associated with use of salicylates after chickenpox disease. Any similar risk associated with the vaccine is merely theoretical.

Two live vaccines (for example, varicella and MMR) may be given on the same day or separated by at least four weeks. But they should not be given less than four weeks apart, because they might interfere with each other. Varicella and inactivated (killed) vaccines may be given together, or at any time in relation to each other.

There is a very small risk that a child who has gotten varicella vaccine could infect a susceptible family member—particularly one with a suppressed immune system. This appears to happen very rarely, and only when the vaccinated child develops a rash. To be safe, anyone with a suppressed immune system should consider avoiding contact with a child who develops a varicella vaccine-related rash.

Combination Vaccines

Several vaccines are sometimes combined into a single shot. These are called combination vaccines. Some combination vaccines are used routinely—DTaP is a combination; so is MMR. There are currently four other combination vaccines available for children. One combines DTaP and Hib vaccines; the second Hib and hepatitis B; the third combines DTaP, hepatitis B, and polio, and the fourth combines measles, mumps, rubella, and varicella. The advantage of combination vaccines is, of course, that your children get the protection of all the component vaccines while getting fewer injections.

Each of these vaccines has certain restrictions, and not all providers carry them. But ask your provider about them if you are interested in reducing the number of shots your child needs.

Chapter 75

Questions and Answers about Childhood Vaccines

Why do children need so many shots?

Some of us may have gotten only three vaccines as children: diphtheria, tetanus, pertussis (DTP), polio, and smallpox. There were no vaccines for measles, chickenpox, mumps, and other diseases—which meant that many of us also got those diseases. Over the years scientists have developed vaccines against more diseases, and we give them to our children to protect them from those diseases. Children don't get smallpox vaccine any more because we have eradicated the disease. Within our lifetimes, we may also eradicate polio, and then that vaccine too will no longer be needed. More combination vaccines may also reduce the number of shots children will need. At the same time, vaccines may be developed to protect us against even more diseases.

Why are vaccines given at such an early age?

Vaccines are given at an early age because the diseases they prevent can strike at an early age. Some diseases are far more serious or common among infants or young children. For example, up to 60% of severe disease caused by *Haemophilus influenzae* type b occurs in children under 12 months of age. Of children under six months of age who get pertussis, 72% must be hospitalized, and 84% of all deaths

---

Text in this chapter is from "Parents' Guide to Childhood Immunizations: Part Four Appendix," Centers for Disease Control and Prevention (CDC), February 6, 2008.

from pertussis are among children less than six months of age. The ages at which vaccines are recommended are not arbitrary. They are chosen to give children the earliest and best protection against disease.

What if my child misses a dose of vaccine?

They can continue the series where they left off. Vaccinations do not have to be repeated when there is a longer-than-recommended interval between doses.

How safe are vaccines?

They are very safe. But like any medicine, they are not perfect. They can cause reactions. Usually these are mild, like a sore arm or slight fever. Serious reactions are very uncommon. Your health care provider will discuss the risks with you before your child gets each vaccine, and will give you a form called a Vaccine Information Statement, which describes the vaccine's benefits and risks. The important thing to remember is that getting vaccines is much safer than getting the diseases they prevent.

Do vaccines always work?

Vaccines work most of the time, but not always. Most childhood vaccinations work between 90% and 100% of the time. Sometimes, though, a child may not respond to certain vaccines, for reasons that aren't entirely understood. This is one reason why it is important for all children to be immunized. A child who does not respond to a vaccine has to depend on the immunity of others around her for protection. If my child is immune to measles, he can't infect your child who failed to respond to measles vaccine. But if my child never got the vaccine, he cannot only get measles himself, he can pass it along to others who are not immune.

What will happen if my child doesn't get his vaccinations?

One of two things could happen:

1. If your child goes through life without ever being exposed to any of these diseases, nothing will happen.

2. If your child is exposed to one of these diseases, there is a good chance he will get it. What happens then depends on the

child and the disease. Most likely he would get ill and have to stay in bed for a few days up to 1–2 weeks. But he could also get very sick and have to go to the hospital. At the very worst, he could die. In addition, he could also spread the disease to other children or adults who are not immune.

What are my child's chances of being exposed to one of these diseases?

Overall, quite low. Some of these diseases have become very rare in the United States (thanks to immunizations), so the chances of exposure are small. Others, such as varicella and pertussis, are still relatively common. Some are rare in the U.S. but common elsewhere in the world, so there is risk not only to travelers, but also to anyone exposed to travelers from other countries visiting here.

If my child's risk of exposure to disease is so low, why should I bother getting him immunized?

This is a good question. One answer, of course, is that even if the risk of getting these diseases is low, it is not zero. If only one child in the whole country gets diphtheria this year, that child has a one in ten chance of dying. Vaccination would have protected him. But there is also another answer. Even if disease rates are low now, if we stopped vaccinating they wouldn't remain low for very long. We know this because it has already happened in several countries, including Great Britain and Japan. For instance, in 1974, about 80% of Japanese children were being vaccinated against pertussis. That year Japan had only 393 pertussis cases and no deaths. But then there was a national scare about the safety of pertussis vaccine, and over the next few years the vaccination rate dropped to about 10%. In 1979, the country suffered a major pertussis epidemic with more than 13,000 cases and 41 deaths.

When routine vaccination was reinstated, disease rates dropped again. Without the protection afforded by a highly immunized population, diseases could make a comeback here too.

What ingredients go into vaccines, and why?

The major ingredient of any vaccine is a killed or weakened form of the disease organism the vaccine is designed to prevent. Therefore, measles vaccine is mostly measles virus. Pneumococcal vaccine is mostly the surface coating from pneumococcal bacteria.

In addition, vaccines can contain the following:

- **Diluents:** A diluent is a liquid used to dilute a vaccine to the proper concentration. It is usually saline or sterile water.

- **Adjuvants:** Adjuvants are chemicals added to vaccines to make them provide stronger immunity. Various forms of aluminum salts are the most commonly used adjuvants in vaccines.

- **Preservatives:** Preservatives are included in some vaccines (mainly ones that come in multi-dose vials that are used more than once) to prevent bacterial growth that could contaminate the vaccine.

- **Stabilizers:** Some vaccines contain stabilizers (for example, gelatin or lactose-sorbitol), to keep them safe and effective under different conditions or different temperatures.

- **Remnants from manufacturing:** Chemicals are often used during the vaccine manufacturing process, and then removed from the final product. For example, formalin might be used to kill a vaccine virus, or antibiotics might be used to prevent bacterial contamination. When these chemicals are removed, a tiny trace may remain. While some of these chemicals might be harmful in large doses, the trace amounts left in vaccines are too small to have a toxic effect.

The package insert that comes with each vial of vaccine lists all the contents of the vaccine and explains why each substance is there.

Chapter 76

Facts about Adolescent Immunization

Are there vaccines that protect against communicable diseases?

Yes. Immunizations against tetanus (lockjaw)-diphtheria-pertussis (whooping cough), meningococcus (a cause of meningitis and other serious infections), influenza (flu), hepatitis B, measles-mumps-rubella (German measles), varicella (chickenpox), and human papilloma virus (HPV) are recommended for all adolescents who have not already received them. In addition, vaccinations against hepatitis A and pneumococcal disease are needed by some adolescents.

Should all adolescents be immunized?

This depends on which vaccines they have received as children. All adolescents should receive a tetanus-diphtheria-pertussis (Tdap) booster, the meningococcal conjugate vaccine, and an annual influenza vaccine. Hepatitis B vaccine and measles, mumps, rubella (German measles) vaccine is indicated for all adolescents who have not been vaccinated previously. Varicella (chickenpox) vaccine is recommended for those not previously vaccinated and who have no reliable history of the disease. Girls and women aged 11–26 years should receive the human papillomavirus (HPV) vaccine to prevent cervical cancer. All

"Adolescent Immunization Questions and Answers," © 2008 National Foundation for Infectious Diseases (www.nfid.org). Reprinted with permission.

adolescents with diabetes or chronic heart, lung, liver, or kidney disorders need protection against pneumococcal disease and should consult their health care providers regarding their need for these vaccines. Hepatitis A vaccine is recommended for adolescents traveling to or working in countries where the disease is common, living in communities with outbreaks of the disease, and living in states that have hepatitis A rates that exceed the national average. It is also recommended for adolescents who have chronic liver disease or clotting-factor disorders, are injection drug users, or are male and have sex with other males.

How often do I need to be immunized?

The first and only dose of meningococcal conjugate vaccine is recommended for adolescents aged 11–18 years. Immunization against tetanus and diphtheria, and pertussis (Tdap vaccine) should be supplemented with one booster of Tdap at 11–12 years of age. Those who deferred Td boosters during 2001 and early 2002 because of vaccine shortages or have not received the Td booster for any other reason should receive Tdap to get back on track. Adolescents not previously vaccinated should receive three doses of hepatitis B vaccine and one or two of measles, mumps, rubella (MMR), depending on how many they have previously received. Two doses of chickenpox vaccine is recommended for adolescents 11–12 years of age if there is no proof of prior chickenpox disease or immunization. Adolescents who received one dose of varicella vaccine during childhood are recommended to receive a second dose. Girls and women aged 11–26 should receive three doses of the HPV vaccine. Influenza vaccine should be administered yearly to adolescents. A single dose of pneumococcal polysaccharide vaccine is recommended for adolescents with certain chronic diseases who are at increased risk for this disease or its complications. Hepatitis A vaccine is administered in two doses.

Are there side effects to these immunizations?

Vaccines are among the safest medical products available. Some common side effects are a sore arm or low grade fever. As with any medical product, there are very small risks that serious problems could occur after getting a vaccine. However, the potential risks associated with the diseases that these vaccines prevent are much greater than the potential risks associated with the vaccines themselves.

Should I have a personal immunization record?

Yes. This record will help you and your health care provider ensure that you are protected against vaccine-preventable diseases. Ask your provider for this record, and be sure to take it with you every time you visit your provider so that it can be reviewed and updated.

Adolescent Immunization Facts

Fact: Vaccines are among the safest medical products available.

Fact: Approximately 6.8 million children and adolescents aged 2–18 years have chronic illnesses, placing them at risk for influenza and pneumococcal diseases and their complications.

Fact: Although no longer a very common disease in the U.S., diphtheria remains a large problem in other countries and can pose a serious threat to those in the U.S. who may not be fully immunized and who travel to other countries or have contact with immigrants or international travelers coming to the U.S.

Fact: Forty to fifty cases of tetanus (lockjaw) occur each year, resulting in approximately five deaths annually in the U.S.

Fact: The majority of the estimated 60,000 new hepatitis B infections each year strike adolescents and young adults. The hepatitis B virus is 100 times more infectious than human immunodeficiency virus (HIV), the virus that causes acquired immunodeficiency syndrome (AIDS).

Fact: The hepatitis B vaccine is recognized as the first anti-cancer vaccine because it can prevent primary liver cancer caused by hepatitis B infection.

Fact: High rates of hepatitis A infection occur among children and adolescents 5–14 years old who live in some parts of the United States, and most cases can be attributed to person-to-person transmission.

Fact: Of the 55 confirmed cases of measles reported in 2005, approximately one-third occurred in people younger than 20 years of age.

Fact: About one-fifth of people infected with the mumps virus do not have any symptoms.

Fact: By age 50, 80% of women will be infected with human papilloma virus (HPV), the virus that causes cervical cancer. There are on average 9,710 new cases and 3,700 deaths from cervical cancer in the United States every year.

Fact: In 2005, approximately 30% of reported pertussis cases were in adolescents.

For More Information

National Foundation for Infectious Diseases
4733 Bethesda Avenue, Suite 750
Bethesda, MD 20814
Phone: 301-656-0003
Fax: 301-907-0878
Website: http://www.nfid.org

Chapter 77

Adult Immunization Recommendations

Influenza Vaccine

- Trivalent inactivated influenza vaccine (TIV)
- Live attenuated influenza vaccine (LAIV)

Vaccination Recommended For

- All persons who want to reduce the likelihood of becoming ill with influenza or of spreading it to others.
- Persons age 50 years and older. [TIV only]
- Persons with medical problems (for example, heart or lung disease, renal, hepatic, hematologic, or metabolic disorder [including diabetes], immunosuppression). [TIV only]
- Persons with any condition that compromises respiratory function or the handling of respiratory secretions or that can increase the risk of aspiration (for example, cognitive dysfunction, spinal cord injury, seizure disorder, or other neuromuscular disorder). [TIV only]
- Persons living in chronic care facilities. [TIV only]
- Persons who work or live with high-risk people.

"Summary of Recommendations for Adult Immunization," November 2008. © 2008 Immunization Action Coalition (www.immunize.org). Reprinted with permission.

- Women who will be pregnant during the influenza season (December–spring). [If currently pregnant, TIV only]

- All health care personnel and other persons who provide direct care to high-risk people.

- Household contacts and out-of-home caregivers of children age 0–5 years.

- Travelers at risk for complications of influenza who go to areas where influenza activity exists or who may be among people from areas of the world where there is current influenza activity (such as on organized tours). [TIV only]

- Students or other persons in institutional settings (residents of dormitories or correctional facilities).

Schedule for Vaccine Administration

- Give one dose every year in the fall or winter.

- Begin vaccination services as soon as vaccine is available and continue until the supply is depleted.

- Continue to give vaccine to unvaccinated adults throughout the influenza season (including when influenza activity is present in the community) and at other times when the risk of influenza exists.

- If two or more of the following live virus vaccines are to be given—LAIV, measles, mumps, rubella [MMR], Varicella [Var], and/or yellow fever vaccine—they should be given on the same day. If they are not, space them by at least 28 days.

Contraindications

- Previous anaphylactic reaction to this vaccine, to any of its components, or to eggs.

- For LAIV only, age 50 years or older, pregnancy, asthma, reactive airway disease, or other chronic disorder of the pulmonary or cardiovascular system; an underlying medical condition, including metabolic disease such as diabetes, renal dysfunction, and hemoglobinopathy; a known or suspected immune deficiency disease, or immunosuppressed state.

Precautions

- Moderate or severe acute illness

- History of Guillain-Barré syndrome (GBS) within six weeks of previous influenza vaccination

Pneumococcal Polysaccharide Saccharide Vaccine (PPSV)

Vaccination Recommended For

- Persons age 65 years and older.

- Persons who have chronic illness or other risk factors, including chronic cardiac or pulmonary disease, chronic liver disease, alcoholism, diabetes, cerebral spinal fluid [CSF] leaks, cigarette smoking, as well as people living in special environments or social settings (including Alaska Natives and certain American Indian populations age 50 through 64 years if recommended by local public health authorities).

- Those at highest risk of fatal pneumococcal infection, including persons who:

  - have anatomic asplenia, functional asplenia, or sickle cell disease;

  - have an immunocompromising condition, including human immunodeficiency virus (HIV) infection, leukemia, lymphoma, Hodgkin disease, multiple myeloma, generalized malignancy, chronic renal failure, or nephrotic syndrome;

  - are receiving immunosuppressive chemotherapy (including corticosteroids);

  - have received an organ or bone marrow transplant;

  - are candidates for or recipients of cochlear implants.

Schedule for Vaccine Administration

- Give one dose if unvaccinated or if previous vaccination history is unknown.

- Give a one-time revaccination at least five years after first dose to persons age 65 years and older if the first dose was given prior to age 65 years or to those at highest risk of fatal pneumococcal infection or rapid antibody loss.

Contraindication: Previous anaphylactic reaction to this vaccine or to any of its components.

Precaution: Moderate or severe acute illness.

Zoster (Shingles) (Zos) Vaccine

Vaccination recommended for persons age 60 years and older.

Schedule for vaccine administration: Give one-time dose if unvaccinated, regardless of previous history of herpes zoster (shingles) or chickenpox

Contraindications: Previous anaphylactic reaction to any component of zoster vaccine (gelatin and neomycin); primary cellular or acquired immunodeficiency; or pregnancy.

Precaution: Moderate or severe acute illness.

Hepatitis B (HepB) Vaccine

Brands may be used interchangeably.

Vaccination Recommended For

- All persons through age 18 years.
- All adults wishing to be protected from hepatitis B virus infection.
- High-risk persons, including household contacts and sex partners of HBs Ag-positive persons; injecting drug users; sexually active persons not in a long-term, mutually monogamous relationship; men who have sex with men; persons with HIV; persons seeking evaluation or treatment for a sexually transmitted disease (STD); patients receiving hemodialysis and patients with renal disease that may result in dialysis; health care personnel and public safety workers who are exposed to blood; clients and staff of institutions for the developmentally disabled; inmates of long-term correctional facilities; and certain international travelers.
- Persons with chronic liver disease.

Note: Provide serologic screening for immigrants from endemic areas. If patient is chronically infected, assure appropriate disease management. Screen sex partners and household members; give HepB at the same visit if not already vaccinated.

Schedule for Vaccine Administration

- Give three doses on a 0-, 1-, 6-month schedule.

- Alternative timing options for vaccination include 0-, 2-, 4-months and 0-, 1-, 4-months.

- There must be at least four weeks between first and second doses, and at least eight weeks between the second and third doses. Overall, there must be at least 16 weeks between first and third doses.

- Schedule for those who have fallen behind: If the series is de-layed between doses, do not start the series over. Continue from where you left off.

- For Twinrix® (hepatitis A and B combination vaccine [GSK]) for patients age 18 years and older only: give three doses on a 0-, 1-, 6-month schedule. There must be at least four weeks between the first and second doses, and at least five months between the second and third doses. An alternative schedule can also be used at 0-, 7-days, 21–30 days, and a booster at 12 months.

Contraindication: Previous anaphylactic reaction to this vaccine or to any of its components.

Precautions: Moderate or severe acute illness; and safety during pregnancy has not been determined, so benefits must be weighed against potential risk.

Hepatitis A (HepA) Vaccine

Brands may be used interchangeably.

Vaccination Recommended For

- All persons wishing to be protected from hepatitis A virus (HAV) infection.

- Persons who travel or work anywhere except the U.S., Western Europe, New Zealand, Australia, Canada, and Japan.

- Persons with chronic liver disease; injecting and non-injecting drug users; men who have sex with men; people who receive clotting-factor concentrates; persons who work with HAV in experimental lab settings (not routine medical laboratories); food handlers when health authorities or private employers determine vaccination to be appropriate.

- Unvaccinated adults age 40 years or younger with recent (within two weeks) exposure to HAV. For persons older than age 40 years with recent (within two weeks) exposure to HAV, immune globulin is preferred over HepA vaccine.

Schedule for Vaccine Administration

- Give two doses.

- The minimum interval between first and second doses is 6 months.

- If second dose is delayed, do not repeat first dose. Just give second dose.

- For Twinrix® (hepatitis A and B combination vaccine [GSK]) for patients age 18 years and older only: give three doses on a 0-, 1-, 6-month schedule. There must be at least four weeks between first and second doses, and at least five months between the second and third doses. An alternative schedule can also be used at 0-, 7-days, 21–30 days, and a booster at twelve months.

Tetanus, Diphtheria, Pertussis (Td, Tdap) Vaccine

Vaccination Recommended For

- All adults who lack written documentation of a primary series consisting of at least three doses of tetanus- and diphtheria-toxoid-containing vaccine.

- A booster dose of tetanus- and diphtheria-toxoid-containing vaccine may be needed for wound management as early as five years after receiving a previous dose, so consult Advisory Committee on Immunization Practices (ACIP) recommendations.

- Using tetanus toxoid (TT) instead of Td or Tdap is not recommended.

- In pregnancy, when indicated, give Td or Tdap in second or third trimester. If not administered during pregnancy, give Tdap in immediate postpartum period.

For Tdap only:

- All adults younger than age 65 years who have not already received Tdap.

- Adults in contact with infants younger than age 12 months (parents, grandparents younger than age 65 years, childcare providers, health care personnel) who have not received a dose of Tdap should be prioritized for vaccination.

- Health care personnel who work in hospitals or ambulatory care settings and have direct patient contact and who have not received Tdap.

Schedule for Vaccine Administration

- For persons who are unvaccinated or behind, complete the primary series with Td (spaced at 0, 1–2 month, 6–12 month intervals). One-time dose of Tdap may be used for any dose if younger than age 65 years.

- Give Td booster every ten years after the primary series has been completed. For adults younger than age 65 years, a one-time dose of Tdap is recommended to replace the next Td.

- Intervals of two years or less between Td and Tdap may be used.

Note: The two Tdap products are licensed for different age groups: Adacel™ (Sanofi) for use in persons age 11–64 years and Boostrix® (GSK) for use in persons age 10–18 years.

Contraindications

- Previous anaphylactic reaction to this vaccine or to any of its components

- For Tdap only, history of encephalopathy within seven days following DTP/DTaP

Precautions

- Moderate or severe acute illness

- Guillain-Barré syndrome within six weeks of receiving a previous dose of tetanus-toxoid-containing vaccine

- Unstable neurologic condition

- History of Arthus reaction following a previous dose of tetanus-and/or diphtheria-toxoid containing vaccine, including MCV

Note: Use of Td/Tdap is not contraindicated in pregnancy. Either vaccine may be given during the second or third trimester at the provider's discretion.

Polio (IPV) Vaccine

Vaccination not routinely recommended for U.S. residents age 18 years and older. Note: Adults living in the U.S. who never received or completed a primary series of polio vaccine need not be vaccinated unless they intend to travel to areas where exposure to wild-type virus is likely (for example, India, Pakistan, Afghanistan, and Nigeria). Previously vaccinated adults can receive one booster dose if traveling to polio endemic areas.

Schedule for vaccine administration: Refer to Advisory Committee on Immunization Practices (ACIP) recommendations regarding unique situations, schedules, and dosing information.

Contraindication: Previous anaphylactic or neurologic reaction to this vaccine or to any of its components.

Precautions: Moderate or severe acute illness; or pregnancy.

Varicella (Var) (Chickenpox) Vaccine

Vaccination recommended for all adults without evidence of immunity.

Note: Evidence of immunity is defined as written documentation of two doses of varicella vaccine; a history of varicella disease or herpes zoster (shingles) based on health care-provider diagnosis; laboratory evidence of immunity; laboratory confirmation of disease; and/or birth in the U.S. before 1980, with the exceptions that follow. Health care personnel (HCP) and pregnant women born in the U.S. before 1980 who do not meet any of the criteria above should be tested. If they are not immune, give the first dose of varicella vaccine immediately (HCP) or postpartum and before hospital discharge (pregnant women). Give the second dose 4–8 weeks later. Routine post-vaccination testing is not recommended.

Schedule for Vaccine Administration

- Give two doses.

- Second dose is given 4–8 weeks after first dose.

- If the second dose is delayed, do not repeat first dose. Just give second dose.

- If two or more of the following live virus vaccines are to be given—LAIV, MMR, Var, and/or yellow fever vaccine—they should be given on the same day. If they are not, space them by at least 28 days.

- May use as postexposure prophylaxis if given within five days.

Contraindications

- Previous anaphylactic reaction to this vaccine or to any of its components

- Pregnancy or possibility of pregnancy within four weeks

- Persons on high-dose immunosuppressive therapy or who are immunocompromised because of malignancy and primary or acquired cellular immunodeficiency, including HIV/acquired immunodeficiency syndrome (AIDS) (although vaccination may be considered if CD4+ T-lymphocyte counts are greater than or equal to 200 cells/μL. See *MMWR* 2007;56,RR-4)

Precautions: Moderate or severe acute illness; and if blood, plasma, and/or immune globulin (IG or VZIG) were given in past 11 months, see ACIP statement "General Recommendations on Immunization" regarding time to wait before vaccinating.

Meningococcal Conjugate Vaccine (MCV) (MPSV)

Vaccination Recommended For

- All persons age 11 through 18 years

- College freshmen living in a dormitory

- Persons with anatomic or functional asplenia or with a terminal complement component deficiency

- Persons who travel to or reside in countries in which meningo-coccal disease is hyperendemic or epidemic (for example, the meningitis belt of sub-Saharan Africa)

- Microbiologists routinely exposed to isolates of *N. meningitidis*

Schedule for Vaccine Administration

- Give one dose.

- If previous vaccine was MPSV, revaccinate after three years if risk continues.

- Revaccination after MCV is not recommended.

- MCV is preferred over MPSV for persons age 55 years and younger, although MPSV is an acceptable alternative.

Contraindication: Previous anaphylactic or neurologic reaction to this vaccine or to any of its components, including diphtheria toxoid (for MCV).

Precautions: Moderate or severe acute illness; and for MCV only, history of Guillain-Barré syndrome (GBS)

Measles, Mumps, Rubella (MMR) Vaccine

Vaccination Recommended For

- Persons born in 1957 or later (especially those born outside the U.S.) should receive at least one dose of MMR if there is no serologic proof of immunity or documentation of a dose given on or after the first birthday.

- Persons in high-risk groups, such as health care personnel (paid, unpaid, or volunteer), students entering college and other post-high school educational institutions, and international travelers, should receive a total of two doses.

- Persons born before 1957 are usually considered immune, but proof of immunity (serology or vaccination) may be desirable for health care personnel.

- Women of childbearing age who do not have acceptable evidence of rubella immunity or vaccination.

Schedule for Vaccine Administration

- Give one or two doses.

- If second dose is recommended, give it no sooner than four weeks after first dose.

- If a pregnant woman is found to be rubella susceptible, give one dose of MMR postpartum.

- If two or more of the following live virus vaccines are to be given—LAIV, MMR, Var, and/or yellow fever vaccine—they should be given on the same day. If they are not, space them by at least 28 days.

- Within 72 hours of measles exposure, give one dose as post-exposure prophylaxis to susceptible adults.

Contraindications

- Previous anaphylactic reaction to this vaccine or to any of its components

- Pregnancy or possibility of pregnancy within four weeks

- Severe immunodeficiency (for example, hematologic and solid tumors; receiving chemotherapy; congenital immunodeficiency; long-term immunosuppressive therapy; or severely symptomatic HIV.) Note: HIV infection is not a contraindication to MMR for those who are not severely immunocompromised (for example, CD4+ T-lymphocyte counts are greater than or equal to 200 cells/μL)

Precautions

- Moderate or severe acute illness.

- If blood, plasma, and/or immune globulin were given in past 11 months, see ACIP statement "General Recommendations on Immunization" regarding time to wait before vaccinating.

- History of thrombocytopenia or thrombocytopenic purpura.

Note: If TST (tuberculosis skin test) and MMR are both needed but not given on same day, delay TST for 4–6 weeks after MMR.

Human Papillomavirus (HPV) Vaccine

Vaccination recommended for all previously unvaccinated women through age 26 years.

Schedule for Vaccine Administration

- Give three doses on a 0-, 2-, 6-month schedule.
- There must be at least four weeks between first and second doses and at least 12 weeks between second and third doses. Overall, there must be at least 24 weeks between first and third doses.

Contraindication: Previous anaphylactic reaction to this vaccine or to any of its components.

Precautions: Moderate or severe acute illness; also, data on vaccination in pregnancy are limited, so vaccination should be delayed until after completion of the pregnancy.

Chapter 78

Problems with Vaccinations

Any vaccine can cause side effects. For the most part these are minor (for example, a sore arm or low-grade fever) and go away within a few days. This chapter describes side-effects of vaccines for contagious diseases licensed in the United States. This information is from the Centers for Disease Control and Prevention (CDC) Vaccine Information Statements, which in turn are derived from the Advisory Committee on Immunization Practices (ACIP) recommendations for each vaccine.

Diphtheria, Tetanus, and Acellular Pertussis (DTaP) Vaccine Side-Effects

Getting diphtheria, tetanus or pertussis disease is much riskier than getting DTaP vaccine. However, a vaccine, like any medicine, is capable of causing serious problems, such as severe allergic reactions. The risk of DTaP vaccine causing serious harm, or death, is extremely small.

Mild Problems (Common)

- Fever (up to about one child in four)

- Redness or swelling where the shot was given (up to about one child in four)

Excerpted from "Possible Side-Effects from Vaccines," Centers for Disease Control and Prevention (CDC), May 19, 2009.

- Soreness or tenderness where the shot was given (up to about one child in four)

These problems occur more often after the fourth and fifth doses of the DTaP series than after earlier doses. Sometimes the fourth or fifth dose of DTaP vaccine is followed by swelling of the entire arm or leg in which the shot was given, for one to seven days (up to about one child in 30).

Other mild problems include: fussiness (up to about one child in three), tiredness or poor appetite (up to about one child in ten), and vomiting (up to about one child in 50). These problems generally occur one to three days after the shot.

Moderate Problems (Uncommon)

- Seizure (jerking or staring) (about one child out of 14,000)

- Non-stop crying, for three hours or more (up to about one child out of 1,000)

- High fever, 105° Fahrenheit (F) or higher (about one child out of 16,000)

Severe Problems (Very Rare)

Serious allergic reaction (less than one out of a million doses); several other severe problems have been reported after DTaP vaccine. These include long-term seizures, coma, lowered consciousness, and permanent brain damage. These are so rare it is hard to tell if they are caused by the vaccine. Controlling fever is especially important for children who have had seizures, for any reason. It is also important if another family member has had seizures. You can reduce fever and pain by giving your child an aspirin-free pain reliever when the shot is given, and for the next 24 hours, following the package instructions.

Hepatitis A Vaccine Side-Effects

A vaccine, like any medicine, could possibly cause serious problems, such as severe allergic reactions. The risk of hepatitis A vaccine causing serious harm, or death, is extremely small. Getting hepatitis A vaccine is much safer than getting the disease.

Mild problems: Soreness where the shot was given (about one out of two adults, and up to one out of six children), headache (about one out of six adults and one out of 25 children), loss of appetite (about one out of 12 children), and tiredness (about one out of 14 adults). If these problems occur, they usually last one or two days.

A **severe problem** is serious allergic reaction that may occur within a few minutes to a few hours of the shot (very rare).

Hepatitis B Vaccine Side-Effects

Hepatitis B is a very safe vaccine. Most people do not have any problems with it.

Mild problems reported: Soreness where the shot was given (up to about one person four), and temperature of 99.9° F or higher (up to about one person in 15).

Severe problems are extremely rare. Severe allergic reactions are believed to occur about once in 1.1 million doses. A vaccine, like any medicine, could cause a serious reaction. But the risk of a vaccine causing serious harm, or death, is extremely small. More than 100 million people have gotten hepatitis B vaccine in the United States.

Haemophilus Influenzae *Type B (Hib) Vaccine Side-Effects*

A vaccine, like any medicine, is capable of causing serious problems, such as severe allergic reactions. The risk of Hib vaccine causing serious harm or death is extremely small. Most people who get Hib vaccine do not have any problems with it.

Mild problems: Redness, warmth, or swelling where the shot was given (up to one out of four children); or fever over 101° F (up to one out of 20 children). If these problems happen, they usually start within a day of vaccination. They may last two to three days.

Human Papillomavirus (HPV) Vaccine Side-Effects

HPV vaccine does not appear to cause any serious side effects. However, a vaccine, like any medicine, could possibly cause serious problems, such as severe allergic reactions. The risk of any vaccine causing serious harm, or death, is extremely small.

Several mild problems may occur with HPV vaccine including: pain at the injection site (about eight people in ten), redness or swelling at the injection site (about one person in four), mild fever (100° F) (about one person in ten), itching at the injection site (about one person in 30), and moderate fever (102° F) (about one person in 65). These symptoms do not last long and go away on their own. Life-threatening allergic reactions from vaccines are very rare. If they do occur, it would be within a few minutes to a few hours after the vaccination. Like all vaccines, HPV vaccine will continue to be monitored for unusual or severe problems.

Influenza (Inactivated) Vaccine Side-Effects

A vaccine, like any medicine, could possibly cause serious problems, such as severe allergic reactions. The risk of a vaccine causing serious harm, or death, is extremely small. Serious problems from influenza vaccine are very rare. The viruses in inactivated influenza vaccine have been killed, so you cannot get influenza from the vaccine.

Mild problems: Soreness, redness, or swelling where the shot was given; fever; and aches. If these problems occur, they usually begin soon after the shot and last one to two days.

Severe Problems

- Life-threatening allergic reactions from vaccines are very rare. If they do occur, it is within a few minutes to a few hours after the shot.

- In 1976, a certain type of influenza (swine flu) vaccine was associated with Guillain-Barré Syndrome (GBS). Since then, flu vaccines have not been clearly linked to GBS. However, if there is a risk of GBS from current flu vaccines, it would be no more than one or two cases per million people vaccinated. This is much lower than the risk of severe influenza, which can be prevented by vaccination.

Influenza (Live) Vaccine Side-Effects

A vaccine, like any medicine, could possibly cause serious problems, such as severe allergic reactions. However, the risk of a vaccine causing serious harm, or death, is extremely small. Live attenuated influenza vaccine (LAIV) viruses rarely spread from person to person. Even if they do, they are not likely to cause illness. LAIV is made from weakened virus and does not cause influenza. The vaccine can cause mild symptoms in people who get it.

Mild problems: Some children and adolescents 2–17 years of age have reported mild reactions, including: runny nose, nasal congestion or cough; headache and muscle aches; fever; wheezing; and abdominal pain or occasional vomiting or diarrhea.

Some adults 18–49 years of age have reported runny nose or nasal congestion; sore throat; cough, chills, tiredness/weakness; and headache. These symptoms did not last long and went away on their own. Although they can occur after vaccination, they may not have been caused by the vaccine.

Severe Problems

- Life-threatening allergic reactions from vaccines are very rare. If they do occur, it is within a few minutes to a few hours after the vaccination.

- If rare reactions occur with any product, they may not be identified until thousands, or millions, of people have used it. Millions of doses of LAIV have been distributed since it was licensed, and no serious problems have been identified. Like all vaccines, LAIV will continue to be monitored for unusual or severe problems.

Measles, Mumps, Rubella (MMR) Vaccine Side-Effects

A vaccine, like any medicine, is capable of causing serious problems, such as severe allergic reactions. The risk of MMR vaccine causing serious harm, or death, is extremely small. Getting MMR vaccine is much safer than getting any of these three diseases. Most people who get MMR vaccine do not have any problems with it.

Mild problems: Fever (up to one person out of six), mild rash (about one person out of 20), and swelling of glands in the cheeks or neck (rare). If these problems occur, it is usually within 7–12 days after the shot. They occur less often after the second dose.

Moderate Problems

- Seizure (jerking or staring) caused by fever (about one out of 3,000 doses)

- Temporary pain and stiffness in the joints, mostly in teenage or adult women (up to one out of four)

- Temporary low platelet count, which can cause a bleeding disorder (about one out of 30,000 doses)

Severe Problems (Very Rare)

- Serious allergic reaction (less than one out of a million doses)

- Several other severe problems have been known to occur after a child gets MMR vaccine. But this happens so rarely, experts cannot be sure whether they are caused by the vaccine or not. These include deafness; long-term seizures, coma, or lowered consciousness; and permanent brain damage

Note: The first dose of MMRV vaccine has been associated with rash and higher rates of fever than MMR and varicella vaccines given separately. Rash has been reported in about one person in 20 and fever in about one person in five. Seizures caused by a fever are also reported more often after MMRV. These usually occur 5–12 days after the first dose.

Meningococcal Vaccine Side-Effects

A vaccine, like any medicine, could possibly cause serious problems, such as severe allergic reactions. The risk of the meningococcal vaccine causing serious harm, or death, is extremely small.

Mild Problems

As many as half the people who get meningococcal vaccines have mild side effects, such as redness or pain where the shot was given. If these problems occur, they usually last for one or two days. They are more common after MCV4 than after MPSV4. A small percentage of people who receive the vaccine develop a fever.

Severe Problems

- Serious allergic reactions, within a few minutes to a few hours of the shot, are very rare.

- A serious nervous system disorder called Guillain-Barré syndrome (or GBS) has been reported among some people who received

MCV4. This happens so rarely that it is currently not possible to tell if the vaccine might be a factor. Even if it is, the risk is very small.

Pneumococcal Conjugate Vaccine (PCV7) Vaccine Side-Effects

In studies (nearly 60,000 doses), pneumococcal conjugate vaccine was associated with only mild reactions including the following:

- Up to about one infant out of four had redness, tenderness, or swelling where the shot was given.

- Up to about one out of three had a fever of over 100.4° F, and up to about one in 50 had a higher fever (over 102.2° F).

- Some children also became fussy or drowsy, or had a loss of appetite.

So far, no moderate or severe reactions have been associated with this vaccine. However, a vaccine, like any medicine, could cause serious problems, such as a severe allergic reaction. The risk of this vaccine causing serious harm, or death, is extremely small.

Pneumococcal Polysaccharide (PPSV23) Vaccine Side-Effects

About half of people who get PPSV have mild side effects, such as redness or pain where the shot is given. Less than one percent develop a fever, muscle aches, or more severe local reactions. A vaccine, like any medicine, could cause a serious reaction. But the risk of a vaccine causing serious harm, or death, is extremely small.

Polio Vaccine (IPV) Side-Effects

Some people who get inactivated polio vaccine (IPV) get a sore spot where the shot was given. The vaccine used today has never been known to cause any serious problems, and most people don't have any problems at all with it. However, a vaccine, like any medicine, could cause serious problems, such as a severe allergic reaction. The risk of a polio shot causing serious harm, or death, is extremely small.

Rabies Vaccine Side-Effects

A vaccine, like any medicine, is capable of causing serious problems, such as severe allergic reactions. The risk of a vaccine causing serious harm, or death, is extremely small. Serious problems from rabies vaccine are very rare.

Mild problems: Soreness, redness, swelling, or itching where the shot was given (30%–74%); and headache, nausea, abdominal pain, muscle aches, dizziness (5%–40%).

Moderate problems: Hives, pain in the joints, fever (about 6% of booster doses); and illness resembling Guillain-Barré syndrome (GBS), with complete recovery (very rare). Other nervous system disorders have been reported after rabies vaccine, but this happens so rarely that it is not known whether they are related to the vaccine.

Note: Several brands of rabies vaccine are available in the United States, and reactions may vary between brands. Your provider can give you more information about a particular brand.

Rotavirus Vaccine Side-Effects

A vaccine, like any medicine, could possibly cause serious problems, such as severe allergic reactions. The risk of rotavirus vaccine causing serious harm, or death, is extremely small. Most babies who get rotavirus vaccine do not have any problems with it.

Mild problems: Babies may be slightly more likely to be irritable, or to have mild, temporary diarrhea or vomiting after getting a dose of rotavirus vaccine than babies who did not get the vaccine. Rotavirus vaccine does not appear to cause any serious side effects.

If rare reactions occur with any new product, they may not be identified until thousands, or millions, of people have used it. Like all vaccines, rotavirus vaccine will continue to be monitored for unusual or severe problems.

Shingles (Herpes Zoster) Vaccine Side-Effects

A vaccine, like any medicine, could possibly cause serious problems, such as severe allergic reactions. However, the risk of a vaccine causing serious harm, or death, is extremely small. No serious problems have been identified with shingles vaccine.

Mild problems: Redness, soreness, swelling, or itching at the site of the injection (about one person in three); and headache (about one person in 70). Like all vaccines, shingles vaccine is being closely monitored for unusual or severe problems.

Smallpox (Vaccinia) Vaccine Side-Effects

A vaccine, like any medicine, could possibly cause serious problems, such as severe allergic reactions. The risk of smallpox vaccine causing serious harm, or death, is very small.

Mild to Moderate Problems

- Mild rash, lasting 2–4 days
- Swelling and tenderness of lymph nodes, lasting 2–4 weeks after the blister has healed
- Fever of over 100° F (about 70% of children, 17% of adults) or over 102° F (about 15%–20% of children, under 2% of adults)
- Secondary blister elsewhere on the body (about one per 1,900)

Moderate to Severe Problems

- Serious eye infection, or loss of vision, due to spread of vaccine virus to the eye
- Rash on entire body (as many as one per 4,000)
- Severe rash on people with eczema (as many as one per 26,000)
- Encephalitis (severe brain reaction), which can lead to permanent brain damage (as many as one per 83,000)
- Severe infection beginning at the vaccination site (as many as one per 667,000, mostly in people with weakened immune systems)
- Death (1–2 per million, mostly in people with weakened immune systems)

For every million people vaccinated, between 14 and 52 could have a life-threatening reaction to smallpox vaccine. People who come in direct contact with the vaccination site of a vaccinated person, or with materials that have touched the site, can also have a reaction. This is from exposure to virus from the vaccination site.

Adult Tetanus and Diphtheria (Td) Vaccine and Combined Tetanus, Diphtheria and Pertussis (Tdap) Vaccine

With a vaccine (as with any medicine) there is always a small risk of a life-threatening allergic reaction or other serious problem. Getting tetanus, diphtheria, or pertussis would be much more likely to lead to severe problems than getting either vaccine.

Mild Problems

Tdap problems that were noticeable, but did not interfere with activities:

- Pain (about three in four adolescents and two in three adults)
- Redness or swelling (about one in five)
- Mild fever of at least 100.4° F (up to about one in 25 adolescents and one in 100 adults)
- Headache (about four in ten adolescents and three in ten adults)
- Tiredness (about one in three adolescents and one in four adults)
- Nausea, vomiting, diarrhea, stomach ache (up to one in four adolescents and one in ten adults)
- Chills, body aches, sore joints, rash, swollen glands (uncommon)

Td problems that were noticeable, but did not interfere with activities include pain (up to about eight in ten), redness or swelling (up to about one in three), mild fever (up to about one in 15), and headache or tiredness (uncommon).

Moderate Problems

Tdap vaccine problems which interfered with activities, but did not require medical attention:

- Pain at the injection site (about one in 20 adolescents and one in 100 adults)

- Redness or swelling (up to about one in 16 adolescents and one in 25 adults)

- Fever over 102° F (about one in 100 adolescents and one in 250 adults)

- Headache (one in 300)

- Nausea, vomiting, diarrhea, stomach ache (up to three in 100 adolescents and one in 100 adults)

Td vaccine problems which interfered with activities, but did not require medical attention:

- Fever over 102° F (rare)

Tdap or Td vaccine problems which interfered with activities, but did not require medical attention:

- Extensive swelling of the arm where the shot was given (up to about three in 100)

Severe Problems

Tdap vaccine problems causing individuals to be unable to perform usual activities which required medical attention included two adults that had nervous system problems after getting the vaccine during clinical trials. These may or may not have been caused by the vaccine. These problems went away on their own and did not cause any permanent harm.

Tdap or Td vaccine problems causing individuals to be unable to perform usual activities which required medical attention included swelling, severe pain, and redness in the arm where the shot was given (rare). A severe allergic reaction could occur after any vaccine (estimated to occur less than once in a million doses).

Varicella (Chickenpox) Vaccine Side-Effects

A vaccine, like any medicine, is capable of causing serious problems, such as severe allergic reactions. The risk of chickenpox vaccine causing serious harm, or death, is extremely small. Getting chickenpox vaccine is much safer than getting chickenpox disease. Most people who get chickenpox vaccine do not have any problems with it. Reactions are usually more likely after the first dose than after the second.

Mild Problems

- Soreness or swelling where the shot was given (about one out of five children and up to one out of three adolescents and adults)

- Fever (one person out of ten, or less)

- Mild rash, up to a month after vaccination (one person out of 25) (It is possible for these people to infect other members of their household, but this is extremely rare.)

Note: The first dose of MMRV vaccine has been associated with rash and higher rates of fever than MMR and varicella vaccines given separately. Rash has been reported in about one person in 20 and fever in about one person in five. Seizures caused by a fever are also reported more often after MMRV. These usually occur 5–12 days after the first dose.

A moderate problem is seizure (jerking or staring) caused by fever (very rare).

A severe problem is pneumonia (very rare). Other serious problems, including severe brain reactions and low blood count, have been reported after chickenpox vaccination. These happen so rarely experts cannot tell whether they are caused by the vaccine or not. If they are, it is extremely rare.

Chapter 79

Vaccine Adverse Event Reporting System

What is VAERS?

The Vaccine Adverse Event Reporting System (VAERS) is a national program that monitors the safety of vaccines after they are licensed. VAERS is managed by the U.S. Centers for Disease Control and Prevention (CDC) and the U.S. Food and Drug Administration (FDA).

Vaccines prevent serious illnesses and even death in persons who receive them. Before a vaccine is licensed, FDA takes steps to make sure the vaccine is safe. FDA requires that a vaccine goes through extensive safety testing. After a vaccine is licensed, VAERS is one of the mechanisms used to monitor for any problems, or adverse events, that happen after vaccination.

Not all events reported to VAERS are caused by the vaccine. Even though careful studies are done before a vaccine is licensed, rare adverse effects may not be found until a vaccine is given to millions of people with different backgrounds and medical histories. By continued monitoring, VAERS helps to make sure that the benefits of vaccines are far greater than the risks.

Anyone who receives a vaccine should be informed about both the benefits and risks of vaccination. Any questions or concerns should be discussed with a health care provider.

Text in this chapter is from "VAERS Vaccine Adverse Event Reporting System," U.S. Department of Health and Human Services (HHS), 2008.

Limitation and Usefulness of VAERS

VAERS is unable to determine that a vaccine caused or did not cause an adverse event. Sometimes people who are vaccinated get sick from another cause unrelated to the vaccine.

Even though VAERS cannot determine that a vaccine caused an adverse event, it can give FDA and CDC important information that might signal a problem. If it looks as though a vaccine might be causing an adverse event, FDA and CDC will investigate further.

Does VAERS provide medical advice?

No, VAERS does not provide medical advice. For medical advice, please contact your health care provider or state health department.

Who can report to VAERS?

- Parents
- Patients
- Health care providers
- Others

FDA and CDC encourage anybody who experiences any problems after vaccination to report to VAERS. Health care providers are required by law to report certain problems.

Why should I report to VAERS?

- Reporting gives valuable information that helps CDC and FDA make sure that vaccines are safe

- Reporting strengthens VAERS so it can be used to assess public health response to vaccines

- Reporting allows for evaluating public health prevention and control measures

Remember, no vaccine (or any medicine) is completely free of risk and adverse events are possible. If you have an adverse event after a vaccine, please report to VAERS. Each report is important

What types of events should I report?

You should report any adverse event that happens after getting a vaccine, even if you are not sure that the vaccine caused the adverse event. It is especially important to report any adverse event that resulted in hospitalization, disability, or death. If you are not sure that a certain type of adverse event should be reported to VAERS, talk with your health care provider.

Health care providers are required by law to report certain adverse events. To get a list of these, please call 800-822-7967 or go to www .vaers.hhs.gov/reportable.htm.

For More Information

National Vaccine Injury Compensation Program
Toll-Free: 800-338-2382
Website: http://www.hrsa.gov/vaccinecompensation

The National Vaccine Injury Compensation Program (VICP) is a separate federal program that provides compensation to individuals whose injuries may have been caused by certain vaccines. Please be aware that reporting an event to VAERS does not constitute filing a claim with the VICP.

Vaccine Adverse Event Reporting System (VAERS)
P.O. Box 1100
Rockville, MD 20849-1100
Toll-Free: 800-822-7967
Website: http://www.vaers.hhs.gov
E-mail: info@vaers.org

Chapter 80

Vaccination Records

Where are my (or my child's) immunization records?

There is no central repository of vaccination records. The only records that exist are the ones you or your parents were given when the vaccines were administered and the ones in the medical record of the doctor or clinic where the vaccines were given. Sometimes schools hold the vaccination records of children who attended, but these records are usually not kept for more than a year or two.

If you cannot locate your personal record or the record from your doctor, it may be necessary to repeat some of the vaccines or arrange blood tests to determine your immunity.

Where can I look for existing immunization records?

Children's Records

- Try calling your local or state health department's immunization program.

- Sometimes schools hold the vaccination records of children who attended, but these records are generally not kept for more than a year or two or, at the longest, until graduation. After a student graduates, records are sent to storage and may not be accessible.

"Vaccination Records: Finding, Interpreting, and Recording," Centers for Disease Control and Prevention (CDC), February 23, 2007.

- Look for family records such as a baby book.

- Check for records with your doctor or public health clinic. Please keep in mind, however, that immunization records are maintained for a limited number of years and then usually only by the medical provider who actually administered the vaccines.

College Student's Records

- Many colleges provide vaccinations (often, certain vaccinations are required for enrollment). Contact your college's medical services department (student health) for further information.

Military Records

- Check your military records.

Tracking Vaccinations

Who is responsible for keeping immunization records?

In most states, it is the responsibility of the parents of school-aged children, not family doctors, to provide vaccination records to the health department and to schools.

Today we move, travel, and change health providers more than we did in previous generations. Also, doctor's offices and clinics store records of children's vaccinations and the dates they were received only for a few years. If you keep an accurate record, you will be more likely to remember when to bring your children in for the next visit. These records also can prove that your children are up to date with their immunizations. In most states, children are not allowed to enter school or childcare unless they can prove that they meet all school immunization requirements.

Your doctor or clinic will be happy to give you an immunization record form for your use. Bring this record with you whenever you take your child to the doctor or clinic, and ask the doctor to sign and date the form each time a vaccination is given. That way, you can be sure that the immunization information is current and correct.

Finally, make sure you know if your doctor participates in an immunization registry. However, keep in mind that very few registries existed prior to the mid-1990s.

Immunization Registries' Role

What are immunization information systems and who benefits from them?

Immunization information systems are computerized information systems that collect vaccination histories and help ensure correct and timely immunizations, especially for children.

Health care providers use registries to:

- obtain a complete, accurate immunization history for a new or continuing patient;
- produce official immunization records;
- reduce paperwork;
- manage vaccine inventories;
- introduce new vaccines or changes in the vaccination schedule;
- help interpret the complex immunization schedule; and
- provide coverage data for health insurance plans and other national organizations.

Communities use registries to:

- identify populations at high risk for vaccine-preventable diseases; and
- target immunization interventions and resources efficiently.

Parents working with their health care provider(s), can use registries systems to:

- be notified when immunizations are due or late;
- obtain an accurate, official immunization history for personal use and for daycare, school, or camp entry requirements;
- consolidate records for all immunizations a child has received;
- help ensure that a child's immunizations are up to date;
- help ensure timely immunization for children if families move or switch health care providers; and
- prevent unnecessary (duplicative) immunization.

Note: No universal registry system now exists. Registries in one state or area may not be compatible with other registries, and information may have to be manually transferred from registry to registry. Also, to protect personal information in registries, this information cannot be directly retrieved by individuals.

Chapter 81

Vaccine Misinformation May Have Tragic Consequences

Decades ago, when thousands of children and adults in the United States contracted smallpox, diphtheria, poliomyelitis, or measles each year, vaccine safety concerns were not very common. People were more afraid of the diseases themselves than of possible side effects of the vaccines.

Today the situation is different; because of vaccines most parents have not encountered these once-dreaded diseases. For instance:

- smallpox has been eradicated;
- poliomyelitis has been eliminated in much of the world;
- measles, rubella, tetanus, diphtheria, *Haemophilus influenzae* type b, and rabies have largely been controlled in the United States and other parts of the world;
- mumps, chickenpox, hepatitis B, and invasive *Streptococcus pneumoniae* are decreasing in the U.S.;
- new vaccines have been developed against rotavirus, meningococcus, human papillomavirus, shingles, and adult and adolescent pertussis; and
- new vaccines are being developed for other diseases.

Most parents today have not seen a child paralyzed by polio, or choking to death from diphtheria, or brain damaged by measles. Fear of vaccine-preventable diseases has diminished while concerns about vaccine safety have increased—even though a number of the vaccines are even safer than decades ago as a result of medical research.

A lack of information or erroneous information about vaccine safety and effectiveness can create confusion among parents who are considering immunizations for their children; this can have tragic consequences.

For instance, pertussis outbreaks in England and Wales, Japan, and Sweden have been attributed to misinformation about pertussis vaccine safety in the late 1970s and 1980s. Measles and mumps outbreaks in many countries followed misinformation about measles vaccine as a cause of autism in the United Kingdom (UK).[8] And, in 2008, three unimmunized children in Minnesota developed invasive disease due to *Haemophilus influenzae*, type B (Hib) infection. One of the children died. Two other children who also developed invasive Hib disease should have been protected by community immunity, but were not.[9]

Vaccine Safety Concerns and Risk Perception

No vaccine is 100% effective; no vaccine is 100% safe. As with any drug, there are risks and side effects with vaccines, although serious side effects are mostly rare. However, there is a much higher standard of safety expected of preventive vaccines than for drugs because:

- Vaccines are generally given to many people most of whom are healthy. People tolerate far less risk from *Haemophilus influenzae* type b vaccines than the antibiotics used to treat the diseases it causes, for example.

- Many vaccines are given to children at the ages when developmental and other problems are being recognized for the first time. Because something happened at about the same time does not mean that one caused the other.

- Some vaccines are mandated by state legislatures in order to protect the health and welfare of the public. Some people think that this violates their civil rights, however.

Research shows that people respond better to some types of risks than others.

Natural risks (such as infectious diseases) are better tolerated than manmade risks (such as vaccine side effects). Also, risks that affect adults are better tolerated than risks affecting our children. Risks that are perceived with unclear benefits may be less tolerated than risks where the benefits are understood.

Take for example, measles and the MMR (measles-mumps-rubella) vaccine. Since these diseases are no longer epidemic in the United States, some parents incorrectly assume that the risk of contracting the disease is lower than the risk of their child experiencing an adverse reaction to MMR. They conclude that there may be little benefit from immunizing their child, hence there may seem to be no reason to take the risk of an adverse event. However, there was a mumps outbreak in the United States in 2006, probably introduced from the epidemic in Great Britain. Most of the 173 cases of measles in the United States in 2008 occurred among unimmunized children; measles introductions that year were largely from Europe. These infections are just a plane ride away.

Perception of risk depends on people's experiences and knowledge. A person who experienced an adverse event after vaccination—or thinks that they know someone who did—will perceive vaccines as riskier than a person who has not. Conversely, one who has survived a vaccine-preventable disease—or a physician who has treated that disease—will likely be an advocate for vaccines.

Although concerns about vaccine safety are valid—and necessary—we must carefully examine each claim about the risks of immunizations:

- Is the claim relying on scientific data (for example, large, controlled studies published in respected scientific journals) or on anecdotes (personal stories of sick persons)?
- Are the claims based on facts or are they personal opinions?

Missing Information

When up-to-date, complete, and scientifically valid information about vaccines is available, parents can make informed decisions. For example, they need to have access to accurate evidence-based information so that they understand the risks of exposure parties, the importance of community immunity, and what the actual risks of complications are. Without this information many may develop a false sense of security and regard immunizations as unimportant.

For example, measles is the most communicable of diseases, has many serious complications, and can cause severe brain damage or be fatal. But when a vaccine-preventable disease such as measles is no longer common in a community, parents may not see the need to vaccinate their children against measles, resulting in low immunization rates.

Unfortunately, when a community has low immunization rates, many children—including some who have been immunized—are placed at risk of harm if measles is introduced into the community. With global travel an everyday occurrence, measles is just a plane ride away. For instance, in March 2004, the Centers for Disease Control and Prevention (CDC) published information about a student flying from India to Cedar Rapids, Iowa, while incubating measles[1] as well as cases of measles among children who had recently been adopted from China.[2]

Like parents, scientists and scientific review groups need data to evaluate vaccine safety concerns. Vaccine safety research often requires very large—often expensive—studies that do not compete well with other types of research funded by the federal government.

Unfortunately, when a vaccine safety concern is suggested, the necessary data to support or reject the hypothesis may not yet have been collected—in fact sometimes this may take several years of research. This often leaves scientific review groups like the Institute of Medicine Vaccine Safety Committee with insufficient data to be able to fully evaluate vaccine safety concerns.

The experience concerning the hypothesis that thimerosal in vaccines caused autism—first suggested in 1999—is illustrative of the dilemma of insufficient data (missing information). In 2001, when the Institute of Medicine's Immunization Safety Review Committee first examined the issue, it stated that at that time the available evidence was inadequate to decide.[3] In other words, the information was missing. By 2004, however, much more scientific data was available and the IOM Committee was able to conclude that the data favored rejection of that hypothesis.[4]

Misinformation (False or Misleading Information)

The timing and widespread use of vaccines make them easy scapegoats to be blamed for all sorts of serious illnesses. Of course not all vaccine safety concerns are misinformation—only those that persist despite the evidence against them. Even when the concern stops being an issue for most in the scientific community, it may remain an issue for many others with vested interests—whether politicians, lawyers, journalists, or the group that concerns health professionals the most: well intentioned but misinformed parents trying to understand and alleviate their child's afflictions. Many media stories use faulty reports and parental concerns to depict a controversy about vaccines, failing to mention that the scientific community does not feel that a controversy exists.

In spite of the substantial evidence now available that allows rejection of the hypotheses that vaccines cause autism, there are some who continue to state that there is a causal association. These claims, once based on missing information, now fall into the category of misinformation.

Unfortunately, the misinformed person with a fixed opinion about vaccines has many sophisticated tools to disseminate misinformation, creating confusion about vaccine safety. Misinformation comes in many packages and may be widely publicized by the media and others causing lowered immunization levels and disease risk.

For example, a misinformed couple in Tennessee, confused about vaccine safety because of what they had read on the internet, decided to delay their daughter's vaccinations. Some time later, the baby girl was stricken with a form of meningitis that could have been prevented by a vaccine.[5]

Misinformation also involves the intentional dissemination of false information. In this case, people are not only confused about vaccine safety but may be against vaccines altogether.

Misinformation about vaccines is frequently encountered on the internet. Some websites, for instance, oppose the immunization of infants and children. They express a variety of claims that are largely unsupported by peer-reviewed scientific literature (See Table 81.1).

Misinformation websites tend to rely on emotionally filled anecdotes about bad things that happened to children or were first recognized—coincidental in time with vaccine administration—while ignoring or distorting scientific studies.[6]

Unfortunately for communities, anti-vaccination movements have also had a negative effect on public health through the years. One study, for example, showed that movements against the whooping cough vaccine caused whooping cough epidemics in several countries.[7]

How can you distinguish good information from misinformation? Misinformation often includes one or more of the following elements:

- **Invalid assumptions:** An invalid assumption is something you treat as if it were known to be true or false, when in fact it is not. For example, some parents regard hepatitis B immunization as unnecessary, assuming that this is a disease for which their children are not at risk. This is an invalid assumption.

Table 81.1. Common Claims Found on Misinformation Web Sites

Claims	Facts
Natural methods of enhancing immunity are better than vaccinations.	The only natural way to be immune is to have the disease. Immunity from a preventive vaccine provides protection against disease when a person is exposed to it in the future. That immunity is usually similar to what is acquired from natural infection, although several doses of a vaccine may have to be given for a child to have a full immune response.
Epidemiology—often used to establish vaccine safety—is not science but number crunching.	Epidemiology is a well-established scientific discipline that, among other things, identifies the cause of diseases and the factors that increase a person's risk for a disease.
Giving multiple vaccines at the same time causes an 'overload' of the immune system.	Vaccination does not overburden a child's immune system; the recommended vaccines use only a small portion of the immune system's memory.
Vaccines are ineffective.	Vaccines have spared millions of people the effects of devastating diseases.
Prior to the use of vaccinations these diseases had begun to decline due to improved nutrition and hygiene.	In the 19th and 20th centuries, some infectious diseases began to be better controlled because of improvements in sanitation, clean water, pasteurized milk, pest control, and so forth. However, vaccine-preventable diseases only began to drop dramatically after the vaccines for those diseases were licensed and were given to large numbers of children.
Vaccines cause illnesses or disorders of unknown cause such as autism, sudden infant death syndrome (SIDS), immune dysfunction, diabetes, neurological disorders, allergic rhinitis, eczema, and asthma.	Scientific evidence does not support these claims.
Contaminated vaccination lots (or hot lots) are more likely to cause an adverse reaction.	The Food and Drug Administration regulates the production of vaccines very carefully to assure the potency, purity, and safety of vaccines.

- **Logical fallacies:** A logical fallacy is a flaw in an argument that makes the argument illogic or invalid. Some common logical fallacies are *ad hominem* arguments (attacking those presenting the argument rather than the argument itself); appeals to pity (trying to win support for one's arguments by appealing to feelings of sympathy or guilt); and arguments from ignorance (claiming that a statement is true only because it has not been proven false, or that it is false only because it has not been proven true) among others.

- **Ad hoc hypotheses:** An ad hoc (literally, for this) hypothesis is an adjustment made to a theory just for the purpose of salvaging it from being refuted. Ad hoc explanations try to explain findings that do not fit the original theory.

- **False experts or experts who lack the needed expertise:** An expert in one field may be completely ignorant in another field. For instance, an expert endocrinologist may be an expert on diabetes but is not likely to be expert about vaccine safety or immunology. Unfortunately, some who may be experts in one field eagerly make claims about things outside their field of expertise.

- **Pseudoscience:** Pseudoscientific claims cannot be verified by other researchers because they are often ambiguous and not measurable. In most cases, these claims are not submitted to peer review (that is, review by experts) before making them public and the methods are usually difficult to understand, making the observations difficult to replicate. Often, data may be represented to show one outcome when another is the case. Other times the methods that are used are likely to give a predetermined outcome. Only data purporting to support the claims is presented while conflicting data are ignored or discarded.

References

1. CDC. Brief Report: Imported Measles Case Associated with Nonmedical Vaccine Exemption–Iowa, March 2004. *MMWR* March 26, 2004/53(11);244–246.

2. CDC. Multistate Investigation of Measles among Adoptees from China–April 9, 2004. *MMWR* April 16, 2004/53(14); 309.

3. Institute of Medicine. *Immunization Safety Review: Thimerosal-Containing Vaccines and Neurodevelopmental Disorders*. Washington, DC: National Academies Press 2001.

4. Institute of Medicine. *Immunization Safety Review: Vaccines and Autism*. Washington, DC: National Academies Press 2004.

5. Snyder B. Vaccines' safety, morality hit home for girl's parents. *The Tennessean*, September 17, 2000.

6. Wolfe RM, Sharp LK, Lipsky MS (2002). Content and Design Attributes of Antivaccination Web Sites. *JAMA*, 287:3245–3248.

7. Gangarosa EJ, Galazka AM, Wolfe CR, et al (1998). Impact of anti-vaccine movements on pertussis control: the untold story. *Lancet*, 351(9099):356–361.

8. Myers MG and Pineda D. 2008. Misinformation and the return of infectious diseases. Chapter 5 in: Do Vaccines cause That?! *A Guide for Evaluating Vaccine Safety Concerns*. I4ph Press, Galveston, Texas.

9. CDC. 2009. Invasive *Haemophilus influenzae* type b disease in five young children–Minnesota, 2008. *MMWR* 58(3):58–60.

Chapter 82

What Would Happen If We Stopped Vaccinations?

In the U.S., vaccines have reduced or eliminated many infectious diseases that once routinely killed or harmed many infants, children, and adults. However, the viruses and bacteria that cause vaccine-preventable disease and death still exist and can be passed on to people who are not protected by vaccines. Vaccine-preventable diseases have many social and economic costs: sick children miss school and can cause parents to lose time from work. These diseases also result in doctor's visits, hospitalizations, and even premature deaths.

Polio

Stopping vaccination against polio will leave people susceptible to infection with the polio virus. Polio virus causes acute paralysis that can lead to permanent physical disability and even death. Before polio vaccine was available, 13,000 to 20,000 cases of paralytic polio were reported each year in the United States. These annual epidemics of polio often left thousands of victims—mostly children—in braces, crutches, wheelchairs, and iron lungs. The effects were life-long.

In 1988 the World Health Assembly unanimously agreed to eradicate polio worldwide. As a result of global polio eradication efforts, the number of cases reported globally has decreased from more than 350,000 cases in 125 countries in 1988 to 2,000 cases of polio in 17 countries in 2006, and only four countries remain endemic (Afghanistan,

Text in this chapter is from "What Would Happen If We Stopped Vaccinations?" Centers for Disease Control and Prevention (CDC), May 24, 2007.

India, Nigeria, Pakistan). To date polio has been eliminated from the Western hemisphere, and the European and Western Pacific regions. Stopping vaccination before eradication is achieved would result in a resurgence of the disease in the United States and worldwide.

Measles

Before measles immunization was available, nearly everyone in the U.S. got measles. An average of 450 measles-associated deaths were reported each year between 1953 and 1963.

In the U.S., up to 20 percent of persons with measles are hospitalized. Seventeen percent of measles cases have had one or more complications, such as ear infections, pneumonia, or diarrhea. Pneumonia is present in about six percent of cases and accounts for most of the measles deaths. Although less common, some persons with measles develop encephalitis (swelling of the lining of the brain), resulting in brain damage.

As many as three of every 1,000 persons with measles will die in the U.S. In the developing world, the rate is much higher, with death occurring in about one of every 100 persons with measles.

Measles is one of the most infectious diseases in the world and is frequently imported into the U.S. In the period 1997–2000, most cases were associated with international visitors or U.S. residents who were exposed to the measles virus while traveling abroad. More than 90 percent of people who are not immune will get measles if they are exposed to the virus.

According to the World Health Organization (WHO), nearly 900,000 measles-related deaths occurred among persons in developing countries in 1999. In populations that are not immune to measles, measles spreads rapidly. If vaccinations were stopped, each year about 2.7 million measles deaths worldwide could be expected.

In the U.S., widespread use of measles vaccine has led to a greater than 99 percent reduction in measles compared with the pre-vaccine era. If we stopped immunization, measles would increase to pre-vaccine levels.

Haemophilus Influenzae *Type b (Hib)* Meningitis

Before Hib vaccine became available, Hib was the most common cause of bacterial meningitis in U.S. infants and children. Before the vaccine was developed, there were approximately 20,000 invasive Hib cases annually. Approximately two-thirds of the 20,000 cases were meningitis, and one-third were other life-threatening invasive Hib diseases such as bacteria in the blood, pneumonia, or inflammation of the epiglottis. About one of every 200 U.S. children under five years of age got an invasive Hib disease. Hib meningitis once killed 600 children each year and left many survivors with deafness, seizures, or mental retardation.

Since introduction of conjugate Hib vaccine in December 1987, the incidence of Hib has declined by 98 percent. From 1994–1998, fewer than ten fatal cases of invasive Hib disease were reported each year.

This preventable disease was a common, devastating illness as recently as 1990; now, most pediatricians just finishing training have never seen a case. If we were to stop immunization, we would likely soon return to the pre-vaccine numbers of invasive Hib disease cases and deaths.

Pertussis (Whooping Cough)

Since the early 1980s, reported pertussis cases have been increasing, with peaks every four years; however, the number of reported cases remains much lower than levels seen in the pre-vaccine era. Compared with pertussis cases in other age groups, infants who are six months old or younger who have pertussis experience the highest rate of hospitalization, pneumonia, seizures, encephalopathy (a degenerative disease of the brain), and death. From 1990 to 1996, 57 persons died from pertussis; 49 of these were less than six months old.

Before pertussis immunizations were available, nearly all children developed whooping cough. In the U.S., prior to pertussis immunization, between 150,000 and 260,000 cases of pertussis were reported each year, with up to 9,000 pertussis-related deaths.

Pertussis can be a severe illness, resulting in prolonged coughing spells that can last for many weeks. These spells can make it difficult for a child to eat, drink, and breathe. Because vomiting often occurs after a coughing spell, infants may lose weight and become dehydrated. In infants, it can also cause pneumonia and lead to brain damage, seizures, and mental retardation.

The newer pertussis vaccine (acellular or DTaP) has been available for use in the United States since 1991 and has been recommended for exclusive use since 1998. These vaccines are effective and associated with fewer mild and moderate adverse reactions when compared with the older (whole-cell DTP) vaccines.

During the 1970s, widespread concerns about the safety of the older pertussis vaccine led to a rapid fall in immunization levels in the

United Kingdom. More than 100,000 cases and 36 deaths due to pertussis were reported during an epidemic in the mid 1970s. In Japan, pertussis vaccination coverage fell from 80 percent in 1974 to 20 percent in 1979. An epidemic occurred in 1979, resulted in more than 13,000 cases and 41 deaths.

Pertussis cases occur throughout the world. If we stopped pertussis immunizations in the U.S., we would experience a massive resurgence of pertussis disease. A study found that, in eight countries where immunization coverage was reduced, incidence rates of pertussis surged to 10–100 times the rates in countries where vaccination rates were sustained.

Pneumococcal

Before pneumococcal conjugate vaccine became available for children, pneumococcus caused 63,000 cases of invasive pneumococcal disease and 6,100 deaths in the U.S. each year. Many children who developed pneumococcal meningitis also developed long-term complications such as deafness or seizures. Since the vaccine was introduced, the incidence of invasive pneumococcal disease in children has been reduced by 75%. Pneumococcal conjugate vaccine also reduces spread of pneumococcus from children to adults. In 2003 alone, there were 30,000 fewer cases of invasive pneumococcal disease caused by strains included in the vaccine, including 20,000 fewer cases in children and adults too old to receive the vaccine. If we were to stop immunization, we would likely soon return to the pre-vaccine numbers of invasive pneumococcal disease cases and deaths.

Rubella (German Measles)

While rubella is usually mild in children and adults, up to 90 percent of infants born to mothers infected with rubella during the first trimester of pregnancy will develop congenital rubella syndrome (CRS), resulting in heart defects, cataracts, mental retardation, and deafness.

In 1964–1965, before rubella immunization was used routinely in the U.S., there was an epidemic of rubella that resulted in an estimated 20,000 infants born with CRS, with 2,100 neonatal deaths and 11,250 miscarriages. Of the 20,000 infants born with CRS, 11,600 were deaf, 3,580 were blind, and 1,800 were mentally retarded.

Due to the widespread use of rubella vaccine, only six CRS cases were provisionally reported in the U.S. in 2000. Because many developing countries do not include rubella in the childhood immunization schedule, many of these cases occurred in foreign-born adults. Since 1996, greater than 50 percent of the reported rubella cases have been among adults. Since 1999, there have been 40 pregnant women infected with rubella.

If we stopped rubella immunization, immunity to rubella would decline and rubella would once again return, resulting in pregnant women becoming infected with rubella and then giving birth to infants with CRS.

Varicella (Chickenpox)

Prior to the licensing of the chickenpox vaccine in 1995, almost all persons in the United States had suffered from chickenpox by adulthood. Each year, the virus caused an estimated four million cases of chickenpox, 11,000 hospitalizations, and 100–150 deaths.

A highly contagious disease, chickenpox is usually mild but can be severe in some persons. Infants, adolescents and adults, pregnant women, and immunocompromised persons are at particular risk for serious complications including secondary bacterial infections, loss of fluids (dehydration), pneumonia, and central nervous system involvement. The availability of the chickenpox vaccine and its subsequent widespread use has had a major impact on reducing cases of chickenpox and related morbidity, hospitalizations, and deaths. In some areas, cases have decreased as much as 90% over prevaccination numbers.

In 2006, routine two-dose vaccination against chickenpox was recommended for all children, adolescents, and adults who do not have evidence of immunity to the disease. In addition to further reducing cases, this strategy will also decrease the risk for exposure to the virus for persons who are unable to be vaccinated because of illness or other conditions and who may develop severe disease. If vaccination against chickenpox were to stop, the disease would eventually return to prevaccination rates, with virtually all susceptible persons becoming infected with the virus at some point in their lives.

Hepatitis B

More than two billion persons worldwide have been infected with the hepatitis B virus at some time in their lives. Of these, 350 million are life-long carriers of the disease and can transmit the virus to others. One million of these people die each year from liver disease and liver cancer.

National studies have shown that about 12.5 million Americans have been infected with hepatitis B virus at some point in their lifetime. One and one quarter million Americans are estimated to have chronic (long-lasting) infection, of whom 20 percent to 30 percent acquired their infection in childhood. Chronic hepatitis B virus infection increases a person's risk for chronic liver disease, cirrhosis, and liver cancer. About 5,000 persons will die each year from hepatitis B-related liver disease resulting in over $700 million in medical and work loss costs.

The number of new infections per year has declined from an average of 450,000 in the 1980s to about 80,000 in 1999. The greatest decline has occurred among children and adolescents due to routine hepatitis B vaccination.

Infants and children who become infected with hepatitis B virus are at highest risk of developing lifelong infection, which often leads to death from liver disease (cirrhosis) and liver cancer. Approximately 25 percent of children who become infected with life-long hepatitis B virus would be expected to die of related liver disease as adults.

CDC estimates that one-third of the life-long hepatitis B virus infections in the United States resulted from infections occurring in infants and young children. About 16,000–20,000 hepatitis B antigen infected women give birth each year in the United States. It is estimated that 12,000 children born to hepatitis B virus infected mothers were infected each year before implementation of infant immunization programs. In addition, approximately 33,000 children (ten years of age and younger) of mothers who are not infected with hepatitis B virus were infected each year before routine recommendation of childhood hepatitis B vaccination.

Diphtheria

Diphtheria is a serious disease caused by a bacterium. This germ produces a poisonous substance or toxin which frequently causes heart and nerve problems. The case fatality rate is 5–10 percent, with higher case-fatality rates (up to 20 percent) in the very young and the elderly.

In the 1920s, diphtheria was a major cause of illness and death for children in the U.S. In 1921, a total of 206,000 cases and 15,520 deaths were reported. With vaccine development in 1923, new cases of diphtheria began to fall in the U.S., until in 2001 only two cases were reported.

Although diphtheria is rare in the U.S., it appears that the bacteria continue to get passed among people. In 1996, ten isolates of the bacteria were obtained from persons in an American Indian community in South Dakota, none of whom had classic diphtheria disease. There was one death reported in 2003 from clinical diphtheria in a 63-year-old male who had never been vaccinated.

There are high rates of susceptibility among adults. Screening tests conducted since 1977 have shown that 41 percent to 84 percent of adults 60 and over lack protective levels of circulating antitoxin against diphtheria.

Although diphtheria is rare in the U.S., it is still a threat. Diphtheria is common in other parts of the world and with the increase in international travel, diphtheria and other infectious diseases are only a plane ride away. If we stopped immunization, the U.S. might experience a situation similar to the Independent States of the former Soviet Union. With the breakdown of the public health services in this area, diphtheria epidemics began in 1990, fueled primarily by persons who were not properly vaccinated. From 1990–1999, more than 150,000 cases and 5,000 deaths were reported.

Tetanus (Lockjaw)

Tetanus is a severe, often fatal disease. The bacteria that cause tetanus are widely distributed in soil and street dust, are found in the waste of many animals, and are very resistant to heat and germ-killing cleaners. From 1922–1926, there were an estimated 1,314 cases of tetanus per year in the U.S. In the late 1940s, the tetanus vaccine was introduced, and tetanus became a disease that was officially counted and tracked by public health officials. In 2000, only 41 cases of tetanus were reported in the U.S.

People who get tetanus suffer from stiffness and spasms of the muscles. The larynx (throat) can close causing breathing and eating difficulties, muscles spasms can cause fractures (breaks) of the spine and long bones, and some people go into a coma, and die. Approximately 20 percent of reported cases end in death.

Tetanus in the U.S. is primarily a disease of adults, but unvaccinated children and infants of unvaccinated mothers are also at risk for tetanus and neonatal tetanus, respectively. From 1995–1997, 33 percent of reported cases of tetanus occurred among persons 60 years of age or older and 60 percent occurred in patients greater than 40 years of age. The National Health Interview Survey found that in 1995, only 36 percent of adults 65 or older had received a tetanus vaccination during the preceding ten years.

Worldwide, tetanus in newborn infants continues to be a huge problem. Every year tetanus kills 300,000 newborns and 30,000 birth mothers who were not properly vaccinated. Even though the number of reported cases is low, an increased number of tetanus cases in younger persons has been observed recently in the U.S. among intravenous drug users, particularly heroin users.

Tetanus is infectious, but not contagious, so unlike other vaccine-preventable diseases, immunization by members of the community will not protect others from the disease. Because tetanus bacteria are widespread in the environment, tetanus can only be prevented by immunization. If vaccination against tetanus were stopped, persons of all ages in the U.S. would be susceptible to this serious disease.

Mumps

Before the mumps vaccine was introduced, mumps was a major cause of deafness in children, occurring in approximately one in 20,000 reported cases. Mumps is usually a mild viral disease. However, rare conditions such as swelling of the brain, nerves, and spinal cord can lead to serious side effects such as paralysis, seizures, and fluid in the brain.

Serious side effects of mumps are more common among adults than children. Swelling of the testes is the most common side effect in males past the age of puberty, occurring in up to 20 percent to 50 percent of men who contract mumps. An increase in miscarriages has been found among women who develop mumps during the first trimester of pregnancy.

An estimated 212,000 cases of mumps occurred in the U.S. in 1964. After vaccine licensure in 1967, reports of mumps decreased rapidly. In 1986 and 1987, there was a resurgence of mumps with 12,848 cases reported in 1987. Since 1989, the incidence of mumps has declined, with 266 reported cases in 2001. This recent decrease is probably due to the fact that children have received a second dose of mumps vaccine (part of the two-dose schedule for measles, mumps, rubella or MMR) and the eventual development of immunity in those who did not gain protection after the first mumps vaccination.

We cannot let our guard down against mumps. A 2006 outbreak among college students, most of whom had received two doses of vaccine, led to over 5500 cases in 15 states. Mumps is highly communicable and it only takes a few unvaccinated to initiate transmission.

Chapter 83

Preventing Transmission of Infections in Hospitals and Nursing Homes

Chapter Contents

Section 83.1

Tips for Surgery Patients to Prevent Antibiotic Resistance

"CDC Campaign to Prevent Antimicrobial Resistance in Healthcare Settings," Centers for Disease Control and Prevention (CDC), November 2003. Reviewed in August 2009 by Dr. David A. Cooke, MD, FACP, Diplomate, American Board of Internal Medicine.

Before Surgery

- Ask your doctor if you need to be vaccinated against diseases that cause respiratory infections, including influenza and pneumonia. Preventing respiratory infections and their complications decreases antibiotic use.

- Ask about the facility's infection control program and any procedures that can help reduce infection risk. Let doctors and nurses know that you are concerned about preventing infections while receiving care.

- If you are diabetic, be sure that you and your doctor discuss the best way to control your blood sugar before, during, and after your hospital stay. High blood sugar increases the risk of infection.

- If you are overweight, losing weight will reduce the risk of infection following surgery.

- If you are a smoker, consider a smoking cessation program. This will reduce your chance of developing a lung infection while in the hospital. It may also improve your healing abilities after surgery.

- Be certain your health care providers are aware of any medications you currently take. This includes all prescription and over-the-counter medications, home remedies, and dietary supplements. You should also mention any food allergies (for example, shellfish) that you have. Ask if there are special instructions about taking your medications before and after the procedure.

While in the Hospital

- Wash your hands carefully after handling any type of soiled material or body fluids. This is especially important after you have gone to the bathroom.

- Let your nurse know if your gowns and linens are soiled.

- Since you are part of your health care team, do not be afraid to remind doctors or nurses to clean their hands. This includes washing their hands with soap and water, or using an alcohol-based hand rub before working with you.

- Some patients are on isolation precautions. This is usually done to protect the patient and others from infectious diseases. If you are in isolation, understand what your isolation means and what you should expect from the hospital staff or visitors. Gloves, gowns, and masks are sometimes appropriate, depending on the illness.

- If you have an intravenous catheter, keep the skin around the dressing clean and dry. Tell your nurse promptly if the dressing is loose or wet.

- Likewise, if you have a dressing on a wound, let your nurse know promptly if it becomes loose or wet.

- If you have any type of catheter or drainage tube, let your nurse know promptly if it becomes loose or dislodged.

- Since intravenous catheters and drainage tubes are all entry points for infection, discuss with your doctor when these devices can be safely removed.

- Carefully follow your doctor's instructions regarding breathing treatments and getting out of bed. Don't be afraid to ask for help, advice, or pain medications.

- Ask your friends and relatives not to visit if they feel ill.

- Ask how to contact your hospital pharmacist to talk about your medications.

- Look at all medications before you take them. If you don't know what they are for, or if they look different than expected, ask why. By asking questions, you may prevent errors. Ask the same questions you would ask your local pharmacist.

- Do not let anyone give you medications without checking your hospital identification (ID) bracelet. This helps prevent you from getting someone else's medications.

After the Hospital

When you are ready to go home:

- Ask for the treatment plan before you leave the hospital.

- Have a health care provider or the hospital pharmacist go over each medication with you and a caregiver.

- Ask which medications you should continue taking.

- Update your medications list from home, if any prescriptions change or if new medications are added.

- Notify your primary health care provider, including your pharmacist, about any medication changes that occurred in the hospital.

Pay attention to symptoms that may indicate an infection: unexpected pain, chills, fever, drainage, or increased inflammation of a surgical wound. Contact your doctor immediately if any of these occur, especially after you have been discharged from a hospital.

Section 83.2

Health Tips for Visiting Nursing Homes and Hospitals

"CDC Features: Health Tips for Visiting Nursing Homes and Hospitals," Centers for Disease Control and Prevention (CDC), December 15, 2008.

The holidays traditionally bring family and friends together for visits, and residents of nursing homes and patients in hospitals especially appreciate seeing friendly, loving faces. If someone you know is under such care, we hope you'll have a chance to see them: their holidays and their spirits will shine brighter.

Be aware, however, that people staying in these facilities may more easily catch illnesses that you bring with you on your visit or get sicker than usual from the illness. So, keep everyone safe and healthy by following these simple tips:

- If you have a cold or the flu, stay home. Nursing home residents and hospital patients can be at higher risk for infection. Therefore, if you aren't feeling well, a phone call is a better way to let them know you care; if possible, you can set up a later time to visit when you are well.

- Clean your hands. Many types of illness, from the common cold to more serious infections like *Clostridium difficile* and vancomycin-resistant enterococci (VRE), are spread when people fail to wash their hands properly. When you visit a nursing home or hospital, wash your hands with soap and water for at least 15–20 seconds or use an alcohol-based hand rub (or sanitizer) before hugging or touching the people you are visiting, and especially after using the restroom and before eating. Make sure your children wash their hands as well. Some rooms are equipped with alcohol-based hand sanitizer dispensers, too; look for them near the door or bathroom. If your loved one must follow doctor-ordered special germ-prevention rules (called contact precautions), follow instructions from the nursing staff and clean your hands when leaving.

- Check visiting hours, and consider calling ahead to plan your visit. Not only will you ensure that you'll have enough time to visit with your loved one without interfering with medical treatments or other activities, but you will also give them time to anticipate and look forward to your visit.

- If you are planning to see someone in specialized care, call ahead to make sure you understand their visiting hours and regulations: they may differ from those in the rest of the facility.

- Children bring a special kind of cheer to nursing homes and hospitals, so certainly bring them along—but check with the facility to make sure children are allowed and under what conditions. You may want to prepare them before the visit by explaining what they might see and answering any questions they may have. If your child is sick, leave him or her with other relatives or friends while you visit.

Holiday visitors can raise the spirits of nursing home residents and hospital patients, and these tips will help everyone enjoy safe and healthy visits.

Section 83.3

Prevention and Control of Influenza in Hospitals

Text in this section is from "Infection Control Guidance for the Prevention and Control of Influenza in Acute Care Facilities," Centers for Disease Control and Prevention (CDC), December 19, 2008.

Prevention and Control Measures

Strategies for the prevention and control of influenza in acute care facilities include the following: annual influenza vaccination of all eligible patients and health care personnel, implementation of standard and droplet precautions for infected individuals, active surveillance and influenza testing for new illness cases, restriction of ill visitors and personnel, rapid administration of influenza antiviral medications for treatment and prevention during outbreaks, and respiratory hygiene/cough etiquette.

Vaccination

All health care personnel and persons at high risk for serious complications of influenza should receive annual influenza vaccination according to current national recommendations.

- Vaccination is the primary measure to prevent infection or development of illness from influenza, and thereby limit transmission of influenza and prevent complications from influenza.

- Inactivated influenza vaccine or live attenuated influenza vaccine (LAIV) may be used to vaccinate most health care personnel.

- Inactivated influenza vaccine may be used for all health care personnel and is preferred for vaccinating health care personnel who have close contact with severely immunosuppressed persons (for example, patients with hematopoietic stem cell transplants) during those periods in which the immunosuppressed person requires care in a protective environment.

- The following persons should not receive inactivated influenza vaccine:
  - Persons known to have anaphylactic hypersensitivity to eggs or to other components of the influenza vaccine without first consulting a physician.
  - Persons with moderate-to-severe acute febrile illness usually should not be vaccinated until their symptoms have abated. However, minor illnesses with or without fever do not contraindicate use of influenza vaccine, particularly among children with mild upper-respiratory tract infection or allergic rhinitis.
  - Persons who are not at high risk for severe influenza complications and who are known to have experienced Guillain-Barré Syndrome within six weeks after a previous influenza vaccination. (Benefit may exceed risk for persons at high risk for severe influenza complications.)
- Live, attenuated vaccine (LAIV) may be given to healthy adults less than 50 years of age who are not pregnant and who do not have contraindications to receiving the nasal vaccine. Health care personnel taking care of immunocompromised patients may receive LAIV. However, if health care personnel who care for severely immunocompromised patients in protected environments receive LAIV, then they should not care for these patients for seven days following immunization.
- The following persons should not receive LAIV:
  - Persons with a history of hypersensitivity, including anaphylaxis, to any of the components of LAIV or to eggs
  - Persons 2–4 years old who have recurrent wheezing and healthy persons 50 years and older
  - Persons with asthma, reactive airways disease or other chronic disorders of the pulmonary or cardiovascular systems
  - Persons with other underlying medical conditions, including such metabolic diseases as diabetes mellitus, renal or hepatic dysfunction and hemoglobinopathies; or persons with known or suspected immunodeficiency diseases or who are receiving immunosuppressive therapies
  - Children or adolescents receiving aspirin or other salicylates (because of the association of Reye syndrome with wild-type influenza infection)

- Persons with a history of Guillain-Barré syndrome
- Pregnant women
- Persons with a fever or significant nasal congestion that may interfere with delivery of the LAIV (Administration of LAIV should be postponed; persons with mild respiratory illness can receive LAIV.)

Infection Control Measures

In addition to influenza vaccination, the following infection control measures are recommended to prevent person-to-person transmission of influenza and to control influenza outbreaks in acute care facilities:

1. **Surveillance:** Conduct active surveillance for respiratory illness and use rapid influenza testing to identify outbreaks early so that infection control measures can be promptly initiated to prevent the spread of influenza in the facility.

2. **Education:** Educate personnel about the importance of influenza vaccination, signs and symptoms of influenza, control measures, and indications for obtaining influenza testing.

3. **Influenza testing:** Perform influenza testing (for example, rapid diagnostic test, immunofluorescence) and viral cultures for influenza when clusters of respiratory illness occur or when influenza is suspected in a patient or health care provider.

4. **Antiviral chemoprophylaxis:** Influenza antiviral chemoprophylaxis may be given to patients and health care personnel in accordance with current recommendations.

5. **Respiratory hygiene/cough etiquette:** Respiratory hygiene/ cough etiquette should be implemented beginning at the first point of contact with a potentially infected person to prevent the transmission of all respiratory tract infections in acute care settings. Respiratory hygiene/cough etiquette includes the following:

    - Posting visual alerts instructing patients and persons who accompany them to inform health care personnel if they have symptoms of respiratory infection.

    - Providing tissues or masks to patients and visitors who are coughing or sneezing so that they can cover their nose and mouth.

- Ensuring that supplies for hand washing are available where sinks are located; providing dispensers of alcohol-based hand rubs in other locations.

- Providing space for coughing persons to sit at least 3–6 feet away from others, if feasible.

6. **Standard precautions:** During the care of any patient, health care personnel should adhere to standard precautions. For patients with symptoms of respiratory infection this includes the following:

   - Wear gloves if hand contact with respiratory secretions or potentially contaminated surfaces is anticipated.

   - Wear a gown if soiling of clothes with a patient's respiratory secretions is anticipated.

   - Change gloves and gowns after each patient encounter and perform hand hygiene.

   - Decontaminate hands before and after touching the patient and after touching the patient's environment or the patient's respiratory secretions, whether or not gloves are worn.

   - When hands are visibly soiled or contaminated with respiratory secretions, wash hands with soap (either plain or antimicrobial) and water.

   - If hands are not visibly soiled, use an alcohol-based hand rub.

7. **Droplet precautions:** In addition to standard precautions, health care personnel should adhere to droplet precautions during the care of a patient with suspected or confirmed influenza for five days after the onset of illness:

   - Place patient in a private room. If a private room is not available, place (cohort) suspected influenza patients with other patients suspected of having influenza; cohort confirmed influenza patients with other patients confirmed to have influenza.

   - Wear a surgical or procedure mask when entering the patient's room. Remove the mask when leaving the patient's room and dispose of the mask in a waste container.

   - If patient movement or transport is necessary, have the patient wear a surgical or procedure mask, if possible.

8. Restrictions for ill visitors and ill health care personnel:
If there is no or only sporadic influenza activity occurring in the surrounding community, do the following:

- Discourage persons with symptoms of a respiratory infection from visiting patients. Post notices to inform the public about visitation restrictions.

- Monitor health care personnel for influenza-like symptoms and consider removing them from duties that involve direct patient contact, especially those who work in high-risk patient care areas (for example, intensive care units [ICUs], nurseries, organ-transplant units). If excluded from duty, they should not provide patient care for five days after the onset of symptoms.

9. Restrictions for ill visitors and ill health care personnel:
If widespread influenza activity is in the surrounding community, take these actions:

- Notify visitors (for example, via posted notices) that adults with respiratory symptoms should not visit the facility for five days and children with symptoms should not visit for ten days following the onset of illness.

- Evaluate health care personnel, especially those in high risk areas (for example, ICUs, nurseries, and organ transplant units) for symptoms of respiratory infection; perform rapid influenza tests to confirm that the causative agent is influenza and to determine whether they should be removed from duties that involve direct patient contact. If excluded, they should not provide patient care for five days following the onset of symptoms. Follow current recommendations for treatment of influenza.

Control of Influenza Outbreaks in Acute Care Settings

When influenza outbreaks occur in acute care settings, the following measures should be taken to limit transmission:

- Perform rapid influenza virus testing of patients and personnel with recent onset of symptoms suggestive of influenza. In addition, obtain viral cultures from a subset of patients to determine the infecting virus type and subtype and to confirm the results of rapid tests since most rapid tests are less sensitive than cultures.

- Implement droplet precautions for all patients with suspected or confirmed influenza.

- Separate suspected or confirmed influenza patients from asymptomatic patients.

- Restrict staff movement from areas of the facility having outbreaks.

- Administer the current season's influenza vaccine to unvaccinated patients and health care personnel. Follow current vaccination recommendations for the use of nasal and intramuscular influenza vaccines.

- Administer influenza antiviral chemoprophylaxis and treatment to patients and health care personnel according to current recommendations.

- Consider antiviral chemoprophylaxis for all health care personnel, regardless of their vaccination status, if the health department determines the outbreak is caused by a variant of influenza virus that is a sub-optimal match with the vaccine.

- Curtail or eliminate elective medical and surgical admissions and restrict cardiovascular and pulmonary surgery to emergency cases during influenza outbreaks, especially those characterized by high attack rates and severe illness, in the community or acute care facility.

Chapter 84

Quarantine and Isolation to Control the Spread of Contagious Diseases

When someone is known to be ill with a contagious disease, they are placed in isolation and receive special care, with precautions taken to protect uninfected people from exposure to the disease.

When someone has been exposed to a contagious disease and it is not yet known if they have caught it, they may be quarantined or separated from others who have not been exposed to the disease. For example, they may be asked to remain at home to prevent further potential spread of the illness. They also receive special care and observation for any early signs of the illness.

How long can quarantine and isolation last? What is done to help the people who experience isolation or quarantine?

The list of diseases for which quarantine is authorized is specified in an Executive Order of the President. Since 1983, this list has included cholera, diphtheria, infectious tuberculosis, plague, smallpox, yellow fever, and viral hemorrhagic fevers (Lassa, Marburg, Ebola, Crimean-Congo, South American, and others not yet isolated or named). The list was last amended in April 2003 to include SARS (severe acute respiratory syndrome).

"Understand Quarantine and Isolation," Centers for Disease Control and Prevention (CDC), September 2007.

Isolation

Isolation would last for the period of communicability of the illness, which varies by disease and the availability of specific treatment. Usually it occurs at a hospital or other health care facility or in the person's home. Typically, the ill person will have his or her own room and those who care for him or her will wear protective clothing and take other precautions, depending on the level of personal protection needed for the specific illness.

In most cases, isolation is voluntary; however, federal, state, and local governments have the authority to require isolation of sick people to protect the public.

Quarantine

Modern quarantine lasts only as long as necessary to protect the public by (1) providing public health care (such as immunization or drug treatment, as required); and (2) ensuring that quarantined persons do not infect others if they have been exposed to a contagious disease.

Modern quarantine is more likely to involve limited numbers of exposed persons in small areas than to involve large numbers of persons in whole neighborhoods or cities.

Quarantined individuals will be sheltered, fed, and cared for at home, in a designated emergency facility, or in a specialized hospital, depending on the disease and the available resources. They will also be among the first to receive all available medical interventions to prevent and control disease, including the following:

- Vaccination
- Antibiotics
- Early and rapid diagnostic testing and symptom monitoring
- Early treatment if symptoms appear

The duration and scope of quarantine measures would vary, depending on their purpose and what is known about the incubation period (how long it takes for symptoms to develop after exposure) of the disease-causing agent.

Examples

A few hours for assessment: Passengers on airplanes, trains, or boats believed to be infected with or exposed to a dangerous contagious disease might be delayed for a few hours while health authorities determine the risk they pose to public health. Some passengers may be asked to provide contact information and then released while others who are ill are transported to where they can receive medical attention. There have been a few instances where state and local public health authorities have imposed a brief quarantine at a public gathering, such as a shelter, while investigating if one or more people may be ill.

- **Enough time to provide preventive treatment or other intervention:** If public health authorities determine that a passenger or passengers on airplanes, trains, or boats are sick with a dangerous contagious disease, the other passengers may be quarantined in a designated facility where they may receive preventive treatment and have their health monitored.

- **For the duration of the incubation period:** If public health officials determine that one or more passenger on airplanes, trains, or boats are infected with a contagious disease and that passengers sitting nearby may have had close contact with the infected passenger(s), those at risk might be quarantined in a designated facility, observed for signs of illness, and cared for under isolation conditions if they become ill.

When would quarantine and isolation be used and by whom?

If people in a certain area were potentially exposed to a contagious disease, this is what would happen: State and local health authorities would let people know that they may have been exposed and would direct them to get medical attention, undergo diagnostic tests, and stay at home, limiting their contact with people who have not been exposed to the disease. Only rarely would federal, state, or local health authorities issue an order for quarantine and isolation. However, both quarantine and isolation may be compelled on a mandatory basis through legal authority as well as conducted on a voluntary basis.

States have the authority to declare and enforce quarantine and isolation within their borders. This authority varies widely, depending on state laws. It derives from the authority of state governments granted by the U.S. Constitution to enact laws and promote regulations to safeguard the health and welfare of people within state borders.

Further, at the national level, the Centers for Disease Control and Prevention (CDC) may detain, medically examine, or conditionally release persons suspected of having certain contagious diseases. This authority applies to individuals arriving from foreign countries, including Canada and Mexico, on airplanes, trains, automobiles, boats, or by foot. It also applies to individuals traveling from one state to another or in the event of inadequate local control.

The CDC regularly uses its authority to monitor passengers arriving in the United States for contagious diseases. In modern times, most quarantine measures have been imposed on a small scale, typically involving small numbers of travelers (airline or cruise ship passengers) who have curable diseases, such as infectious tuberculosis or cholera. No instances of large-scale quarantine have occurred in the U.S. since the "Spanish Flu" pandemic of 1918–1919.

Based on years of experience working with state and local partners, the CDC anticipates that the need to use its federal authority to involuntarily quarantine a person would occur only in rare situations—for example, if a person posed a threat to public health and refused to cooperate with a voluntary request.

Definitions

Communicable disease: An infectious disease that is contagious and which can be transmitted from one source to another by infectious bacteria or viral organisms.

Contagious disease: A very communicable disease capable of spreading rapidly from one person to another by contact or close proximity.

Infectious disease: A disease caused by a microorganism and therefore potentially infinitely transferable to new individuals. May or may not be communicable. Example of non communicable is disease caused by toxins from food poisoning or infection caused by toxins in the environment, such as tetanus.

Part Six

Additional Help and Information

Chapter 85

Glossary of Terms Related to Contagious Diseases

adjuvant: A substance sometimes included in a vaccine formulation to enhance the immune-stimulating properties of the vaccine.

antibiotics: Medicines that damage or kill bacteria and are used to treat some bacterial diseases.[1]

antibody: A molecule produced by a B cell in response to an antigen. When an antibody attaches to an antigen, it helps destroy the microbe bearing the antigen.

antigen: A molecule on a microbe that identifies it as foreign to the immune system and stimulates the immune system to attack it.

artificially acquired immunity: Immunity provided by vaccines, as opposed to naturally acquired immunity, which is acquired from exposure to a disease-causing organism.

attenuation: The weakening of a microbe so that it can be used in a live vaccine.

B cells: Small white blood cells crucial to the immune defenses. Also known as B lymphocytes, they come from bone marrow and develop

---

Terms in this chapter are from "Understanding Vaccines," National Institute of Allergy and Infectious Disease (NIAID), January 2008. Terms marked with a [1] are excerpted from "Microbes: Glossary of Terms," NIAID, July 14, 2008. Terms marked with a [2] are from "Understand Quarantine and Isolation," Centers for Disease Control and Prevention (CDC), September 2007.

into blood cells called plasma cells, which are the source of anti-bodies.[1]

bacteria: Microscopic organisms composed of a single cell and lacking a defined nucleus and membrane-enclosed internal compartments.

booster shot: Supplementary dose of a vaccine, usually smaller than the first dose, that is given to maintain immunity.

clinical trial: An experiment that tests the safety and effectiveness of a vaccine or drug in humans.

communicable disease: An infectious disease that is contagious and which can be transmitted from one source to another by infectious bacteria or viral organisms.[2]

complement protein: A molecule that circulates in the blood whose actions complement the work of antibodies. Complement proteins destroy antibody-coated microbes.

conjugate vaccine: A vaccine in which proteins that are easily recognizable to the immune system are linked to the molecules that form the outer coat of disease-causing bacteria to promote an immune response. Conjugate vaccines are designed primarily for very young children because their immune systems cannot recognize the outer coats of certain bacteria.

contagious disease: A very communicable disease capable of spreading rapidly from one person to another by contact or close proximity.[2]

cytotoxic T cells or killer T cells: A subset of T cells that destroy body cells infected by viruses or bacteria.

disease: A state in which a function or part of the body is no longer in a healthy condition.[1]

DNA vaccine or naked DNA vaccine: A vaccine that uses a microbe's genetic material, rather than the whole organism or its parts, to stimulate an immune response.

edible vaccines: Foods genetically engineered to produce antigens to specific microbes and safely trigger an immune response to them.

epidemic: A disease outbreak that affects many people in a region at the same time.[1]

formalin: A solution of water and formaldehyde, used in toxoid vaccines to inactivate bacterial toxins.

genetic material: Molecules of DNA (deoxyribonucleic acid) or RNA (ribonucleic acid) that carry the directions that cells or viruses use to perform a specific function, such as making a particular protein molecule.

***Haemophilus influenzae* type b (Hib):** A bacterium found in the respiratory tract that causes acute respiratory infections, including pneumonia, and other diseases such as meningitis.

helper T cells: A subset of T cells that function as messengers. They are essential for turning on antibody production, activating cytotoxic T cells, and initiating many other immune functions.

herd immunity or community immunity: The resistance to a particular disease gained by a community when a critical number of people are vaccinated against that disease.

HIV: Human immunodeficiency virus, the virus that causes acquired immunodeficiency syndrome (AIDS).

immune: Have a high degree of resistance to or protection from a disease.

immune system: A collection of specialized cells and organs that protect the body against infectious diseases.

immunization: Vaccination or other process that induces protection (immunity) against infection or disease caused by a microbe.[1]

infection: A state in which disease-causing microbes have invaded or multiplied in body tissues.[1]

infectious diseases: Diseases caused by microbes that can be passed to or among humans by several methods.[1]

inflammation: An immune system process that stops the progression of disease-causing microbes, often seen at the site of an injury like a cut. Signs include redness, swelling, pain, and heat.[1]

inactivated vaccine or killed vaccine: A vaccine made from a whole virus or bacteria inactivated with chemicals or heat.

live, attenuated vaccine: A vaccine made from microbes that have been weakened in the laboratory so that they can't cause disease.

lymph node: A small bean-shaped organ of the immune system, distributed widely throughout the body and linked by lymphatic vessels. Lymph nodes are gathering sites of B, T, and other immune cells.

lymphocyte: A white blood cell central to the immune system's response to foreign microbes. B cells and T cells are lymphocytes.

macrophage: A large and versatile immune cell that devours and kills invading microbes and other intruders. Macrophages stimulate other immune cells by presenting them with small pieces of the invaders.

memory cells: A subset of T cells and B cells that have been exposed to antigens and can then respond more readily and rapidly when the immune system encounters the same antigens again.

microbe: A microscopic organism. Microbes include bacteria, viruses, fungi, and single-celled plants and animals.

microorganisms: Microscopic organisms, including bacteria, viruses, fungi, plants, and animals.[1]

molecule: A building block of a cell. Some examples are proteins, fats, and carbohydrates.

mutate: To change a gene or unit of hereditary material that results in a new inheritable characteristic.

naturally acquired immunity: Immunity produced by antibodies passed from mother to fetus (passive), or by the body's own antibody and cellular immune response to a disease-causing organism (active).

pandemics: Diseases that affect many people in different regions around the world.[1]

parasites: Plants or animals that live, grow, and feed on or within another living organism.[1]

passive immunity: Immunity acquired through transfer of antibody or lymphocytes from an immune donor.

pathogens: Disease-causing organisms.[1]

pertussis or whooping cough: A respiratory infection caused by the toxic bacterium *Bordetella pertussis*. The wracking coughs characteristic of this disease are sometimes so intense the victims, usually infants, vomit or turn blue from lack of air.

plasma cell: A cell produced by a dividing B cell that is entirely devoted to producing and secreting antibodies.

polysaccharide: A long, chain-like molecule made up of a linked sugar molecule. The outer coats of some bacteria are made of polysaccharides.

preclinical testing: Required laboratory testing of a vaccine before it can be given to people in clinical trials. Preclinical testing is done in cell cultures and in animals.

rotavirus: A group of viruses that can cause digestive problems and diarrhea in young children.[1]

rubella or German measles: A viral disease often affecting children and spread through the air by coughs or sneezes. Symptoms include a characteristic rash, low-grade fever, aching joints, runny nose, and reddened eyes. If a pregnant woman gets rubella during her first three months of pregnancy, her baby is at risk of having serious birth defects or dying.

subunit vaccine: A vaccine that uses one or more components of a disease-causing organism, rather than the whole, to stimulate an immune response.

T cell or T lymphocyte: A white blood cell that directs or participates in immune defenses.

tissue: A group of similar cells joined to perform the same function.

toxin: Agent produced by plants and bacteria, normally very damaging to cells.

toxoid or inactivated toxin: A toxin, such as those produced by certain bacteria, that has been treated by chemical means, heat, or irradiation and is no longer capable of causing disease.

toxoid vaccine: A vaccine containing a toxoid, used to protect against toxins produced by certain bacteria.

vaccines: Substances that contain parts of antigens from an infectious organism. By stimulating an immune response (but not disease), they protect the body against subsequent infection by that organism.[1]

vector: In vaccine technology, a bacterium or virus that cannot cause disease in humans and is used in genetically engineered vaccines to transport genes coding for antigens into the body to induce an immune response.

virulent: Toxic, causing disease.

virus: A very small microbe that does not consist of cells but is made up of a small amount of genetic material surrounded by a membrane or protein shell. Viruses cannot reproduce by themselves. To reproduce, viruses must infect a cell and use the cell's resources and molecular machinery to make more viruses.

Chapter 86

Directory of Organizations with Information about Contagious Diseases

Government Organizations

Agency for Healthcare Research and Quality (AHRQ)
540 Gaither Rd., Suite 2000
Rockville, MD 20850
Toll-Free: 800-358-9295
Phone: 301-427-1364
Fax: 301-427-1430
Website: http://www.ahrq.gov
E-mail: info@ahrq.gov

CDC Division of STD Prevention (DSTDP)
1600 Clifton Rd.
Atlanta, GA 30333
Toll-Free: 800-CDC-INFO
(232-4636)
Toll-Free TTY: 888-232-6348
Website: http://www.cdc.gov/std
E-mail: dstd@cdc.gov

CDC Division of Viral Hepatitis
1600 Clifton Rd.
Atlanta, GA 30333
Toll-Free: 800-CDC-INFO
(232-4636)
Toll-Free TTY: 888-232-6348
Phone: 404-718-8596
(M–F, 8:00 am–5:00 pm)
Fax: 404-718-8588
Website: http://www.cdc.gov/
hepatitis
E-mail: info@cdcnpin.org

Resources in this chapter were compiled from several sources deemed reliable; all contact information was verified and updated in August 2009.

CDC National Prevention Information Network (NPIN)
P.O. Box 6003
Rockville, MD 20849
Toll-Free: 800-458-5231
Toll-Free Fax: 888-282-7681
Toll-Free TTY: 800-243-7012
Phone: 404-679-3860
Website: http://www.cdcnpin.org
E-mail: info@cdcnpin.org

CDC Vaccines and Immunizations
1600 Clifton Rd.
Atlanta, GA 30333
Toll-Free: 800-CDC-INFO
(232-4636)
Toll-Free TTY: 888-232-6348
Website: http://www.cdc.gov/
vaccines
E-mail: info@cdcnpin.org

Centers for Disease Control and Prevention (CDC)
1600 Clifton Rd.
Atlanta, GA 30333
Toll-Free: 800-CDC-INFO
(232-4636)
Toll-Free TTY: 888-232-6348
Fax: 770-488-4760
Website: http://www.cdc.gov
E-mail: cdcinfo@cdc.gov

FDA MedWatch
5600 Fishers Lane
Rockville, MD 20857
Toll-Free: 800-332-1088
Toll-Free Fax: 800-332-0178
Website: http://www.fda.gov/
medwatch

Federal Trade Commission (FTC)
Consumer Response Center
600 Pennsylvania Ave., NW
Washington, DC 20580
Toll-Free: 877-FTC-HELP
(877-382-4357)
Toll-Free TDD/TTY: 866-653-4261
Website: http://www.ftc.gov

Health Resources and Services Administration (HRSA)
Information Center
P.O. Box 2910
Merrifield, VA 22116
Toll-Free: 888-275-4772
Toll-Free TTY: 877-489-4772
Fax: 703-821-2098
Website: http://www.hrsa.gov
E-mail: ask@hrsa.gov

Healthfinder®
National Health Information
Center
P.O. Box 1133
Washington, DC 20013
Toll-Free: 800-336-4797
Phone: 301-565-4167
Fax: 301-984-4256
Website: http://
www.healthfinder.gov
E-mail: healthfinder@nhic.org

MedlinePlus
National Library of Medicine
8600 Rockville Pike
Bethesda, MD 20894
Toll-Free: 888-346-3656
Phone: 302-594-5983
Website: http://
www.medlineplus.gov

National Cancer Institute (NCI)
NCI Public Inquiries Office
6116 Executive Blvd., Rm. 3036A
Bethesda, MD 20892
Toll-Free: 800-4-CANCER
(422-6237)
Toll-Free TTY: 800-332-8615
Website: http://www.cancer.gov
E-mail:
cancergovstaff@mail.nih.gov

National Center for Complementary and Alternative Medicine (NCCAM)
P.O. Box 7923
Gaithersburg, MD 20898
Bethesda, MD 20892
Toll-Free: 888-644-6226
Toll-Free TTY: 866-464-3615
Phone: 301-519-3153
Fax: 866-464-3616
Website: http://nccam.nih.gov
E-mail: info@nccam.nih.gov

National Diabetes Information Clearinghouse
1 Information Way
Bethesda, MD 20892-3560
Toll-Free: 800-860-8747
Phone: 301-654-3327
Fax: 703-738-4929
Website: http://
diabetes.niddk.nih.gov
E-mail: ndic@info.niddk.nih.gov

National Health Information Center
P.O. Box 1133
Washington, DC 20013
Toll-Free: 800-336-4797
Phone: 301-565-4167
Fax: 301-984-4256
Website: http://www.health.gov/
NHIC
E-mail: nhicinfo@health.org

National Heart, Lung, and Blood Institute (NHLBI)
P.O. Box 30105
Bethesda, MD 20824
Phone: 301-592-8573
TTY: 240-629-3255
Fax: 240-629-3246
Website: http://
www.nhlbi.nih.gov
E-mail: nhlbiinfo@nhlbi.nih.gov

National Institute of Allergy and Infectious Diseases (NIAID)
6610 Rockledge Drive, MSC 6612
Bethesda, MD 20892
Toll-Free: 866-284-4107
Phone: 301-496-5717
Toll-Free TDD: 800-877-8339
Fax: 301-402-3573
Website: http://
www3.niaid.nih.gov

National Institute of Child Health and Human Development (NICHD)

Information Resource
Center
P.O. Box 3006
Rockville, MD 20847
Toll-Free: 800-370-2943
Toll-Free TTY: 888-320-6942
Fax: 301-984-1473
Website: http://
www.nichd.nih.gov
E-mail: nichdinformation
ResourceCenter@mail.nih.gov

National Institute of Diabetes and Digestive and Kidney Diseases (NIDDK)

Office of Communications
and Public Liaison
Building 31
Room 9A06
31 Center Drive
MSC 2560
Bethesda, MD 20892
Toll-Free: 800-891-5390
Phone: 301-496-3583
Website: http://
www2.niddk.nih.gov
E-mail: dwebmaster
@extra.niddk.nih.gov

National Institute of Neurological Disorders and Stroke (NINDS)

P.O. Box 5801
Bethesda, MD 20824
Toll-Free: 800-352-9424
Phone: 301-496-5751
TTY: 301-496-5981
Website: http://
www.ninds.nih.gov
E-mail: braininfo@ninds.nih.gov

National Institute on Aging (NIA)

Building 31, Rm. 5C27
31 Center Dr., MSC 2292
Bethesda, MD 20892
Toll-Free: 800-222-2225
Toll-Free TTY: 800-222-4225
Phone: 301-496-1752
Fax: 301-496-1072
Website: http://www.nia.nih.gov

National Institutes of Health (NIH)

9000 Rockville Pike
Bethesda, MD 20892
Phone: 301-496-4000
TTY: 301-402-9612
Website: http://www.nih.gov
E-mail: NIHinfo@od.nih.gov

National Vaccine Injury Compensation Program

Parklawn Bldg., Room 8A-35
5600 Fishers Lane
Rockville, MD 20857
Toll-Free: 800-338-2382
Website: http://www.hrsa.gov/
vaccinecompensation

National Women's Health Information Center (NWHIC)

8270 Willow Oaks Corporate Dr.
Fairfax, VA 22031
Toll-Free: 800-994-9662
Toll-Free TDD: 888-220-5446
Website: http://
www.womenshealth.gov, or
http://www.4woman.gov

Office of Dietary Supplements (ODS)

Room 3B01, MSC 7517
6100 Executive Blvd.
Bethesda, MD 20892
Phone: 301-435-2920
Fax: 301-480-1845
Website: http://
dietary-supplements.info.nih.gov
E-mail: ods@nih.gov

U.S. Food and Drug Administration (FDA)

10903 New Hampshire Ave.
Silver Spring, MD 20993
Toll-Free: 888-463-6332
Phone: 301-827-4420
Fax: 301-443-9767
Website: http://www.fda.gov

U.S. Department of Health and Human Services (HHS)

200 Independence Ave., SW
Washington, DC 20201
Toll-Free: 877-696-6775
Phone: 202-619-0257
Website: http://www.hhs.gov

U.S. Environmental Protection Agency (EPA)

1200 Pennsylvania Ave., NW
Washington, DC 20460
Phone: 202-272-0167
TTY: 202-272-0165
Website: http://www.epa.gov

U.S. National Library of Medicine

8600 Rockville Pike
Bethesda, MD 20894
Toll-Free: 888-346-3656
Toll-Free TDD: 800-735-2258
Phone: 301-594-5983
Fax: 301-402-1384
Website: http://www.nlm.nih.gov
E-mail: custserv@nlm.nih.gov

Vaccine Adverse Event Reporting System (VAERS)

P.O. Box 1100
Rockville, MD 20849
Toll-Free: 800-822-7967
Website: http://
www.vaers.hhs.gov
E-mail: info@vaers.org

Private Organizations

American Academy of Allergy, Asthma & Immunology
555 E. Wells St., Suite 1100
Milwaukee, WI 53202
Phone: 414-272-6071
Website: http://www.aaaai.org

American Academy of Family Physicians
P.O. Box 11210
Shawnee Mission, KS 66207
Toll-Free: 800-274-2237
Phone: 913-906-6000
Website: http://www.aafp.org
E-mail: fp@aafp.org

American Association of Blood Banks (AABB)
8101 Glenbrook Rd.
Bethesda, MD 20814
Phone: 301-907-6977
Fax: 301-907-6895
Website: http://www.aabb.org
E-mail: aabb@aabb.org

American Cancer Society (ACS)
13599 Clifton Rd., NE
Atlanta, GA 30329
Toll-Free: 800-227-2345
Toll-Free TTY: 866-228-4327
Website: http://www.cancer.org

American Liver Foundation
75 Maiden Lane, Suite 603
New York, NY 10038
Toll-Free: 800-GO-LIVER
(465-4837), or 888-4HEP-USA
(443-7872)
Phone: 212-668-1000
Fax: 212-483-8179
Website: http://www.liverfoundation.org
E-mail: info@liverfoundation.org

American Lung Association (ALA)
1301 Pennsylvania Ave, NW
Suite 800
Washington, DC 20004
Toll-Free: 800-586-4872 (for location of nearest ALA group)
Toll-Free: 800-548-8252 (to speak with a lung health professional)
Phone: 212-315-8700
Website: http://www.lungusa.org

American Medical Association (AMA)
515 N. State St.
Chicago, IL 60610
Toll-Free: 800-621-8335
Phone: 312-464-5000
Fax: 312-464-5600
Website: http://www.ama-assn.org

American Social Health Association (ASHA)
P.O. Box 13827
Research Triangle Park,
NC 27709
Toll-Free: 800-783-9822
Phone: 919-361-8400
Fax: 919-361-8425
Website: http://www.ashastd.org

Hepatitis Foundation International
504 Blick Drive
Silver Spring, MD 20904
Toll-Free: 800-891-0707
Phone: 301-622-4200
Fax: 301-622-4702
Website: http://
www.hepatitisfoundation.org
E-mail: hfi@comcast.net

Immunization Safety Review Committee
Institute of Medicine
500 Fifth St. NW
Washington, DC 20001
Phone: 202-334-2352
Fax: 202-334-1412
Website: http://www.iom.edu/
imsafety
E-mail: iowww@nas.edu

National Foundation for Infectious Diseases
4733 Bethesda Ave., Suite 750
Bethesda, MD 20814
Phone: 301-656-0003
Fax: 301-907-0878
Website: http://www.nfid.org

National Network for Immunization Information
301 University Blvd.
Galveston, TX 77555
Phone: 409-772-0199
Fax: 409-772-5208
Website: http://
www.immunizationinfo.org
E-mail: nnii@i4ph.org

National Patient Advocate Foundation
725 15th St. NW, 10th Fl.
Washington, DC 20005
Phone: 202-347-8009
Fax: 202-347-5579
Website: http://www.npaf.org

Nemours Foundation
Center for Children's Health
Media
1600 Rockland Rd.
Wilmington, DE 19803
Phone: 302-651-4000
Website: http://
www.kidshealth.org, or http://
www.teenshealth.org
E-mail: info@kidshealth.org

World Health Organization (WHO)
Avenue Appia 20
1211 Geneva 27
Switzerland
Phone: (00 41 22) 791-21-11
Website: http://www.who.int

Index

Index

H

Health Reference Series

Complete Catalog

List price $93 per volume. School and library price $84 per volume.

Adolescent Health Sourcebook, 2nd Edition

Basic Consumer Health Information about the Physical, Mental, and Emotional Growth and Development of Adolescents, Including Medical Care, Nutritional and Physical Activity Requirements, Puberty, Sexual Activity, Acne, Tanning, Body Piercing, Common Physical Illnesses and Disorders, Eating Disorders, Attention Deficit Hyperactivity Disorder, Depression, Bullying, Hazing, and Adolescent Injuries Related to Sports, Driving, and Work

Along with Substance Abuse Information about Nicotine, Alcohol, and Drug Use, a Glossary, and Directory of Additional Resources

Edited by Joyce Brennfleck Shannon. 655 pages. 2007. 978-0-7808-0943-7.

"A particularly good resource for both parents and teens. The concise presentation of the material in brief and well-organized chapters creates an easy volume to browse."
—School Library Journal, Jun '07

"I don't believe there are any other books written in such easy to understand language that encompass such a breadth of topics. This is a complete revision of the book and is an excellent resource for parents and teens."
—Doody's Review Service, 2007

Adult Health Concerns Sourcebook

Basic Consumer Health Information about Medical and Mental Concerns of Adults, Including Facts about Choosing Healthcare Providers, Navigating Insurance Options, Maintaining Wellness, Preventing Cancer, Heart Disease, Stroke, Diabetes, and Osteoporosis, and Understanding Aging-Related Health Concerns, Including Menopause, Cognitive Changes, and Changes in the Coronary and Vascular Systems

Along with Tips on Caring for Aging Parents and Dealing with Health-Related Work and Travel Issues, a Glossary, and a Directory of Resources for Additional Help and Information

Edited by Sandra J. Judd. 648 pages. 2008. 978-0-7808-0999-4.

"Provides a thorough list of topics that are important to adult health and for caregivers."
—CHOICE, Nov '08

"Written in easy-to-understand language . . . the content is well-organized and is intended to aid adults in making health care-related decisions."
—AORN Journal, Dec '08

AIDS Sourcebook, 4th Edition

Basic Consumer Health Information about Human Immunodeficiency Virus (HIV) and Acquired Immunodeficiency Syndrome (AIDS), Featuring Updated Statistics and Facts about Risks, Prevention, Screening, Diagnosis, Treatments, Side Effects, and Complications, and Including a Section about the Impact of HIV/AIDS on the Health of Women, Children, and Adolescents

Along with Tips on Managing Life with AIDS, Reports on Current Research Initiatives and Clinical Trials, a Glossary of Related Terms, and Resource Directories for Further Help and Information

Edited by Ivy L. Alexander. 680 pages. 2008. 978-0-7808-0997-0.

SEE ALSO *Contagious Diseases Sourcebook, 2nd Edition*

Alcoholism Sourcebook, 2nd Edition

Basic Consumer Health Information about Alcohol Use, Abuse, and Dependence, Featuring Facts about the Physical, Mental, and Social Health Effects of Alcohol Addiction, Including Alcoholic Liver Disease, Pancreatic Disease, Cardiovascular Disease, Neurological Disorders, and the Effects of Drinking during Pregnancy

Along with Information about Alcohol Treatment, Medications, and Recovery Programs, in Addition to Tips for Reducing the Prevalence of Underage Drinking, Statistics about Alcohol Use, a Glossary of Related Terms, and Directories of Resources for More Help and Information

Edited by Amy L. Sutton. 625 pages. 2007. 978-0-7808-0942-0.

"A comprehensive look at the adverse effects of alcohol on people of all ages . . . It serves to whet the reader's appetite to continue learning using other resources. It is practical, easy to read, and enlightening, and is the first book a lay person should consult to learn about alcoholism."
—*Doody's Review Service, 2007*

"Should be a basic acquisition for any serious public or college-level library including health reference titles for general-interest readers."
—*California Bookwatch, Feb '07*

SEE ALSO *Drug Abuse Sourcebook, 2nd Edition*

Allergies Sourcebook, 3rd Edition

Basic Consumer Health Information about Allergic Disorders, Such as Anaphylaxis, Hives, Eczema, Rhinitis, Sinusitis, and Conjunctivitis, and Their Triggers, Including Pollen, Mold, Dust Mites, Animal Dander, Insects, Chemicals, Food, Food Additives, and Medications

Along with Advice about the Diagnosis and Treatment of Allergy Symptoms, a Glossary of Related Terms, a Directory of Resources for Help and Information, and Suggestions for Additional Reading

Edited by Amy L. Sutton. 588 pages. 2007. 978-0-7808-0950-5.

SEE ALSO *Asthma Sourcebook, 2nd Edition*

Alzheimer Disease Sourcebook, 4th Edition

Basic Consumer Health Information about Alzheimer Disease, Other Dementias, and Related Disorders, Including Multi-Infarct Dementia, Dementia with Lewy Bodies, Fronto-temporal Dementia (Pick Disease), Wernicke-Korsakoff Syndrome (Alcohol-Related Dementia), AIDS Dementia Complex, Huntington Disease, Creutzfeldt-Jacob Disease, and Delirium

Along with Information about Coping with Memory Loss and Forgetfulness, Maintaining

Skills, and Long-Term Planning for People with Dementia, and Suggestions Addressing Common Caregiver Concerns, Updated Information about Current Research Efforts, a Glossary of Related Terms, and Directories of Sources for Additional Help and Information

Edited by Karen Bellenir. 603 pages. 2008. 978-0-7808-1001-3.

"An invaluable resource for persons who have received a diagnosis, for caregivers, and for family members dealing with this insidious disease. It is recommended for public, community college, and ready-reference sections in academic libraries."
—*ARBAonline, Jul '08*

SEE ALSO *Brain Disorders Sourcebook, 2nd Edition*

Arthritis Sourcebook, 2nd Edition

Basic Consumer Health Information about Osteoarthritis, Rheumatoid Arthritis, Other Rheumatic Disorders, Infectious Forms of Arthritis, and Diseases with Symptoms Linked to Arthritis, Featuring Facts about Diagnosis, Pain Management, and Surgical Therapies

Along with Coping Strategies, Research Updates, a Glossary, and Resources for Additional Help and Information

Edited by Amy L. Sutton. 567 pages. 2004. 978-0-7808-0667-2.

"This easy-to-read volume is recommended for consumer health collections within public or academic libraries."
—*E-Streams, May '05*

"As expected, this updated edition continues the excellent reputation of this series in providing sound, usable health information. . . . Highly recommended."
—*American Reference Books Annual, 2005*

Asthma Sourcebook, 2nd Edition

Basic Consumer Health Information about the Causes, Symptoms, Diagnosis, and Treatment of Asthma in Infants, Children, Teenagers, and Adults, Including Facts about Different Types of Asthma, Common Co-Occurring Conditions, Asthma Management Plans, Triggers, Medications, and Medication Delivery Devices

Along with Asthma Statistics, Research Updates, a Glossary, a Directory of Asthma-Related Resources, and More

Edited by Karen Bellenir. 581 pages. 2006. 978-0-7808-0866-9.

Attention Deficit Disorder Sourcebook

Basic Consumer Health Information about Attention Deficit/Hyperactivity Disorder in Children and Adults, Including Facts about Causes, Symptoms, Diagnostic Criteria, and Treatment Options Such as Medications, Behavior Therapy, Coaching, and Homeopathy

Along with Reports on Current Research Initiatives, Legal Issues, and Government Regulations, and Featuring a Glossary of Related Terms, Internet Resources, and a List of Additional Reading Material

Edited by Dawn D. Matthews. 447 pages. 2002. 978-0-7808-0624-5.

"Recommended reference source."
—*Booklist, Jan '03*

SEE ALSO *Learning Disabilities Sourcebook, 3rd Edition*

Autism and Pervasive Developmental Disorders Sourcebook

Basic Consumer Health Information about Autism Spectrum and Pervasive Developmental Disorders, Such as Classical Autism, Asperger Syndrome, Rett Syndrome, and Childhood Disintegrative Disorder, Including Information about Related Genetic Disorders and Medical Problems and Facts about Causes, Screening Methods, Diagnostic Criteria, Treatments and Interventions, and Family and Education Issues

Along with a Glossary of Related Terms, Tips for Evaluating the Validity of Health Claims, and a Directory of Resources for Additional Help and Information

Edited by Sandra J. Judd. 603 pages. 2007. 978-0-7808-0953-6.

"Recommended for public libraries"
—*SciTech Book News, Mar '08*

SEE ALSO *Learning Disabilities Sourcebook, 3rd Edition*

Back and Neck Disorders Sourcebook, 2nd Edition

Basic Consumer Health Information about Spinal Pain, Spinal Cord Injuries, and Related Disorders, Such as Degenerative Disk Disease, Osteoarthritis, Scoliosis, Sciatica, Spina Bifida, and Spinal Stenosis, and Featuring Facts about Maintaining Spinal Health, Self-Care, Pain Management, Rehabilitative Care, Chiropractic Care, Spinal Surgeries, and Complementary Therapies

Along with Suggestions for Preventing Back and Neck Pain, a Glossary of Related Terms, and a Directory of Resources

Edited by Amy L. Sutton. 607 pages. 2004. 978-0-7808-0738-9.

"Recommended. ...An easy to use, comprehensive medical reference book."
—*E-Streams, Sep '05*

"For anyone who has back or neck problems, this book is ideal. Its easy-to-understand language and variety of topics makes this sourcebook a worthwhile read. The price...is reasonable for the amount of information contained in the book"
—*Occupational Therapy in Health Care, 2007*

Blood and Circulatory Disorders Sourcebook, 2nd Edition

Basic Consumer Health Information about the Blood and Circulatory System and Related Disorders, Such as Anemia and Other Hemoglobin Diseases, Cancer of the Blood and Associated Bone Marrow Disorders, Clotting and Bleeding Problems, and Conditions That Affect the Veins, Blood Vessels, and Arteries, Including Facts about the Donation and Transplantation of Bone Marrow, Stem Cells, and Blood and Tips for Keeping the Blood and Circulatory System Healthy

Along with a Glossary of Related Terms and Resources for Additional Help and Information

Edited by Amy L. Sutton. 634 pages. 2005. 978-0-7808-0746-4.

"Highly recommended pick for basic consumer health reference holdings at all levels."
—*The Bookwatch, Aug '05*

Brain Disorders Sourcebook, 2nd Edition

Basic Consumer Health Information about Acquired and Traumatic Brain Injuries, Infections of the Brain, Epilepsy and Seizure Disorders, Cerebral Palsy, and Degenerative Neurological Disorders, Including Amyotrophic Lateral Sclerosis (ALS), Dementias, Multiple Sclerosis, and More

Along with Information on the Brain's Structure and Function, Treatment and Rehabilitation Options, Reports on Current Research Initiatives, a Glossary of Terms Related to Brain Disorders and Injuries, and a Directory of Sources for Further Help and Information

Edited by Sandra J. Judd. 600 pages. 2005. 978-0-7808-0744-0.

"This easy-to-read volume provides up-to-date health information... Recommended for consumer health collections within public or academic libraries."

—*E-Streams, Feb '06*

SEE ALSO *Alzheimer Disease Sourcebook, 4th Edition*

Breast Cancer Sourcebook, 3rd Edition

Basic Consumer Health Information about Breast Health and Breast Cancer, Including Facts about Environmental, Genetic, and Other Risk Factors, Prevention Efforts, Screening and Diagnostic Methods, Surgical Treatment Options and Other Care Choices, Complementary and Alternative Therapies, and Post-Treatment Concerns

Along with Statistical Data, News about Research Advances, a Glossary of Related Terms, and Directories of Resources for Additional Information and Support

Edited by Karen Bellenir. 606 pages. 2009. 978-0-7808-1030-3.

SEE ALSO *Cancer Sourcebook for Women, 3rd Edition, Women's Health Concerns Sourcebook, 3rd Edition*

Breastfeeding Sourcebook

Basic Consumer Health Information about the Benefits of Breastmilk, Preparing to Breastfeed, Breastfeeding as a Baby Grows, Nutrition, and More, Including Information on Special Situations and Concerns Such as Mastitis, Illness, Medications, Allergies, Multiple Births, Prematurity, Special Needs, and Adoption

Along with a Glossary and Resources for Additional Help and Information

Edited by Jenni Lynn Colson. 367 pages. 2002. 978-0-7808-0332-9.

SEE ALSO *Pregnancy and Birth Sourcebook, 2nd Edition*

Burns Sourcebook

Basic Consumer Health Information about Various Types of Burns and Scalds, Including Flame, Heat, Cold, Electrical, Chemical, and Sun Burns

Along with Information on Short-Term and Long-Term Treatments, Tissue Reconstruction, Plastic Surgery, Prevention Suggestions, and First Aid

Edited by Allan R. Cook. 604 pages. 1999. 978-0-7808-0204-9.

"This is an exceptional addition to the series and is highly recommended for all consumer health collections, hospital libraries, and academic medical centers."

—*E-Streams, Mar '00*

"This key reference guide is an invaluable addition to all health care and public libraries in confronting this ongoing health issue."

—*American Reference Books Annual, 2000*

SEE ALSO *Dermatological Disorders Sourcebook, 2nd Edition*

Cancer Sourcebook, 5th Edition

Basic Consumer Health Information about Major Forms and Stages of Cancer, Featuring Facts about Head and Neck Cancers, Lung Cancers, Gastrointestinal Cancers, Genitourinary Cancers, Lymphomas, Blood Cell Cancers, Endocrine Cancers, Skin Cancers, Bone Cancers, Metastatic Cancers, and More

Along with Facts about Cancer Treatments, Cancer Risks and Prevention, a Glossary of Related Terms, Statistical Data, and a Directory of Resources for Additional Information

Edited by Karen Bellenir. 1105 pages. 2007. 978-0-7808-0947-5.

"The 5th, updated edition of *Cancer Sourcebook* should be in every public and health lending library collection... An unparalleled discussion essential for any health collections considering an all-in-one basic general reference."

—*California Bookwatch, Aug '07*

SEE ALSO *Breast Cancer Sourcebook, 3rd Edition, Cancer Sourcebook for Women, 3rd Edition, Cancer Survivorship Sourcebook, Leukemia Sourcebook*

Cancer Sourcebook for Women, 3rd Edition

Basic Consumer Health Information about Leading Causes of Cancer in Women, Featuring Facts about Gynecologic Cancers and Related Concerns, Such as Breast Cancer, Cervical Cancer, Endometrial Cancer, Uterine Sarcoma, Vaginal Cancer, Vulvar Cancer, and Common Non-Cancerous Gynecologic Conditions, in Addition to Facts about Lung Cancer, Colorectal Cancer, and Thyroid Cancer in Women

Along with Information about Cancer Risk Factors, Screening and Prevention, Treatment Options, and Tips on Coping with Life after Cancer Treatment, a Glossary of Cancer Terms, and a Directory of Resources for Additional Help and Information

Edited by Amy L. Sutton. 687 pages. 2006. 978-0-7808-0867-6.

"This excellent book provides the general public with information compiled in a way that will help them to gain the knowledge they need. 4 Stars!"

—*Doody's Review Service, Dec '06*

"An indispensable reference for health consumers and cancer patients. Recommended for public libraries and academic libraries with a medical department."

—*E-Streams, Sep '08*

Cancer Survivorship Sourcebook

Basic Consumer Health Information about the Physical, Educational, Emotional, Social, and Financial Needs of Cancer Patients from Diagnosis, through Cancer Treatment, and Beyond, Including Facts about Researching Specific Types of Cancer and Learning about Clinical Trials and Treatment Options, and

Featuring Tips for Coping with the Side Effects of Cancer Treatments and Adjusting to Life after Cancer Treatment Concludes

Along with Suggestions for Caregivers, Friends, and Family Members of Cancer Patients, a Glossary of Cancer Care Terms, and Directories of Related Resources

Edited by Karen Bellenir. 633 pages. 2007. 978-0-7808-0985-7.

"Well organized and comprehensive in coverage, the book speaks to issues encountered both during and after cancer treatment. Recommended for consumer health and public libraries."

—*Library Journal, Aug 1 '07*

"*Cancer Survivorship Sourcebook* will be useful to anyone who has a friend or loved one with a cancer diagnosis."

—*American Reference Books Annual, 2008*

SEE ALSO *Cancer Sourcebook, 5th Edition*

Cardiovascular Diseases and Disorders Sourcebook, 3rd Edition

Basic Consumer Health Information about Heart and Vascular Diseases and Disorders, Such as Angina, Heart Attacks, Arrhythmias, Cardiomyopathy, Valve Disease, Atherosclerosis, and Aneurysms, with Information about Managing Cardiovascular Risk Factors and Maintaining Heart Health, Medications and Procedures Used to Treat Cardiovascular Disorders, and Concerns of Special Significance to Women

Along with Reports on Current Research Initiatives, a Glossary of Related Medical Terms, and a Directory of Sources for Further Help and Information

Edited by Sandra J. Judd. 687 pages. 2005. 978-0-7808-0739-6.

"This updated sourcebook is still the best first stop for comprehensive introductory information on cardiovascular diseases."

—*American Reference Books Annual, 2006*

"Recommended for public libraries and libraries supporting health care professionals."

—*E-Streams, Sep '05*

Caregiving Sourcebook

Basic Consumer Health Information for Caregivers, Including a Profile of Caregivers, Caregiving Responsibilities and Concerns, Tips for Specific Conditions, Care Environments, and the Effects of Caregiving

Along with Facts about Legal Issues, Financial Information, and Future Planning, a Glossary, and a Listing of Additional Resources

Edited by Joyce Brennfleck Shannon. 583 pages. 2001. 978-0-7808-0331-2.

"Essential for most collections."
—Library Journal, Apr 1 '02

"An ideal addition to the reference collection of any public library. Health sciences information professionals may also want to acquire the Caregiving Sourcebook for their hospital or academic library for use as a ready reference tool by health care workers interested in aging and caregiving."
—E-Streams, Jan '02

Child Abuse Sourcebook, 2nd Edition

Basic Consumer Health Information about the Physical, Sexual, and Emotional Abuse of Children, Neglect, Münchhausen Syndrome by Proxy (MSBP), and Shaken Baby Syndrome, and Featuring Facts about Withholding Medical Care, Corporal Punishment, Child Maltreatment in Youth Sports, and Parental Substance Abuse

Along with Information about Child Protective Services, Foster Care, Adoption, Parenting Challenges, Abuse Prevention Programs, and Intervention, Treatment, and Recovery Guidelines, a Glossary of Related Terms, and Resources for Additional Help and Information

Edited by Joyce Brennfleck Shannon. 600 pages. 2009. 978-0-7808-1037-2.

SEE ALSO Domestic Violence Sourcebook, 3rd Edition

Childhood Diseases and Disorders Sourcebook, 2nd Edition

Basic Consumer Health Information about the Physical, Mental, and Developmental Health of Pre-Adolescent Children, Including Facts about Infectious Diseases, Asthma, Allergies, Diabetes, and Other Acute and Chronic Conditions Affecting the Gastrointestinal Tract, Ears, Nose, Throat, Liver, Kidneys, Heart, Blood, Brain, Muscles, Bones, and Skin

Along with Reports on Recommended Childhood Vaccinations, Wellness Guidelines, a Glossary of Related Medical Terms, and a List of Resources for Parents

Edited by Sandra J. Judd. 694 pages. 2009. 978-0-7808-1031-0.

SEE ALSO Healthy Children Sourcebook

Colds, Flu and Other Common Ailments Sourcebook

Basic Consumer Health Information about Common Ailments and Injuries, Including Colds, Coughs, the Flu, Sinus Problems, Headaches, Fever, Nausea and Vomiting, Menstrual Cramps, Diarrhea, Constipation, Hemorrhoids, Back Pain, Dandruff, Dry and Itchy Skin, Cuts, Scrapes, Sprains, Bruises, and More

Along with Information about Prevention, Self-Care, Choosing a Doctor, Over-the-Counter Medications, Folk Remedies, and Alternative Therapies, and Including a Glossary of Important Terms and a Directory of Resources for Further Help and Information

Edited by Chad T. Kimball. 622 pages. 2001. 978-0-7808-0435-7.

"A good starting point for research on common illnesses. It will be a useful addition to public and consumer health library collections."
—American Reference Books Annual, 2002

"Will prove valuable to any library seeking to maintain a current, comprehensive reference collection of health resources. . . Excellent reference."
—The Bookwatch, Aug '01

Communication Disorders Sourcebook

Basic Information about Deafness and Hearing Loss, Speech and Language Disorders, Voice Disorders, Balance and Vestibular Disorders, and Disorders of Smell, Taste, and Touch

Edited by Linda M. Ross. 533 pages. 1996. 978-0-7808-0077-9.

Complementary and Alternative Medicine Sourcebook, 3rd Edition

Basic Consumer Health Information about Complementary and Alternative Medical Therapies, Including Acupuncture, Ayurveda, Traditional Chinese Medicine, Herbal Medicine, Homeopathy, Naturopathy, Biofeedback, Hypnotherapy, Yoga, Art Therapy, Aromatherapy, Clinical Nutrition, Vitamin and Mineral Supplements, Chiropractic, Massage, Reflexology, Crystal Therapy, Therapeutic Touch, and More

Along with Facts about Alternative and Complementary Treatments for Specific Conditions Such as Cancer, Diabetes, Osteoarthritis, Chronic Pain, Menopause, Gastrointestinal Disorders, Headaches, and Mental Illness, a Glossary, and a Resource List for Additional Help and Information

Edited by Sandra J. Judd. 630 pages. 2006. 978-0-7808-0864-5.

Congenital Disorders Sourcebook, 2nd Edition

Basic Consumer Health Information about Nonhereditary Birth Defects and Disorders Related to Prematurity, Gestational Injuries, Congenital Infections, and Birth Complications, Including Heart Defects, Hydrocephalus, Spina Bifida, Cleft Lip and Palate, Cerebral Palsy, and More

Along with Facts about the Prevention of Birth Defects, Fetal Surgery and Other Treatment Options, Research Initiatives, a Glossary of Related Terms, and Resources for Additional Information and Support

Edited by Sandra J. Judd. 619 pages. 2007. 978-0-7808-0945-1.

SEE ALSO *Pregnancy and Birth Sourcebook, 2nd Edition*

Contagious Diseases Sourcebook, 2nd Edition

Basic Consumer Health Information about Diseases Spread from Person to Person through Direct Physical Contact, Airborne Transmissions, Sexual Contact, or Contact with Blood or Other Body Fluids, Including Pneumococcal, Staphylococcal, and Streptococcal Diseases, Colds, Influenza, Lice, Measles, Mumps, Tuberculosis, and Others

Along with Facts about Self-Care and Over-the-Counter Medications, Antibiotics and Drug Resistance, Disease Prevention, Vaccines, and Bioterrorism, a Glossary, and a Directory of Resources for More Information

Edited by Joyce Brennfleck Shannon. 600 pages. 2009. 978-0-7808-1075-4.

SEE ALSO *AIDS Sourcebook, 4th Edition, Hepatitis Sourcebook*

Cosmetic and Reconstructive Surgery Sourcebook, 2nd Edition

Basic Consumer Information about Plastic Surgery and Non-Surgical Appearance-Enhancing Procedures, Including Facts about Botulinum Toxin, Collagen Replacement, Dermabrasion,

Chemical Peels, Eyelid Surgery, Nose Reshaping, Lip Augmentation, Liposuction, Breast Enlargement and Reduction, Tummy Tucking, and Other Skin, Hair, Facial, and Body Shaping Procedures

Along with Information about Reconstructive Procedures for Congenital Disorders, Disfiguring Diseases, Burns, and Traumatic Injuries, a Glossary of Related Terms, and a Directory of Additional Resources

Edited by Karen Bellenir. 483 pages. 2007. 978-0-7808-0951-2.

"A practical guide for health care consumers and health care workers. . . . This easy-to-read reference guide would be useful for novice and veteran health care consumers, surgical technology students, nursing students, and perioperative nurses new to plastic and reconstructive surgery. It also may be helpful for medical-surgical nurses as a guide for patient teaching in their practices."

—*AORN Journal, Aug '08*

SEE ALSO *Surgery Sourcebook, 2nd Edition*

Death and Dying Sourcebook, 2nd Edition

Basic Consumer Health Information about End-of-Life Care and Related Perspectives and Ethical Issues, Including End-of-Life Symptoms and Treatments, Pain Management, Quality-of-Life Concerns, the Use of Life Support, Patients' Rights and Privacy Issues, Advance Directives, Physician-Assisted Suicide, Caregiving, Organ and Tissue Donation, Autopsies, Funeral Arrangements, and Grief

Along with Statistical Data, Information about the Leading Causes of Death, a Glossary, and Directories of Support Groups and Other Resources

Edited by Joyce Brennfleck Shannon. 626 pages. 2006. 978-0-7808-0871-3.

Dental Care and Oral Health Sourcebook, 3rd Edition

Basic Consumer Health Information about Dental Care and Oral Health Throughout the Lifespan, Including Facts about Cavities, Bad Breath, Cold and Canker Sores, Dry Mouth,

Toothaches, Gum Disease, Malocclusion, Temporomandibular Joint and Muscle Disorders, Oral Cancers, and Dental Emergencies

Along with Information about Mouth Hygiene, Crowns, Bridges, Implants, and Fillings, Surgical, Orthodontic, and Cosmetic Dental Procedures, Pain Management, Health Conditions that Impact Oral Care, a Glossary of Related Terms, and a Directory of Additional Resources

Edited by Amy L. Sutton. 619 pages. 2008. 978-0-7808-1032-7.

Depression Sourcebook, 2nd Edition

Basic Consumer Health Information about Unipolar Depression, Bipolar Disorder, Dysthymia, Seasonal Affective Disorder, Postpartum Depression, and Other Depressive Disorders, Including Facts about Populations at Special Risk, Coexisting Medical Conditions, Symptoms, Treatment Options, and Suicide Prevention

Along with Statistical Data, a Glossary of Related Terms, and a Directory of Resources for Additional Help and Information

Edited by Sandra J. Judd. 646 pages. 2008. 978-0-7808-1003-7.

"Recommended for public libraries."
—*ARBAonline, Nov '08*

SEE ALSO *Mental Health Disorders Sourcebook, 4th Edition*

Dermatological Disorders Sourcebook, 2nd Edition

Basic Consumer Health Information about Conditions and Disorders Affecting the Skin, Hair, and Nails, Such as Acne, Rosacea, Rashes, Dermatitis, Pigmentation Disorders, Birthmarks, Skin Cancer, Skin Injuries, Psoriasis, Scleroderma, and Hair Loss, Including Facts about Medications and Treatments for Dermatological Disorders and Tips for Maintaining Healthy Skin, Hair, and Nails

Along with Information about How Aging Affects the Skin, a Glossary of Related Terms, and a Directory of Resources for Additional Help and Information

Edited by Amy L. Sutton. 617 pages. 2006. 978-0-7808-0795-2.

"Helpfully brings together. . . sources in one convenient place, saving the user hours of research time."
—*American Reference Books Annual, 2006*

SEE ALSO *Burns Sourcebook*

Diabetes Sourcebook, 4th Edition

Basic Consumer Health Information about Type 1 and Type 2 Diabetes Mellitus, Gestational Diabetes, Monogenic Forms of Diabetes, and Insulin Resistance, with Guidelines for Lifestyle Modifications and the Medical Management of Diabetes, Including Facts about Insulin, Insulin Delivery Devices, Oral Diabetes Medications, Self-Monitoring of Blood Glucose, Meal Planning, Physical Activity Recommendations, Foot Care, and Treatment Options for People with Kidney Failure

Along with a Section about Diabetes Complications and Co-Occurring Conditions, a Glossary of Related Terms, and Directories of Resources for Additional Help and Information

Edited by Karen Bellenir. 627 pages. 2008. 978-0-7808-1005-1.

"Completely and comprehensively covering almost everything a student or physician would need to know.... well worth the investment."
—*Internet Bookwatch, Dec '08*

SEE ALSO *Endocrine and Metabolic Disorders Sourcebook, 2nd Edition*

Diet and Nutrition Sourcebook, 3rd Edition

Basic Consumer Health Information about Dietary Guidelines and the Food Guidance System, Recommended Daily Nutrient Intakes, Serving Proportions, Weight Control, Vitamins and Supplements., Nutrition Issues for Different Life Stages and Lifestyles, and the Needs of People with Specific Medical Concerns, Including Cancer, Celiac Disease, Diabetes, Eating Disorders, Food Allergies, and Cardiovascular Disease

Along with Facts about Federal Nutrition Support Programs, a Glossary of Nutrition and Dietary Terms, and Directories of Additional Resources for More Information about Nutrition

Edited by Joyce Brennfleck Shannon. 605 pages. 2006. 978-0-7808-0800-3.

"A valuable resource tool for any individual."
—*Journal of Dental Hygiene, Apr '07*

"From different recommended eating habits to reduce disease and common ailments to nutrition advice for those with specific conditions, *Diet and Nutrition Sourcebook* is especially important because so much is changing in this area, and so rapidly."
—*California Bookwatch, Jun '06*

SEE ALSO *Digestive Diseases and Disorders Sourcebook, Eating Disorders Sourcebook, 2nd Edition, Gastrointestinal Diseases and Disorders Sourcebook, 2nd Edition, Vegetarian Sourcebook*

Digestive Diseases and Disorders Sourcebook

Basic Consumer Health Information about Diseases and Disorders that Impact the Upper and Lower Digestive System, Including Celiac Disease, Constipation, Crohn's Disease, Cyclic Vomiting Syndrome, Diarrhea, Diverticulosis and Diverticulitis, Gallstones, Heartburn, Hemorrhoids, Hernias, Indigestion (Dyspepsia), Irritable Bowel Syndrome, Lactose Intolerance, Ulcers, and More

Along with Information about Medications and Other Treatments, Tips for Maintaining a Healthy Digestive Tract, a Glossary, and Directory of Digestive Diseases Organizations

Edited by Karen Bellenir. 323 pages. 2000. 978-0-7808-0327-5.

"An excellent addition to all public or patient-research libraries."
—*American Reference Books Annual, 2001*

"Recommended reference source."
—*Booklist, May '00*

SEE ALSO *Diet and Nutrition Sourcebook, 3rd Edition, Gastrointestinal Diseases and Disorders Sourcebook, 2nd Edition*

Disabilities Sourcebook

Basic Consumer Health Information about Physical and Psychiatric Disabilities, Including Descriptions of Major Causes of Disability, Assistive and Adaptive Aids, Workplace Issues, and Accessibility Concerns

645

Along with Information about the Americans with Disabilities Act, a Glossary, and Resources for Additional Help and Information

Edited by Dawn D. Matthews. 602 pages. 2000. 978-0-7808-0389-3.

"A must for libraries with a consumer health section."
—*American Reference Books Annual, 2002*

"A much needed addition to the Omnigraphics *Health Reference Series*. A current reference work to provide people with disabilities, their families, caregivers or those who work with them, a broad range of information in one volume, has not been available until now. . . . It is recommended for all public and academic library reference collections."
—*E-Streams, May '01*

"An excellent source book in easy-to-read format covering many current topics; highly recommended for all libraries."
—*CHOICE, Jan '01*

▨

Disease Management Sourcebook

Basic Consumer Health Information about Coping with Chronic and Serious Illnesses, Navigating the Health Care System, Communicating with Health Care Providers, Assessing Health Care Quality, and Making Informed Health Care Decisions, Including Facts about Second Opinions, Hospitalization, Surgery, and Medications

Along with a Section about Children with Chronic Conditions, Information about Legal, Financial, and Insurance Issues, a Glossary of Related Terms, and Directories of Additional Resources

Edited by Joyce Brennfleck Shannon. 621 pages. 2008. 978-0-7808-1002-0.

"Consumers need to know how to manage their health care the same way they manage anything else in their lives. The text is very readable and is written for the layperson and consumer. The cost is not prohibitive. This book should be in all collections of health care libraries and public libraries."
—*ARBAonline, Jul '08*

"The information is very current, and the selection of font and layout make the book easy to read. A hardback that will stand up to much usage, this is an excellent resource for consumers. . . . Recommended. General readers."
—*CHOICE, Nov '08*

"Intended for lay readers, this resource clarifies the many confusing and overwhelming details associated with chronic disease care. Meticulous and clearly explained, the book even includes diagrams intended to ease comprehension of over-the-counter medication labels. An essential guide to navigating the health-care rapids."
—*Library Journal, Aug '08*

▨

Domestic Violence Sourcebook, 3rd Edition

Basic Consumer Health Information about Warning Signs, Risk Factors, and Health Consequences of Intimate Partner Violence, Sexual Violence and Rape, Stalking, Human Trafficking, Child Maltreatment, Teen Dating Violence, and Elder Abuse

Along with Facts about Victims and Perpetrators, Strategies for Violence Prevention, and Emergency Interventions, Safety Plans, and Financial and Legal Tips for Victims, a Glossary of Related Terms, and Directories of Resources for Additional Information and Support

Edited by Joyce Brennfleck Shannon. 600 pages. 2009. 978-0-7808-1038-9.

SEE ALSO *Child Abuse Sourcebook, 2nd Edition*

▨

Drug Abuse Sourcebook, 2nd Edition

Basic Consumer Health Information about Illicit Substances of Abuse and the Misuse of Prescription and Over-the-Counter Medications, Including Depressants, Hallucinogens, Inhalants, Marijuana, Stimulants, and Anabolic Steroids

Along with Facts about Related Health Risks, Treatment Programs, Prevention Programs, a Glossary of Abuse and Addiction Terms, a Glossary of Drug-Related Street Terms, and a Directory of Resources for More Information

Edited by Catherine Ginther. 581 pages. 2004. 978-0-7808-0740-2.

"Commendable for organizing useful, normally scattered government and association-produced data into a logical sequence."
—*American Reference Books Annual, 2006*

SEE ALSO *Alcoholism Sourcebook, 2nd Edition*

Ear, Nose, and Throat Disorders Sourcebook, 2nd Edition

Basic Consumer Health Information about Disorders of the Ears, Hearing Loss, Vestibular Disorders, Nasal and Sinus Problems, Throat and Vocal Cord Disorders, and Otolaryngologic Cancers, Including Facts about Ear Infections and Injuries, Genetic and Congenital Deafness, Sensorineural Hearing Disorders, Tinnitus, Vertigo, Ménière Disease, Rhinitis, Sinusitis, Snoring, Sore Throats, Hoarseness, and More

Along with Reports on Current Research Initiatives, a Glossary of Related Medical Terms, and a Directory of Sources for Further Help and Information

Edited by Sandra J. Judd. 631 pages. 2007. 978-0-7808-0872-0.

Eating Disorders Sourcebook, 2nd Edition

Basic Consumer Health Information about Anorexia Nervosa, Bulimia, Binge Eating, Compulsive Exercise, Female Athlete Triad, and Other Eating Disorders, Including Facts about Body Image and Other Cultural and Age-Related Risk Factors, Prevention Efforts, Adverse Health Effects, Treatment Options, and the Recovery Process

Along with Guidelines for Healthy Weight Control, a Glossary, and Directories of Additional Resources

Edited by Joyce Brennfleck Shannon. 557 pages. 2007. 978-0-7808-0948-2.

SEE ALSO *Diet and Nutrition Sourcebook, 3rd Edition, Mental Health Disorders Sourcebook, 4th Edition*

Emergency Medical Services Sourcebook

Basic Consumer Health Information about Preventing, Preparing for, and Managing Emergency Situations, When and Who to Call for Help, What to Expect in the Emergency Room, the Emergency Medical Team, Patient Issues, and Current Topics in Emergency Medicine

Along with Statistical Data, a Glossary, and Sources of Additional Help and Information

Edited by Jenni Lynn Colson. 472 pages. 2002. 978-0-7808-0420-3.

SEE ALSO *Injury and Trauma Sourcebook*

Endocrine and Metabolic Disorders Sourcebook, 2nd Edition

Basic Consumer Health Information about Hormonal and Metabolic Disorders that Affect the Body's Growth, Development, and Functioning, Including Disorders of the Pancreas, Ovaries and Testes, and Pituitary, Thyroid, Parathyroid, and Adrenal Glands, with Facts about Growth Disorders, Addison Disease, Cushing Syndrome, Conn Syndrome, Diabetic Disorders, Multiple Endocrine Neoplasia, Inborn Errors of Metabolism, and More

Along with Information about Endocrine Functioning, Diagnostic and Screening Tests, a Glossary of Related Terms, and Directories of Additional Resources

Edited by Joyce Brennfleck Shannon. 597 pages. 2007. 978-0-7808-0952-9.

SEE ALSO *Diabetes Sourcebook, 4th Edition*

Environmental Health Sourcebook, 2nd Edition

Basic Consumer Health Information about the Environment and Its Effect on Human Health, Including the Effects of Air Pollution, Water Pollution, Hazardous Chemicals, Food Hazards, Radiation Hazards, Biological Agents, Household Hazards, Such as Radon, Asbestos, Carbon Monoxide, and Mold, and Information about Associated Diseases and Disorders, Including Cancer, Allergies, Respiratory Problems, and Skin Disorders

Along with Information about Environmental Concerns for Specific Populations, a Glossary of Related Terms, and Resources for Further Help and Information

Edited by Dawn D. Matthews. 650 pages. 2003. 978-0-7808-0632-0.

"Recommended for teenage and adult students and readers, and for public and academic libraries, as well as any library focusing on consumer health."
—*E-Streams, May '04*

"This recently updated edition continues the level of quality and the reputation of the numerous other volumes in Omnigraphics' Health Reference Series."
—*American Reference Books Annual, 2004*

Ethnic Diseases Sourcebook

Basic Consumer Health Information for Ethnic and Racial Minority Groups in the United States, Including General Health Indicators and Behaviors, Ethnic Diseases, Genetic Testing, the Impact of Chronic Diseases, Women's Health, Mental Health Issues, and Preventive Health Care Services

Along with a Glossary and a Listing of Additional Resources

Edited by Joyce Brennfleck Shannon. 648 pages. 2001. 978-0-7808-0336-7.

"Not many books have been written on this topic to date, and the *Ethnic Diseases Sourcebook* is a strong addition to the list. It will be an important introductory resource for health consumers, students, health care personnel, and social scientists. It is recommended for public, academic, and large hospital libraries."
—*American Reference Books Annual, 2002*

"Will prove valuable to any library seeking to maintain a current, comprehensive reference collection of health resources. . . . An excellent source of health information about genetic disorders which affect particular ethnic and racial minorities in the U.S."
—*The Bookwatch, Aug '01*

Eye Care Sourcebook, 3rd Edition

Basic Consumer Health Information about Eye Care and Eye Disorders, Including Facts about the Diagnosis, Prevention, and Treatment of Refractive Disorders, Cataracts, Glaucoma, Macular Degeneration, and Problems Affecting the Cornea, Retina, and Lacrimal Glands

Along with Advice about Preventing Eye Injuries and Tips for Living with Low Vision or Blindness, a Glossary of Related Terms, and Directories of Resources for More Help and Information

Edited by Amy L. Sutton. 646 pages. 2008. 978-0-7808-1000-6.

Family Planning Sourcebook

Basic Consumer Health Information about Planning for Pregnancy and Contraception, Including Traditional Methods, Barrier Methods, Hormonal Methods, Permanent Methods, Future Methods, Emergency Contraception, and Birth Control Choices for Women at Each Stage of Life

Along with Statistics, a Glossary, and Sources of Additional Information

Edited by Amy Marcaccio Keyzer. 503 pages. 2001. 978-0-7808-0379-4.

"Recommended for public, health, and undergraduate libraries as part of the circulating collection."
—*E-Streams, Mar '02*

"Will prove valuable to any library seeking to maintain a current, comprehensive reference collection of health resources. . . . Excellent reference."

—*The Bookwatch, Aug '01*

SEE ALSO *Pregnancy and Birth Sourcebook, 2nd Edition*

Fitness and Exercise Sourcebook, 3rd Edition

Basic Consumer Health Information about the Physical and Mental Benefits of Fitness, Including Cardiorespiratory Endurance, Muscular Strength, Muscular Endurance, and Flexibility, with Facts about Sports Nutrition and Exercise-Related Injuries and Tips about Physical Activity and Exercises for People of All Ages and for People with Health Concerns

Along with Advice on Selecting and Using Exercise Equipment, Maintaining Exercise Motivation, a Glossary of Related Terms, and a Directory of Resources for More Help and Information

Edited by Amy L. Sutton. 635 pages. 2007. 978-0-7808-0946-8.

"Updates the consumer information on the physical and mental benefits of physical activity throughout the lifespan offered in earlier editions. . . . Recommended. All readers; all levels."

—*CHOICE, Oct '07*

"An exceptionally well-rounded coverage perfect for any concerned about developing and understanding a fitness program."

—*California Bookwatch, Jun '07*

SEE ALSO *Sports Injuries Sourcebook, 3rd Edition*

Food Safety Sourcebook

Basic Consumer Health Information about the Safe Handling of Meat, Poultry, Seafood, Eggs, Fruit Juices, and Other Food Items, and Facts about Pesticides, Drinking Water, Food Safety Overseas, and the Onset, Duration, and Symptoms of Foodborne Illnesses, Including Types of Pathogenic Bacteria, Parasitic Protozoa, Worms, Viruses, and Natural Toxins

Along with the Role of the Consumer, the Food Handler, and the Government in Food Safety; a Glossary, and Resources for Additional Help and Information

Edited by Dawn D. Matthews. 327 pages. 1999. 978-0-7808-0326-8.

"Recommended reference source."

—*Booklist, May '00*

"This book takes the complex issues of food safety and foodborne pathogens and presents them in an easily understood manner. [It does] an excellent job of covering a large and often confusing topic."

— *American Reference Books Annual, 2000*

Forensic Medicine Sourcebook

Basic Consumer Information for the Layperson about Forensic Medicine, Including Crime Scene Investigation, Evidence Collection and Analysis, Expert Testimony, Computer-Aided Criminal Identification, Digital Imaging in the Courtroom, DNA Profiling, Accident Reconstruction, Autopsies, Ballistics, Drugs and Explosives Detection, Latent Fingerprints, Product Tampering, and Questioned Document Examination

Along with Statistical Data, a Glossary of Forensics Terminology, and Listings of Sources for Further Help and Information

Edited by Annemarie S. Muth. 574 pages. 1999. 978-0-7808-0232-2.

"Given the expected widespread interest in its content and its easy to read style, this book is recommended for most public and all college and university libraries."

—*E-Streams, Feb '01*

"A wealth of information, useful statistics, references are up-to-date and extremely complete. This wonderful collection of data will help students who are interested in a career in any type of forensic field. It is a great resource for attorneys who need information about types of expert witnesses needed in a particular case. It also offers useful information for fiction and nonfiction writers whose work involves a crime. A fascinating compilation. All levels."

—*CHOICE, Jan '00*

"There are several items that make this book attractive to consumers who are seeking certain forensic data. . . . This is a useful current

source for those seeking general forensic medical answers."
—*American Reference Books Annual, 2000*

Gastrointestinal Diseases and Disorders Sourcebook, 2nd Edition

Basic Consumer Health Information about the Upper and Lower Gastrointestinal (GI) Tract, Including the Esophagus, Stomach, Intestines, Rectum, Liver, and Pancreas, with Facts about Gastroesophageal Reflux Disease, Gastritis, Hernias, Ulcers, Celiac Disease, Diverticulitis, Irritable Bowel Syndrome, Hemorrhoids, Gastrointestinal Cancers, and Other Diseases and Disorders Related to the Digestive Process

Along with Information about Commonly Used Diagnostic and Surgical Procedures, Statistics, Reports on Current Research Initiatives and Clinical Trials, a Glossary, and Resources for Additional Help and Information

Edited by Sandra J. Judd. 654 pages. 2006. 978-0-7808-0798-3.

"The text is designed for the general reader seeking information on prevention, disease warning signs, diagnostic and therapeutic questions. . . . It is an excellent resource for the general reader to conveniently locate credible, coordinated and indexed information. . . . The sourcebook will prove very helpful for patients, caregivers and should be available in every physician waiting room."
—*Doody's Review Service, 2006*

SEE ALSO *Diet and Nutrition Sourcebook, 3rd Edition, Digestive Diseases and Disorders Sourcebook*

Genetic Disorders Sourcebook, 4th Edition

Basic Consumer Health Information about Hereditary Diseases and Disorders, Including Facts about the Human Genome, Genetic Inheritance Patterns, Disorders Associated with Specific Genes, Such as Sickle Cell Disease, Hemophilia, and Cystic Fibrosis, Chromosome Disorders, Such as Down Syndrome, Fragile X Syndrome, and Turner Syndrome, and Complex Diseases and Disorders Resulting from the Interaction of Environmental and Genetic Factors, Such as Allergies, Cancer, and Obesity

Along with Facts about Genetic Testing, Suggestions for Parents of Children with Special Needs, Reports on Current Research Initiatives, a Glossary of Genetic Terminology, and Resources for Additional Help and Information

Edited by Sandra J. Judd. 600 pages. 2009. 978-0-7808-1076-1.

Head Trauma Sourcebook

Basic Information for the Layperson about Open-Head and Closed-Head Injuries, Treatment Advances, Recovery, and Rehabilitation

Along with Reports on Current Research Initiatives

Edited by Karen Bellenir. 414 pages. 1997. 978-0-7808-0208-7.

Headache Sourcebook

Basic Consumer Health Information about Migraine, Tension, Cluster, Rebound and Other Types of Headaches, with Facts about the Cause and Prevention of Headaches, the Effects of Stress and the Environment, Headaches during Pregnancy and Menopause, and Childhood Headaches

Along with a Glossary and Other Resources for Additional Help and Information

Edited by Dawn D. Matthews. 342 pages. 2002. 978-0-7808-0337-4.

"Highly recommended for academic and medical reference collections."
—*Library Bookwatch, Sep '02*

SEE ALSO *Pain Sourcebook, 3rd Edition*

Healthy Aging Sourcebook

Basic Consumer Health Information about Maintaining Health through the Aging Process, Including Advice on Nutrition, Exercise, and Sleep, Help in Making Decisions about Midlife Issues and Retirement, and Guidance Concerning Practical and Informed Choices in Health Consumerism

Along with Data Concerning the Theories of Aging, Different Experiences in Aging by Minority Groups, and Facts about Aging Now and Aging in the Future; and Featuring a Glossary, a Guide to Consumer Help, Additional Suggested Reading, and Practical Resource Directory

Edited by Jenifer Swanson. 537 pages. 1999. 978-0-7808-0390-9.

"Recommended reference source."
—Booklist, Feb '00

SEE ALSO *Physical and Mental Issues in Aging Sourcebook*

Healthy Children Sourcebook

Basic Consumer Health Information about the Physical and Mental Development of Children between the Ages of 3 and 12, Including Routine Health Care, Preventative Health Services, Safety and First Aid, Healthy Sleep, Dental Care, Nutrition, and Fitness, and Featuring Parenting Tips on Such Topics as Bedwetting, Choosing Day Care, Monitoring TV and Other Media, and Establishing a Foundation for Substance Abuse Prevention

Along with a Glossary of Commonly Used Pediatric Terms and Resources for Additional Help and Information.

Edited by Chad T. Kimball. 624 pages. 2003. 978-0-7808-0247-6.

"Should be required reading for parents and teachers."
—E-Streams, Jun '04

"It is hard to imagine that any other single resource exists that would provide such a comprehensive guide of timely information on health promotion and disease prevention for children aged 3 to 12."
—American Reference Books Annual, 2004

"This easy-to-read volume is a tremendous resource."
—AORN Journal, May '05

SEE ALSO *Childhood Diseases and Disorders Sourcebook, 2nd Edition*

Healthy Heart Sourcebook for Women

Basic Consumer Health Information about Cardiac Issues Specific to Women, Including Facts about Major Risk Factors and Prevention, Treatment and Control Strategies, and Important Dietary Issues

Along with a Special Section Regarding the Pros and Cons of Hormone Replacement Therapy and Its Impact on Heart Health, and Additional Help, Including Recipes, a Glossary, and a Directory of Resources

Edited by Dawn D. Matthews. 321 pages. 2000. 978-0-7808-0329-9.

"A good reference source and recommended for all public, academic, medical, and hospital libraries."
—Medical Reference Services Quarterly, Summer '01

"Contains very important information about coronary artery disease that all women should know. The information is current and presented in an easy-to-read format. The book will make a good addition to any library."
—American Medical Writers Association Journal, Summer '00

SEE ALSO *Cardiovascular Diseases and Disorders Sourcebook, 3rd Edition, Women's Health Concerns Sourcebook, 3rd Edition*

Hepatitis Sourcebook

Basic Consumer Health Information about Hepatitis A, Hepatitis B, Hepatitis C, and Other Forms of Hepatitis, Including Autoimmune Hepatitis, Alcoholic Hepatitis, Nonalcoholic Steatohepatitis, and Toxic Hepatitis, with Facts about Risk Factors, Screening Methods, Diagnostic Tests, and Treatment Options

Along with Information on Liver Health, Tips for People Living with Chronic Hepatitis, Reports on Current Research Initiatives, a Glossary of Terms Related to Hepatitis, and a Directory of Sources for Further Help and Information

Edited by Sandra J. Judd. 570 pages. 2006. 978-0-7808-0749-5.

"The breadth of information found in this one book would not be readily found in another source. Highly recommended."
—American Reference Books Annual, 2006

SEE ALSO *Contagious Diseases Sourcebook*

Household Safety Sourcebook

Basic Consumer Health Information about Household Safety, Including Information about Poisons, Chemicals, Fire, and Water Hazards in the Home

Along with Advice about the Safe Use of Home Maintenance Equipment, Choosing Toys and Nursery Furniture, Holiday and Recreation Safety, a Glossary, and Resources for Further Help and Information

Edited by Dawn D. Matthews. 587 pages. 2002. 978-0-7808-0338-1.

"As a sourcebook on household safety this book meets its mark. It is encyclopedic in scope and covers a wide range of safety issues that are commonly seen in the home."
—*E-Streams, Jul '02*

■

Hypertension Sourcebook

Basic Consumer Health Information about the Causes, Diagnosis, and Treatment of High Blood Pressure, with Facts about Consequences, Complications, and Co-Occurring Disorders, Such as Coronary Heart Disease, Diabetes, Stroke, Kidney Disease, and Hypertensive Retinopathy, and Issues in Blood Pressure Control, Including Dietary Choices, Stress Management, and Medications

Along with Reports on Current Research Initiatives and Clinical Trials, a Glossary, and Resources for Additional Help and Information

Edited by Dawn D. Matthews and Karen Bellenir. 588 pages. 2004. 978-0-7808-0674-0.

"Academic, public, and medical libraries will want to add the *Hypertension Sourcebook* to their collections."
—*E-Streams, Aug '05*

"The strength of this source is the wide range of information given about hypertension."
—*American Reference Books Annual, 2005*

SEE ALSO *Stroke Sourcebook, 2nd Edition*

■

Immune System Disorders Sourcebook, 2nd Edition

Basic Consumer Health Information about Disorders of the Immune System, Including Immune System Function and Response, Diagnosis of Immune Disorders, Information about Inherited Immune Disease, Acquired Immune Disease, and Autoimmune Diseases, Including Primary Immune Deficiency, Acquired Immunodeficiency Syndrome (AIDS), Lupus, Multiple Sclerosis, Type 1 Diabetes, Rheumatoid Arthritis, and Graves' Disease

Along with Treatments, Tips for Coping with Immune Disorders, a Glossary, and a Directory of Additional Resources

Edited by Joyce Brennfleck Shannon. 643 pages. 2005. 978-0-7808-0748-8.

"Highly recommended for academic and public libraries."
—*American Reference Books Annual, 2006*

"The updated second edition is a 'must' for any consumer health library seeking a solid resource covering the treatments, symptoms, and options for immune disorder sufferers. . . . An excellent guide."
—*MBR Bookwatch, Jan '06*

SEE ALSO *AIDS Sourcebook, 4th Edition, Arthritis Sourcebook, 2nd Edition*

■

Infant and Toddler Health Sourcebook

Basic Consumer Health Information about the Physical and Mental Development of Newborns, Infants, and Toddlers, Including Neonatal Concerns, Nutrition Recommendations, Immunization Schedules, Common Pediatric Disorders, Assessments and Milestones, Safety Tips, and Advice for Parents and Other Caregivers

Along with a Glossary of Terms and Resource Listings for Additional Help

Edited by Jenifer Swanson. 570 pages. 2000. 978-0-7808-0246-9.

"As a reference for the general public, this would be useful in any library."
—*E-Streams, May '01*

"Recommended reference source."
—*Booklist, Feb '01*

■

Infectious Diseases Sourcebook

Basic Consumer Health Information about Non-Contagious Bacterial, Viral, Prion, Fungal, and Parasitic Diseases Spread by Food and Water, Insects and Animals, or Environmental Contact, Including Botulism, E. Coli, Encephalitis, Legionnaires' Disease, Lyme Disease, Malaria, Plague, Rabies, Salmonella, Tetanus, and Others, and Facts about Newly Emerging Diseases, Such as Hantavirus, Mad Cow Disease, Monkeypox, and West Nile Virus

Along with Information about Preventing Disease Transmission, the Threat of Bioterrorism, and Current Research Initiatives, with a Glossary and Directory of Resources for More Information

Edited by Karen Bellenir. 610 pages. 2004. 978-0-7808-0675-7.

"This reference continues the excellent tradition of the *Health Reference Series* in consolidating a wealth of information on a selected topic into a format that is easy to use and accessible to the general public."
—*American Reference Books Annual, 2005*

"Recommended for public and academic libraries."
—*E-Streams, Jan '05*

■

Injury and Trauma Sourcebook

Basic Consumer Health Information about the Impact of Injury, the Diagnosis and Treatment of Common and Traumatic Injuries, Emergency Care, and Specific Injuries Related to Home, Community, Workplace, Transportation, and Recreation

Along with Guidelines for Injury Prevention, a Glossary, and a Directory of Additional Resources

Edited by Joyce Brennfleck Shannon. 675 pages. 2002. 978-0-7808-0421-0.

"Practitioners should be aware of guides such as this in order to facilitate their use by patients and their families."
—*Doody's Health Sciences Book Review Journal, Sep-Oct '02*

"Recommended reference source."
—*Booklist, Sep '02*

"Highly recommended for academic and medical reference collections."
—*Library Bookwatch, Sep '02*

SEE ALSO *Emergency Medical Services Sourcebook, Sports Injuries Sourcebook, 3rd Edition*

■

Learning Disabilities Sourcebook, 3rd Edition

Basic Consumer Health Information about Dyslexia, Auditory and Visual Processing Disorders, Communication Disorders, Dyscalculia, Dysgraphia, and Other Conditions That Impede Learning, Including Attention Deficit/ Hyperactivity Disorder, Autism Spectrum Disorders, Hearing and Visual Impairments, Chromosome-Based Disorders, and Brain Injury

Along with Facts about Brain Function, Assessment, Therapy and Remediation, Accommodations, Assistive Technology, Legal Protections, and Tips about Family Life, School Transitions, and Employment Strategies, a Glossary of Related Terms, and Directories of Additional Resources

Edited by Joyce Brennfleck Shannon. 613 pages. 2009. 978-0-7808-1039-6.

SEE ALSO *Attention Deficit Disorder Sourcebook, Autism and Pervasive Developmental Disorders Sourcebook*

■

Leukemia Sourcebook

Basic Consumer Health Information about Adult and Childhood Leukemias, Including Acute Lymphocytic Leukemia (ALL), Chronic Lymphocytic Leukemia (CLL), Acute Myelogenous Leukemia (AML), Chronic Myelogenous Leukemia (CML), and Hairy Cell Leukemia, and Treatments Such as Chemotherapy, Radiation Therapy, Peripheral Blood Stem Cell and Marrow Transplantation, and Immunotherapy

Along with Tips for Life During and After Treatment, a Glossary, and Directories of Additional Resources

Edited by Joyce Brennfleck Shannon. 564 pages. 2003. 978-0-7808-0627-6.

"Unlike other medical books for the layperson, . . . the language does not talk down to the reader. . . . This volume is highly recommended for all libraries."
—*American Reference Books Annual, 2004*

"A fine title which ranges from diagnosis to alternative treatments, staging, and tips for life during and after diagnosis."
—*The Bookwatch, Dec '03*

SEE ALSO *Cancer Sourcebook, 5th Edition*

■

Liver Disorders Sourcebook

Basic Consumer Health Information about the Liver and How It Works; Liver Diseases, Including Cancer, Cirrhosis, Hepatitis, and Toxic and Drug Related Diseases; Tips for Maintaining a Healthy Liver; Laboratory Tests, Radiology Tests, and Facts about Liver Transplantation

Along with a Section on Support Groups, a Glossary, and Resource Listings

Edited by Joyce Brennfleck Shannon. 580 pages. 2000. 978-0-7808-0383-1.

SEE ALSO Gastrointestinal Diseases and Disorders Sourcebook, 2nd Edition, Hepatitis Sourcebook

Lung Disorders Sourcebook

Basic Consumer Health Information about Emphysema, Pneumonia, Tuberculosis, Asthma, Cystic Fibrosis, and Other Lung Disorders, Including Facts about Diagnostic Procedures, Treatment Strategies, Disease Prevention Efforts, and Such Risk Factors as Smoking, Air Pollution, and Exposure to Asbestos, Radon, and Other Agents

Along with a Glossary and Resources for Additional Help and Information

Edited by Dawn D. Matthews. 657 pages. 2002. 978-0-7808-0339-8.

SEE ALSO Respiratory Disorders Sourcebook, 2nd Edition

Medical Tests Sourcebook, 3rd Edition

Basic Consumer Health Information about X-Rays, Blood Tests, Stool and Urine Tests, Biopsies, Mammography, Endoscopic Procedures, Ultrasound Exams, Computed Tomography, Magnetic Resonance Imaging (MRI), Nuclear Medicine, Genetic Testing, Home-Use Tests, and More

Along with Facts about Preventive Care and Screening Test Guidelines, Screening and Assessment Tests Associated with Such Specific Concerns as Cancer, Heart Disease, Allergies, Diabetes, Thyroid Disfunction, and Infertility, a Glossary of Related Terms, and a Directory of Resources for Additional Help and Information

Edited by Karen Bellenir. 627 pages. 2008. 978-0-7808-1040-2

Men's Health Concerns Sourcebook, 3rd Edition

Basic Consumer Health Information about Wellness in Men and Gender-Related Differences in Health, With Facts about Heart Disease, Cancer, Traumatic Injury, and Other Leading Causes of Death in Men, Reproductive Concerns, Sexual Dysfunction, Disorders of the Prostate, Penis, and Testes, Sex-Linked Genetic Disorders, and Other Medical and Mental Concerns of Men

Along with Statistical Data, a Glossary of Related Terms, and a Directory of Resources for Additional Information

Edited by Sandra J. Judd. 600 pages. 2009. 978-0-7808-1033-4.

SEE ALSO Prostate and Urological Disorders Sourcebook

Mental Health Disorders Sourcebook, 4th Edition

Basic Consumer Health Information about the Causes and Symptoms of Mental Health Problems, Including Depression, Bipolar Disorder, Anxiety Disorders, Posttraumatic Stress Disorder, Obsessive-Compulsive Disorder, Eating Disorders, Addictions, and Personality and Psychotic Disorders

Along with Information about Medications and Treatments, Mental Health Concerns in Children, Adolescents, and Adults, Tips on Living with Mental Health Disorders, a Glossary of Related Terms, and a Directory of Resources for Additional Help and Information

Edited by Amy L. Sutton. 600 pages. 2009. 978-0-7808-1041-9.

SEE ALSO Depression Sourcebook, 2nd Edition, Stress-Related Disorders Sourcebook, 2nd Edition

Mental Retardation Sourcebook

Basic Consumer Health Information about Mental Retardation and Its Causes, Including

Down Syndrome, Fetal Alcohol Syndrome, Fragile X Syndrome, Genetic Conditions, Injury, and Environmental Sources

Along with Preventive Strategies, Parenting Issues, Educational Implications, Health Care Needs, Employment and Economic Matters, Legal Issues, a Glossary, and a Resource Listing for Additional Help and Information

Edited by Joyce Brennfleck Shannon. 627 pages. 2000. 978-0-7808-0377-0.

"Public libraries will find the book useful for reference and as a beginning research point for students, parents, and caregivers."
—American Reference Books Annual, 2001

"The strength of this work is that it compiles many basic fact sheets and addresses for further information in one volume. It is intended and suitable for the general public."
—E-Streams, Nov '00

"An invaluable overview."
—Reviewer's Bookwatch, Jul '00

Movement Disorders Sourcebook, 2nd Edition

Basic Consumer Health Information about the Symptoms and Causes of Movement Disorders, Including Parkinson Disease, Amyotrophic Lateral Sclerosis, Cerebral Palsy, Muscular Dystrophy, Multiple Sclerosis, Myasthenia, Myoclonus, Spina Bifida, Dystonia, Essential Tremor, Choreatic Disorders, Huntington Disease, Tourette Syndrome, and Other Disorders That Cause Slowed, Absent, or Excessive Movements

Along with Information about Surgical and Nonsurgical Interventions, Physical Therapies, Strategies for Independent Living, a Glossary of Related Terms, and a Directory of Resources for Additional Help and Information

Edited by Amy L. Sutton. 600 pages. 2009. 978-0-7808-1034-1.

SEE ALSO Multiple Sclerosis Sourcebook, Muscular Dystrophy Sourcebook

Multiple Sclerosis Sourcebook

Basic Consumer Health Information about Multiple Sclerosis (MS) and Its Effects on Mobility, Vision, Bladder Function, Speech,

Swallowing, and Cognition, Including Facts about Risk Factors, Causes, Diagnostic Procedures, Pain Management, Drug Treatments, and Physical and Occupational Therapies

Along with Guidelines for Nutrition and Exercise, Tips on Choosing Assistive Equipment, Information about Disability, Work, Financial, and Legal Issues, a Glossary of Related Terms, and a Directory of Additional Resources

Edited by Joyce Brennfleck Shannon. 553 pages. 2007. 978-0-7808-0998-7.

SEE ALSO Movement Disorders Sourcebook, 2nd Edition

Muscular Dystrophy Sourcebook

Basic Consumer Health Information about Congenital, Childhood-Onset, and Adult-Onset Forms of Muscular Dystrophy, Such as Duchenne, Becker, Emery-Dreifuss, Distal, Limb-Girdle, Facioscapulohumeral (FSHD), Myotonic, and Ophthalmoplegic Muscular Dystrophies, Including Facts about Diagnostic Tests, Medical and Physical Therapies, Management of Co-Occurring Conditions, and Parenting Guidelines

Along with Practical Tips for Home Care, a Glossary, and Directories of Additional Resources

Edited by Joyce Brennfleck Shannon. 552 pages. 2004. 978-0-7808-0676-4.

"This book is highly recommended for public and academic libraries as well as health care offices that support the information needs of patients and their families."
—E-Streams, Apr '05

"Excellent reference."
—The Bookwatch, Jan '05

SEE ALSO Movement Disorders Sourcebook, 2nd Edition

Obesity Sourcebook

Basic Consumer Health Information about Diseases and Other Problems Associated with Obesity, and Including Facts about Risk Factors, Prevention Issues, and Management Approaches

Along with Statistical and Demographic Data, Information about Special Populations,

Research Updates, a Glossary, and Source Listings for Further Help and Information

Edited by Wilma Caldwell and Chad T. Kimball. 360 pages. 2001. 978-0-7808-0333-6.

"The book synthesizes the reliable medical literature on obesity into one easy-to-read and useful resource for the general public."
—*American Reference Books Annual, 2002*

"Well suited for the health reference collection of a public library or an academic health science library that serves the general population."
—*E-Streams, Sep '01*

Osteoporosis Sourcebook

Basic Consumer Health Information about Primary and Secondary Osteoporosis and Juvenile Osteoporosis and Related Conditions, Including Fibrous Dysplasia, Gaucher Disease, Hyperthyroidism, Hypophosphatasia, Myeloma, Osteopetrosis, Osteogenesis Imperfecta, and Paget's Disease

Along with Information about Risk Factors, Treatments, Traditional and Non-Traditional Pain Management, a Glossary of Related Terms, and a Directory of Resources

Edited by Allan R. Cook. 568 pages. 2001. 978-0-7808-0239-1.

"This resource is recommended as a great reference source for public, health, and academic libraries, and is another triumph for the editors of Omnigraphics."
—*American Reference Books Annual, 2002*

"Will prove valuable to any library seeking to maintain a current, comprehensive reference collection of health resources. . . . From prevention to treatment and associated conditions, this provides an excellent survey."
—*The Bookwatch, Aug '01*

SEE ALSO *Healthy Aging Sourcebook, Women's Health Concerns Sourcebook, 3rd Edition*

Pain Sourcebook, 3rd Edition

Basic Consumer Health Information about Acute and Chronic Pain, Including Nerve Pain, Bone Pain, Muscle Pain, Cancer Pain, and Disorders Characterized by Pain, Such as Arthritis, Temporomandibular Muscle and Joint (TMJ) Disorder, Carpal Tunnel Syndrome,

Headaches, Heartburn, Sciatica, and Shingles, and Facts about Diagnostic Tests and Treatment Options for Pain, Including Over-the-Counter and Prescription Drugs, Physical Rehabilitation, Injection and Infusion Therapies, Implantable Technologies, and Complementary Medicine

Along with Tips for Living with Pain, a Glossary of Related Terms, and a Directory of Additional Resources

Edited by Joyce Brennfleck Shannon. 644 pages. 2008. 978-0-7808-1006-8.

"Excellent for ready-reference users and can be used for beginning students in health fields . . . appropriate for the consumer health collection in both public and academic libraries."
—*ARBAonline, Nov '08*

Pediatric Cancer Sourcebook

Basic Consumer Health Information about Leukemias, Brain Tumors, Sarcomas, Lymphomas, and Other Cancers in Infants, Children, and Adolescents, Including Descriptions of Cancers, Treatments, and Coping Strategies

Along with Suggestions for Parents, Caregivers, and Concerned Relatives, a Glossary of Cancer Terms, and Resource Listings

Edited by Edward J. Prucha. 575 pages. 1999. 978-0-7808-0245-2.

"An excellent source of information. Recommended for public, hospital, and health science libraries with consumer health collections."
—*E-Streams, Jun '00*

"A valuable addition to all libraries specializing in health services and many public libraries."
—*American Reference Books Annual, 2000*

SEE ALSO *Childhood Diseases and Disorders Sourcebook, 2nd Edition, Healthy Children Sourcebook*

Physical and Mental Issues in Aging Sourcebook

Basic Consumer Health Information on Physical and Mental Disorders Associated with the Aging Process, Including Concerns about Cardiovascular Disease, Pulmonary Disease, Oral Health, Digestive Disorders, Musculoskeletal and Skin Disorders, Metabolic

Changes, Sexual and Reproductive Issues, and Changes in Vision, Hearing, and Other Senses

Along with Data about Longevity and Causes of Death, Information on Acute and Chronic Pain, Descriptions of Mental Concerns, a Glossary of Terms, and Resource Listings for Additional Help

Edited by Jenifer Swanson. 660 pages. 1999. 978-0-7808-0233-9.

"This is a treasure of health information for the layperson."
— *CHOICE Health Sciences Supplement, May '00*

"Recommended for public libraries."
— *American Reference Books Annual, 2000*

SEE ALSO *Healthy Aging Sourcebook*

Podiatry Sourcebook, 2nd Edition

Basic Consumer Health Information about Disorders, Diseases, and Deformities that Affect the Foot and Ankle, Including Sprains, Corns, Calluses, Bunions, Plantar Warts, Plantar Fasciitis, Neuromas, Clubfoot, Flat Feet, Achilles Tendonitis, and Much More

Along with Information about Selecting a Foot Care Specialist, Foot Fitness, Shoes and Socks, Diagnostic Tests and Corrective Procedures, Financial Assistance for Corrective Devices, a Glossary of Related Terms, and a Directory of Resources for Additional Help and Information

Edited by Ivy L. Alexander. 516 pages. 2007. 978-0-7808-0944-4.

"An excellent resource. . . . Although there have been various types of 'foot books' published in the past, none are as comprehensive as this one. 5 Stars (out of 5)!"
— *Doody's Review Service, 2007*

"Perfect for both health libraries and general-interest lending collections."
— *Internet Bookwatch, Jul '07*

Pregnancy and Birth Sourcebook, 3rd Edition

Basic Consumer Health Information about Pregnancy and Fetal Development, Including Facts about Fertility and Conception, Physical

and Emotional Changes during Pregnancy, Prenatal Care and Diagnostic Tests, High-Risk Pregnancies and Complications, Labor, Delivery, and the Postpartum Period

Along with Tips on Maintaining Health and Wellness during Pregnancy and Caring for Newborn Infants, a Glossary of Related Terms, and Directories of Resources for Additional Help and Information

Edited by Amy L. Sutton. 600 pages. 2009. 978-0-7808-1074-7.

SEE ALSO *Breastfeeding Sourcebook, Congenital Disorders Sourcebook, 2nd Edition, Family Planning Sourcebook, Women's Health Concerns Sourcebook, 3rd Edition*

Prostate and Urological Disorders Sourcebook

Basic Consumer Health Information about Urogenital and Sexual Disorders in Men, Including Prostate and Other Andrological Cancers, Prostatitis, Benign Prostatic Hyperplasia, Testicular and Penile Trauma, Cryptorchidism, Peyronie Disease, Erectile Dysfunction, and Male Factor Infertility, and Facts about Commonly Used Tests and Procedures, Such as Prostatectomy, Vasectomy, Vasectomy Reversal, Penile Implants, and Semen Analysis

Along with a Glossary of Andrological Terms and a Directory of Resources for Additional Information

Edited by Karen Bellenir. 604 pages. 2006. 978-0-7808-0797-6.

"Certain to be a popular pick among library reference holdings. . . . No prior knowledge is assumed for any of the conditions or terms herein, making it a most accessible general-interest reference."
— *California Bookwatch, Apr '06*

SEE ALSO *Men's Health Concerns Sourcebook, 3rd Edition, Urinary Tract and Kidney Diseases and Disorders Sourcebook, 2nd Edition*

Prostate Cancer Sourcebook

Basic Consumer Health Information about Prostate Cancer, Including Information about the Associated Risk Factors, Detection, Diagnosis, and Treatment of Prostate Cancer

Along with Information on Non-Malignant Prostate Conditions, and Featuring a Section

Listing Support and Treatment Centers and a Glossary of Related Terms

Edited by Dawn D. Matthews. 340 pages. 2001. 978-0-7808-0324-4.

"Recommended reference source."
—*Booklist, Jan '02*

"A valuable resource for health care consumers seeking information on the subject.... All text is written in a clear, easy-to-understand language that avoids technical jargon. Any library that collects consumer health resources would strengthen their collection with the addition of the *Prostate Cancer Sourcebook*."
—*American Reference Books Annual, 2002*

SEE ALSO *Cancer Sourcebook, 5th Edition, Men's Health Concerns Sourcebook, 3rd Edition*

Rehabilitation Sourcebook

Basic Consumer Health Information about Rehabilitation for People Recovering from Heart Surgery, Spinal Cord Injury, Stroke, Orthopedic Impairments, Amputation, Pulmonary Impairments, Traumatic Injury, and More, Including Physical Therapy, Occupational Therapy, Speech/Language Therapy, Massage Therapy, Dance Therapy, Art Therapy, and Recreational Therapy

Along with Information on Assistive and Adaptive Devices, a Glossary, and Resources for Additional Help and Information

Edited by Dawn D. Matthews. 519 pages. 2000. 978-0-7808-0236-0.

"This is an excellent resource for public library reference and health collections."
—*American Reference Books Annual, 2001*

"Recommended reference source."
—*Booklist, May '00*

Respiratory Disorders Sourcebook, 2nd Edition

Basic Consumer Health Information about Infectious, Inflammatory, and Chronic Conditions Affecting the Lungs and Respiratory System, Including Pneumonia, Bronchitis, Influenza, Tuberculosis, Sarcoidosis, Asthma, Cystic Fibrosis, Chronic Obstructive Pulmonary Disease, Lung Abscesses, Pulmonary Embolism, Occupational Lung Diseases, and Other Bacterial, Viral, and Fungal Infections

Along with Facts about the Structure and Function of the Lungs and Airways, Methods of Diagnosing Respiratory Disorders, and Treatment and Rehabilitation Options, a Glossary of Related Terms, and a Directory of Resources for Additional Help and Information

Edited by Sandra L. Judd. 638 pages. 2008. 978-0-7808-1007-5.

"A great addition for public and school libraries because it provides concise health information ... readers can start with this reference source and get satisfactory answers before proceeding to other medical reference tools for more in depth information ... A good guide for health education on lung disorders."
—*ARBAonline, Nov '08*

SEE ALSO *Lung Disorders Sourcebook*

Sexually Transmitted Diseases Sourcebook, 4th Edition

Basic Consumer Health Information about Chlamydial Infections, Gonorrhea, Hepatitis, Herpes, HIV/AIDS, Human Papillomavirus, Pubic Lice, Scabies, Syphilis, Trichomoniasis, Vaginal Infections, and Other Sexually Transmitted Diseases, Including Facts about Risk Factors, Symptoms, Diagnosis, Treatment, and the Prevention of Sexually Transmitted Infections

Along with Updates on Current Research Initiatives, a Glossary of Related Terms, and Resources for Additional Help and Information

Edited by Laura Larsen. 600 pages. 2009. 978-0-7808-1073-0.

SEE ALSO *AIDS Sourcebook, 4th Edition, Contagious Diseases Sourcebook, 2nd Edition, Men's Health Concerns Sourcebook, 3rd Edition, Women's Health Concerns Sourcebook, 3rd Edition*

Sleep Disorders Sourcebook, 2nd Edition

Basic Consumer Health Information about Sleep and Sleep Disorders, Including Insomnia, Sleep Apnea, Restless Legs Syndrome, Narcolepsy, Parasomnias, and Other Health Problems That Affect Sleep, Plus Facts about Diagnostic Procedures, Treatment Strategies,

Sleep Medications, and Tips for Improving Sleep Quality

Along with a Glossary of Related Terms and Resources for Additional Help and Information

Edited by Amy L. Sutton. 567 pages. 2005. 978-0-7808-0743-3.

"This book will be useful for just about everybody, especially the 40 million Americans with sleep disorders."
—*American Reference Books Annual, 2006*

"A welcome addition to public libraries and consumer health libraries."
—*Medical Reference Services Quarterly, Summer '06*

Smoking Concerns Sourcebook

Basic Consumer Health Information about Nicotine Addiction and Smoking Cessation, Featuring Facts about the Health Effects of Tobacco Use, Including Lung and Other Cancers, Heart Disease, Stroke, and Respiratory Disorders, Such as Emphysema and Chronic Bronchitis

Along with Information about Smoking Prevention Programs, Suggestions for Achieving and Maintaining a Smoke-Free Lifestyle, Statistics about Tobacco Use, Reports on Current Research Initiatives, a Glossary of Related Terms, and Directories of Resources for Additional Help and Information

Edited by Karen Bellenir. 595 pages. 2004. 978-0-7808-0323-7.

"Provides everything needed for the student or general reader seeking practical details on the effects of tobacco use."
—*The Bookwatch, Mar '05*

"Public libraries and consumer health care libraries will find this work useful."
—*American Reference Books Annual, 2005*

SEE ALSO *Respiratory Disorders Sourcebook, 2nd Edition*

Sports Injuries Sourcebook, 3rd Edition

Basic Consumer Health Information about Sprains and Strains, Fractures, Growth Plate Injuries, Overtraining Injuries, and Injuries to

the Head, Face, Shoulders, Elbows, Hands, Spinal Column, Knees, Ankles, and Feet, and with Facts about Heat-Related Illness, Steroids and Sport Supplements, Protective Equipment, Diagnostic Procedures, Treatment Options, and Rehabilitation*

Along with a Glossary of Related Terms and a Directory of Resources for Additional Help and Information

Edited by Sandra J. Judd. 623 pages. 2007. 978-0-7808-0949-9.

SEE ALSO *Fitness and Exercise Sourcebook, 3rd Edition*

Stress-Related Disorders Sourcebook, 2nd Edition

Basic Consumer Health Information about Stress and Stress-Related Disorders, Including Types of Stress, Sources of Acute and Chronic Stress, the Impact of Stress on the Body's Systems, and Mental and Emotional Health Problems Associated with Stress, Such as Depression, Anxiety Disorders, Substance Abuse, Posttraumatic Stress Disorder, and Suicide

Along with Advice about Getting Help for Stress-Related Disorders, Information about Stress Management Techniques, a Glossary of Stress-Related Terms, and a Directory of Resources for Additional Help and Information

Edited by Amy L. Sutton. 608 pages. 2007. 978-0-7808-0996-3.

"Accessible to the lay reader. Highly recommended for medical and psychiatric collections."
—*Library Journal, Mar '08*

"Well-written for a general readership, the 2 nd Edition of *Stress-Related Disorders Sourcebook* is a useful addition to the health reference literature."
—*American Reference Books Annual, 2008*

SEE ALSO *Mental Health Disorders Sourcebook, 4th Edition*

Stroke Sourcebook, 2nd Edition

Basic Consumer Health Information about Stroke, Including Ischemic, Hemorrhagic, and Mini Strokes, as Well as Risk Factors, Prevention Guidelines, Diagnostic Tests, Medications and

Surgical Treatments, and Complications of Stroke

Along with Rehabilitation Techniques and Innovations, Tips on Staying Healthy and Maintaining Independence after Stroke, a Glossary of Related Terms, and a Directory of Resources for Stroke Survivors and Their Families

Edited by Amy L. Sutton. 626 pages. 2008. 978-0-7808-1035-8.

"An encyclopedic handbook on stroke that is written in a language the layperson can understand. . . . This is one of the most helpful, readable books on stroke. This volume is highly recommended and should be in every medical, hospital and public library; in addition, every family practitioner should have a copy in his or her office."

—*ARBAonline Dec '08*

SEE ALSO *Hypertension Sourcebook*

Surgery Sourcebook, 2nd Edition

Basic Consumer Health Information about Common Inpatient and Outpatient Surgeries, Including Critical Care and Trauma, Gastrointestinal, Gynecologic and Obstetric, Cardiac and Vascular, Neurologic, Ophthalmologic, Orthopedic, Reconstructive and Cosmetic, and Other Major and Minor Surgeries

Along with Information about Anesthesia and Pain Relief Options, Risks and Complications, Postoperative Recovery Concerns, and Innovative Surgical Techniques and Tools, a Glossary of Related Terms, and a Directory of Additional Resources

Edited by Amy L. Sutton. 645 pages. 2008. 978-0-7808-1004-4.

"Large public libraries and medical libraries would benefit from this material in their reference collections."

—*ARBAonline Aug '08*

SEE ALSO *Cosmetic and Reconstructive Surgery Sourcebook, 2nd Edition*

Thyroid Disorders Sourcebook

Basic Consumer Health Information about Disorders of the Thyroid and Parathyroid Glands, Including Hypothyroidism, Hyperthyroidism,

Graves Disease, Hashimoto Thyroiditis, Thyroid Cancer, and Parathyroid Disorders, Featuring Facts about Symptoms, Risk Factors, Tests, and Treatments

Along with Information about the Effects of Thyroid Imbalance on Other Body Systems, Environmental Factors That Affect the Thyroid Gland, a Glossary, and a Directory of Additional Resources

Edited by Joyce Brennfleck Shannon. 573 pages. 2005. 978-0-7808-0745-7.

"Recommended for consumer health collections."

—*American Reference Books Annual, 2006*

"Highly recommended pick for basic consumer health reference holdings at all levels."

—*The Bookwatch, Aug '05*

SEE ALSO *Endocrine and Metabolic Disorders Sourcebook, 2nd Edition*

Transplantation Sourcebook

Basic Consumer Health Information about Organ and Tissue Transplantation, Including Physical and Financial Preparations, Procedures and Issues Relating to Specific Solid Organ and Tissue Transplants, Rehabilitation, Pediatric Transplant Information, the Future of Transplantation, and Organ and Tissue Donation

Along with a Glossary and Listings of Additional Resources

Edited by Joyce Brennfleck Shannon. 610 pages. 2002. 978-0-7808-0322-0.

"Recommended for libraries with an interest in offering consumer health information."

—*E-Streams, Jul '02*

"This is a unique and valuable resource for patients facing transplantation and their families."

—*Doody's Review Service, Jun '02*

Traveler's Health Sourcebook

Basic Consumer Health Information for Travelers, Including Physical and Medical Preparations, Transportation Health and Safety, Essential Information about Food and Water, Sun Exposure, Insect and Snake Bites, Camping and Wilderness Medicine, and Travel with Physical or Medical Disabilities

Along with International Travel Tips, Vaccination Recommendations, Geographical Health Issues, Disease Risks, a Glossary, and a Listing of Additional Resources

Edited by Joyce Brennfleck Shannon. 619 pages. 2000. 978-0-7808-0384-8.

"Recommended reference source."
—*Booklist, Feb '01*

"This book is recommended for any public library, any travel collection, and especially any collection for the physically disabled."
—*American Reference Books Annual, 2001*

SEE ALSO Worldwide Health Sourcebook

Urinary Tract and Kidney Diseases and Disorders Sourcebook, 2nd Edition

Basic Consumer Health Information about the Urinary System, Including the Bladder, Urethra, Ureters, and Kidneys, with Facts about Urinary Tract Infections, Incontinence, Congenital Disorders, Kidney Stones, Cancers of the Urinary Tract and Kidneys, Kidney Failure, Dialysis, and Kidney Transplantation

Along with Statistical and Demographic Information, Reports on Current Research in Kidney and Urologic Health, a Summary of Commonly Used Diagnostic Tests, a Glossary of Related Terms, and a Directory of Resources for Additional Help and Information

Edited by Ivy L. Alexander. 621 pages. 2005. 978-0-7808-0750-1.

"A good choice for a consumer health information library or for a medical library needing information to refer to their patients."
—*American Reference Books Annual, 2006*

SEE ALSO Prostate and Urological Disorders Sourcebook

Vegetarian Sourcebook

Basic Consumer Health Information about Vegetarian Diets, Lifestyle, and Philosophy, Including Definitions of Vegetarianism and Veganism, Tips about Adopting Vegetarianism, Creating a Vegetarian Pantry, and Meeting Nutritional Needs of Vegetarians, with Facts Regarding Vegetarianism's Effect on Pregnant and Lactating Women, Children, Athletes, and Senior Citizens

Along with a Glossary of Commonly Used Vegetarian Terms and Resources for Additional Help and Information

Edited by Chad T. Kimball. 337 pages. 2002. 978-0-7808-0439-5.

"Organizes into one concise volume the answers to the most common questions concerning vegetarian diets and lifestyles. This title is recommended for public and secondary school libraries."
—*E-Streams, Apr '03*

"Invaluable reference for public and school library collections alike."
—*Library Bookwatch, Apr '03*

"The articles in this volume are easy to read and come from authoritative sources. The book does not necessarily support the vegetarian diet but instead provides the pros and cons of this important decision. . . . Recommended for public libraries and consumer health libraries."
—*American Reference Books Annual, 2003*

SEE ALSO Diet and Nutrition Sourcebook, 3rd Edition

Women's Health Concerns Sourcebook, 3rd Edition

Basic Consumer Health Information about Issues and Trends in Women's Health and Health Conditions of Special Concern to Women, Including Endometriosis, Uterine Fibroids, Menstrual Irregularities, Menopause, Sexual Dysfunction, Infertility, Cancer in Women, and Other Such Chronic Disorders as Lupus, Fibromyalgia, and Thyroid Disease

Along with Statistical Data, Tips for Maintaining Wellness, a Glossary, and a Directory of Resources for Further Help and Information

Edited by Sandra J. Judd. 600 pages. 2009. 978-0-7808-1036-5.

SEE ALSO Breast Cancer Sourcebook, 3rd Edition, Cancer Sourcebook for Women, 3rd Edition, Healthy Heart Sourcebook for Women, Osteoporosis Sourcebook

---

Workplace Health and Safety Sourcebook

Basic Consumer Health Information about Workplace Health and Safety, Including the Effect of Workplace Hazards on the Lungs,

Skin, Heart, Ears, Eyes, Brain, Reproductive Organs, Musculoskeletal System, and Other Organs and Body Parts

Along with Information about Occupational Cancer, Personal Protective Equipment, Toxic and Hazardous Chemicals, Child Labor, Stress, and Workplace Violence

Edited by Chad T. Kimball. 610 pages. 2000. 978-0-7808-0231-5.

"As a reference for the general public, this would be useful in any library."
—*E-Streams, Jun '01*

"Provides helpful information for primary care physicians and other caregivers interested in occupational medicine. . . . General readers; professionals."
—*CHOICE, May '01*

Worldwide Health Sourcebook

Basic Information about Global Health Issues, Including Malnutrition, Reproductive Health, Disease Dispersion and Prevention, Emerging Diseases, Risky Health Behaviors, and the Leading Causes of Death

Along with Global Health Concerns for Children, Women, and the Elderly, Mental Health Issues, Research and Technology Advancements, and Economic, Environmental, and Political Health Implications, a Glossary, and a Resource Listing for Additional Help and Information

Edited by Joyce Brennfleck Shannon. 597 pages. 2001. 978-0-7808-0330-5.

"Named an Outstanding Academic Title."
—*CHOICE, Jan '02*

"Yet another handy but also unique compilation in the extensive *Health Reference Series*, this is a useful work because many of the international publications reprinted or excerpted are not readily available. Highly recommended."
—*CHOICE, Nov '01*

SEE ALSO *Traveler's Health Sourcebook*

Teen Health Series

Complete Catalog

List price $69 per volume. School and library price $62 per volume.

Abuse and Violence Information for Teens

Health Tips about the Causes and Consequences of Abusive and Violent Behavior
Including Facts about the Types of Abuse and Violence, the Warning Signs of Abusive and Violent Behavior, Health Concerns of Victims, and Getting Help and Staying Safe

Edited by Sandra Augustyn Lawton. 411 pages. 2008. 978-0-7808-1008-2.

"**A useful resource for schools and organizations providing services to teens and may also be a starting point in research projects.**"
—*Reference and Research Book News, Aug '08*

"**Violence is a serious problem for teens. . . . This resource gives teens the information they need to face potential threats and get help— either for themselves or for their friends.**"
—*ARBAonline, Aug '08*

Accident and Safety Information for Teens

Health Tips about Medical Emergencies, Traumatic Injuries, and Disaster Preparedness
Including Facts about Motor Vehicle Accidents, Burns, Poisoning, Firearms, Natural Disasters, National Security Threats, and More

Edited by Karen Bellenir. 420 pages. 2008. 978-0-7808-1046-4.

SEE ALSO *Sports Injuries Information for Teens, 2nd Edition*

Alcohol Information for Teens, 2nd Edition

Health Tips about Alcohol and Alcoholism
Including Facts about Alcohol's Effects on the Body, Brain, and Behavior, the Consequences of Underage Drinking, Alcohol Abuse Prevention and Treatment, and Coping with Alcoholic Parents

Edited by Lisa Bakewell. 400 pages. 2009. 978-0-7808-1043-3.

SEE ALSO *Drug Information for Teens, 2nd Edition*

Allergy Information for Teens

Health Tips about Allergic Reactions Such as Anaphylaxis, Respiratory Problems, and Rashes
Including Facts about Identifying and Managing Allergies to Food, Pollen, Mold, Animals, Chemicals, Drugs, and Other Substances

Edited by Karen Bellenir. 410 pages. 2006. 978-0-7808-0799-0.

"**This is a comprehensive, readable text on the subject of allergic diseases in teenagers. 5 Stars (out of 5)!**"
—*Doody's Review Service, Jun '06*

"**This authoritative and useful self-help title is a solid addition to YA collections, whether for personal interest or reports.**"
—*School Library Journal, Jul '06*

Asthma Information for Teens

Health Tips about Managing Asthma and Related Concerns
Including Facts about Asthma Causes, Triggers, Symptoms, Diagnosis, and Treatment

Edited by Karen Bellenir. 386 pages. 2005. 978-0-7808-0770-9.

"**Highly recommended for medical libraries, public school libraries, and public libraries.**"
—*American Reference Books Annual, 2006*

"**Although this volume is nearly 400 pages long, it is so clearly written and well organized that even hesitant readers will be able to find the facts they need, whether for reports or personal information. . . . A succinct but complete resource.**"
—*School Library Journal, Sep '05*

Body Information for Teens
Health Tips about Maintaining Well-Being for a Lifetime
Including Facts about the Development and Functioning of the Body's Systems, Organs, and Structures and the Health Impact of Lifestyle Choices

Edited by Sandra Augustyn Lawton. 458 pages. 2007. 978-0-7808-0443-2.

Cancer Information for Teens, 2nd Edition
Health Tips about Cancer Awareness, Symptoms, Prevention, Diagnosis, and Treatment
Including Facts about Common Cancers Affecting Teens, Causes, Detection, Coping Strategies, Clinical Trials, Nutrition and Exercise, Cancer in Friends or Family, and More

Edited by Karen Bellenir and Lisa Bakewell. 400 pages. 2009. 978-0-7808-1085-3.

Complementary and Alternative Medicine Information for Teens
Health Tips about Non-Traditional and Non-Western Medical Practices
Including Information about Acupuncture, Chiropractic Medicine, Dietary and Herbal Supplements, Hypnosis, Massage Therapy, Prayer and Spirituality, Reflexology, Yoga, and More

Edited by Sandra Augustyn Lawton. 407 pages. 2007. 978-0-7808-0966-6.

"This volume covers CAM specifically for teenagers but of general use also. It should be a welcome addition to both public and academic libraries."
—*American Reference Books Annual, 2008*

"This volume provides a solid foundation for further investigation of the subject, making it useful for both public and high school libraries."
—*VOYA: Voice of Youth Advocates, Jun '07*

Diabetes Information for Teens
Health Tips about Managing Diabetes and Preventing Related Complications
Including Information about Insulin, Glucose Control, Healthy Eating, Physical Activity, and Learning to Live with Diabetes

Edited by Sandra Augustyn Lawton. 410 pages. 2006. 978-0-7808-0811-9.

"A comprehensive instructional guide for teens. . . . some of the material may also be directed towards parents or teachers. 5 stars (out of 5)!"
—*Doody's Review Service, 2006*

"Students dealing with their own diabetes or that of a friend or family member or those writing reports on the topic will find this a valuable resource."
—*School Library Journal, Aug '06*

"This text is directed to the teen population and would be an excellent library resource for a health class or for the teacher as a reference for class preparation. It can, however, serve a much wider audience. The clinical educator on diabetes may find it valuable to educate the newly diagnosed client regardless of age. It also would be an excellent reference and education tool for a preventive medicine seminar on diabetes."
—*Physical Therapy, Mar '07*

Diet Information for Teens, 2nd Edition
Health Tips about Diet and Nutrition
Including Facts about Dietary Guidelines, Food Groups, Nutrients, Healthy Meals, Snacks, Weight Control, Medical Concerns Related to Diet, and More

Edited by Karen Bellenir. 432 pages. 2006. 978-0-7808-0820-1.

"A very quick and pleasant read in spite of the fact that it is very detailed in the information it gives. . . . A book for anyone concerned about diet and nutrition."
—*American Reference Books Annual, 2007*

SEE ALSO Eating Disorders Information for Teens, 2nd Edition

Drug Information for Teens, 2nd Edition
Health Tips about the Physical and Mental Effects of Substance Abuse
Including Information about Marijuana, Inhalants, Club Drugs, Stimulants, Hallucinogens,

Opiates, Prescription and Over-the-Counter Drugs, Herbal Products, Tobacco, Alcohol, and More

Edited by Sandra Augustyn Lawton. 468 pages. 2006. 978-0-7808-0862-1.

"As with earlier installments in Omnigraphics' *Teen Health Series*, *Drug Information for Teens* is designed specifically to meet the needs and interests of middle and high school students. . . . Strongly recommended for both academic and public libraries."
—*American Reference Books Annual, 2007*

"Solid thoughtful advice is given about how to handle peer pressure, drug-related health concerns, and treatment strategies."
—*School Library Journal, Dec '06*

SEE ALSO *Alcohol Information for Teens, 2nd Edition, Tobacco Information for Teens*

Eating Disorders Information for Teens, 2nd Edition

Health Tips about Anorexia, Bulimia, Binge Eating, And Other Eating Disorders
Including Information about Risk Factors, Diagnosis and Treatment, Prevention, Related Health Concerns, and Other Issues

Edited by Sandra Augustyn Lawton. 377 pages. 2009. 978-0-7808-1044-0.

SEE ALSO *Diet Information for Teens, 2nd Edition*

Fitness Information for Teens, 2nd Edition

Health Tips about Exercise, Physical Well-Being, and Health Maintenance
Including Facts about Conditioning, Stretching, Strength Training, Body Shape and Body Image, Sports Nutrition, and Specific Activities for Athletes and Non-Athletes

Edited by Lisa Bakewell. 432 pages. 2009. 978-0-7808-1045-7.

SEE ALSO *Diet Information for Teens, 2nd Edition, Sports Injuries Information for Teens, 2nd Edition*

Learning Disabilities Information for Teens

Health Tips about Academic Skills Disorders and Other Disabilities That Affect Learning
Including Information about Common Signs of Learning Disabilities, School Issues, Learning to Live with a Learning Disability, and Other Related Issues

Edited by Sandra Augustyn Lawton. 400 pages. 2006. 978-0-7808-0796-9.

"This book provides a wealth of information for any reader interested in the signs, causes, and consequences of learning disabilities, as well as related legal rights and educational interventions. . . . Public and academic libraries should want this title for both students and general readers."
—*American Reference Books Annual, 2006*

Mental Health Information for Teens, 2nd Edition

Health Tips about Mental Wellness and Mental Illness
Including Facts about Mental and Emotional Health, Depression and Other Mood Disorders, Anxiety Disorders, Conduct Disorder, Self-Injury, Psychosis, Schizophrenia, and More

Edited by Karen Bellenir. 424 pages. 2006. 978-0-7808-0863-8.

"This excellent overview of the psychological disorders that affect teens provides clear definitions and descriptions, and discusses resources, therapies, coping mechanisms, and medications."
—*School Library Journal Curriculum Connections, Fall '07*

"A well done reference for a specific, often under-represented group."
—*Doody's Review Service, 2006*

SEE ALSO *Stress Information for Teens*

Pregnancy Information for Teens

Health Tips about Teen Pregnancy and Teen Parenting
Including Facts about Prenatal Care, Pregnancy Complications, Labor and Delivery,

Postpartum Care, Pregnancy-Related Lifestyle Concerns, and More

Edited by Sandra Augustyn Lawton. 434 pages. 2007. 978-0-7808-0984-0.

SEE ALSO *Sexual Health Information for Teens, 2nd Edition*

Sexual Health Information for Teens, 2nd Edition
Health Tips about Sexual Development, Reproduction, Contraception, and Sexually Transmitted Infections
Including Facts about Puberty, Sexuality, Birth Control, Chlamydia, Gonorrhea, Herpes, Human Papillomavirus, Syphilis, and More

Edited by Sandra Augustyn Lawton. 430 pages. 2008. 978-0-7808-1010-5.

"This offering represents the most up-to-date information available on an array of topics including abstinence-only sexual education and pregnancy-prevention methods. . . . The range of coverage—from puberty and anatomy to sexually transmitted diseases—is thorough and extensive. Each chapter includes a bibliographic citation, and the three back sections containing additional resources, further reading, and the index are all first-rate. . . . This volume will be well used by students in need of the facts, whether for educational or personal reasons."
—*School Library Journal, Nov '08*

SEE ALSO *Pregnancy Information for Teens*

Skin Health Information for Teens, 2nd Edition
Health Tips about Dermatological Concerns and Skin Cancer Risks
Including Facts about Acne, Warts, Allergies, and Other Conditions and Lifestyle Choices, Such as Tanning, Tattooing, and Piercing, That Affect the Skin, Nails, Scalp, and Hair

Edited by Edited by Kim Wohlenhaus. 400 pages. 2009. 978-0-7808-1042-6.

Sleep Information for Teens
Health Tips about Adolescent Sleep Requirements, Sleep Disorders, and the Effects of Sleep Deprivation

Including Facts about Why People Need Sleep, Sleep Patterns, Circadian Rhythms, Dreaming, Insomnia, Sleep Apnea, Narcolepsy, and More

Edited by Karen Bellenir. 355 pages. 2008. 978-0-7808-1009-9.

SEE ALSO *Body Information for Teens*

Sports Injuries Information for Teens, 2nd Edition
Health Tips about Acute, Traumatic, and Chronic Injuries in Adolescent Athletes
Including Facts about Sprains, Fractures, and Overuse Injuries, Treatment, Rehabilitation, Sport-Specific Safety Guidelines, Fitness Suggestions, and More

Edited by Karen Bellenir. 429 pages. 2008. 978-0-7808-1011-2.

"An engaging selection of informative articles about the prevention and treatment of sports injuries. . . The value of this book is that the articles have been vetted and are often augmented with inserts of useful facts, definitions of technical terms, and quick tips. Sensitive topics like injuries to genitalia are discussed openly and responsibly. This revised edition contains updated articles and defines sport more broadly than the first edition."
—*School Library Journal, Nov '08*

"This work will be useful in the young adult collections of public libraries as well as high school libraries. . . . A useful resource for student research."
—*ARBAonline, Aug '08*

SEE ALSO *Accident and Safety Information for Teens*

Stress Information for Teens
Health Tips about the Mental and Physical Consequences of Stress
Including Information about the Different Kinds of Stress, Symptoms of Stress, Frequent Causes of Stress, Stress Management Techniques, and More

Edited by Sandra Augustyn Lawton. 392 pages. 2008. 978-0-7808-1012-9.

"Understanding what stress is, what causes it, how the body and the mind are impacted by it, and what teens can do are the general categories addressed here. . . . The chapters are brief but informative, and the list of community-help organizations is exhaustive. Report writers will find information quickly and easily, as will those who have personal concerns. The print is clear and the format is readable, making this an accessible resource for struggling readers and researchers."

—*School Library Journal, Dec '08*

"The articles selected will specifically appeal to young adults and are designed to answer their most common questions."

—*ARBAonline, Aug '08*

SEE ALSO *Mental Health Information for Teens, 2nd Edition*

having to read the entire book. . . . The book is packed full of statistics, with sources to help students look up more."

—*School Library Journal, Sep '07*

"Pulls together a wide variety of authoritative sources to provide a comprehensive overview of tobacco use for this age group. . . . This reasonably priced reference title should be considered a necessary purchase for all public libraries and school media centers, along with academic libraries supporting teacher education."

—*American Reference Books Annual, 2008*

SEE ALSO *Drug Information for Teens, 2nd Edition*

Suicide Information for Teens

Health Tips about Suicide Causes and Prevention

Including Facts about Depression, Risk Factors, Getting Help, Survivor Support, and More

Edited by Joyce Brennfleck Shannon. 368 pages. 2005. 978-0-7808-0737-2.

"Highly Recommended for libraries serving teenagers as well as those who work with them."

—*E-Streams, Apr '06*

SEE ALSO *Mental Health Information for Teens, 2nd Edition*

Tobacco Information for Teens

Health Tips about the Hazards of Using Cigarettes, Smokeless Tobacco, and Other Nicotine Products

Including Facts about Nicotine Addiction, Immediate and Long-Term Health Effects of Tobacco Use, Related Cancers, Smoking Cessation, Tobacco Use Prevention, and Tobacco Use Statistics

Edited by Karen Bellenir. 440 pages. 2007. 978-0-7808-0976-5.

"A comprehensive resource. Each chapter is written to stand alone, so students can dip in and use the information in each section for reports or to answer personal questions without

667

Health Reference Series

Adolescent Health Sourcebook, 2nd Edition

Adult Health Concerns Sourcebook

AIDS Sourcebook, 4th Edition

Alcoholism Sourcebook, 2nd Edition

Allergies Sourcebook, 3rd Edition

Alzheimer Disease Sourcebook, 4th Edition

Arthritis Sourcebook, 2nd Edition

Asthma Sourcebook, 2nd Edition

Attention Deficit Disorder Sourcebook

Autism & Pervasive Developmental Disorders
Sourcebook

Back & Neck Sourcebook, 2nd Edition

Blood & Circulatory Disorders Sourcebook, 2nd
Edition

Brain Disorders Sourcebook, 2nd Edition

Breast Cancer Sourcebook, 3rd Edition

Breastfeeding Sourcebook

Burns Sourcebook

Cancer Sourcebook, 5th Edition

Cancer Sourcebook for Women, 3rd Edition

Cancer Survivorship Sourcebook

Cardiovascular Diseases & Disorders
Sourcebook, 3rd Edition

Caregiving Sourcebook

Child Abuse Sourcebook

Childhood Diseases & Disorders Sourcebook,
2nd Edition

Colds, Flu & Other Common Ailments
Sourcebook

Communication Disorders Sourcebook

Complementary & Alternative Medicine
Sourcebook, 3rd Edition

Congenital Disorders Sourcebook, 2nd Edition

Contagious Diseases Sourcebook

Cosmetic & Reconstructive Surgery
Sourcebook, 2nd Edition

Death & Dying Sourcebook, 2nd Edition

Dental Care & Oral Health Sourcebook, 3rd
Edition

Depression Sourcebook, 2nd Edition

Dermatological Disorders Sourcebook, 2nd Edition

Diabetes Sourcebook, 4th Edition

Diet & Nutrition Sourcebook, 3rd Edition

Digestive Diseases & Disorder Sourcebook

Disabilities Sourcebook

Disease Management Sourcebook

Domestic Violence Sourcebook, 3rd Edition

Drug Abuse Sourcebook, 2nd Edition

Ear, Nose & Throat Disorders Sourcebook, 2nd
Edition

Eating Disorders Sourcebook, 2nd Edition

Emergency Medical Services Sourcebook

Endocrine & Metabolic Disorders Sourcebook,
2nd Edition

Environmental Health Sourcebook, 2nd Edition

Ethnic Diseases Sourcebook

Eye Care Sourcebook, 3rd Edition

Family Planning Sourcebook

Fitness & Exercise Sourcebook, 3rd Edition

Food Safety Sourcebook

Forensic Medicine Sourcebook

Gastrointestinal Diseases & Disorders
Sourcebook, 2nd Edition

Genetic Disorders Sourcebook, 3rd Edition

Head Trauma Sourcebook

Headache Sourcebook

Health Insurance Sourcebook

Healthy Aging Sourcebook

Healthy Children Sourcebook

Healthy Heart Sourcebook for Women

Hepatitis Sourcebook

Household Safety Sourcebook

Hypertension Sourcebook

Immune System Disorders Sourcebook, 2nd
Edition

Infant & Toddler Health Sourcebook

Infectious Diseases Sourcebook

Injury & Trauma Sourcebook